Colorectal Cancer

METHODS IN MOLECULAR MEDICINE™

John M. Walker, SERIES EDITOR

METHODS IN MOLECULAR MEDICINE™

Colorectal Cancer

Methods and Protocols

Edited by

Steven M. Powell, MD

*University of Virginia Health System,
Charlottesville, VA*

Humana Press ✴ **Totowa, New Jersey**

This publication is printed on acid-free paper. ∞
ANSI Z39.48-1984 (American Standards Institute) Permanence of Paper for Printed Library Materials.

Cover design by Patricia F. Cleary.
Cover illustration: From Fig. 2A in Chapter 1 "Microdissection of Histologic Sections: *Manual and Laser Capture Microdissection Techniques*," by Christopher A. Moskaluk.

For additional copies, pricing for bulk purchases, and/or information about other Humana titles, contact Humana at the above address or at any of the following numbers: Tel.: 973-256-1699; Fax: 973-256-8341; E-mail: humana@humanapr.com; Website: http://humanapress.com

Photocopy Authorization Policy:
Authorization to photocopy items for internal or personal use, or the internal or personal use of specific clients, is granted by Humana Press Inc., provided that the base fee of US $10.00 per copy, plus US $00.25 per page, is paid directly to the Copyright Clearance Center at 222 Rosewood Drive, Danvers, MA 01923. For those organizations that have been granted a photocopy license from the CCC, a separate system of payment has been arranged and is acceptable to Humana Press Inc. The fee code for users of the Transactional Reporting Service is [0-89603-767-3/01 $10.00 + $00.25].

Printed in the United States of America. 10 9 8 7 6 5 4 3 2 1

Library of Congress Cataloging in Publication Data

Main entry under title: Methods in molecular medicine™.

Colorectal cancer: methods and protocols/edited by Steven M. Powell.
        p. ; cm. —(Methods in molecular medicine; 50)
    Includes bibliographical references and index.
    ISBN 0-89603-767-3 (alk. paper)
    1. Colon (Anatomy)—Cancer—Diagnosis—Laboratory manuals. 2.
    Rectum—Cancer—Diagnosis—Laboratory manuals. I. Powell, Steven M. II. Series.
    [DNLM: 1. Colorectal Neoplasms—pathology. 2. Colorectal Neoplasms—diagnosis. WI
    529 C7191 2000]
    RC280.C6 C668 2000
    616.99'4347—dc21

00-022073

Preface

The contents of *Colorectal Cancer: Methods and Protocols* aim to instruct investigators in all the key genetic, cellular, and molecular biological methods of analyzing colorectal tumors. The focused techniques and assays are described in sufficient detail to allow researchers to start an experiment on colon tumors and proceed from beginning to end as if the expert in the field who has performed these studies were guiding them at the bench. Of note, most of the chapters in this volume are written by those scientists who pioneered these methods and assays in their respective fields.

The chapters in *Colorectal Cancer: Methods and Protocols* describe "state of the art" methods to analyze colorectal tumors, ranging from gross microdissection of specimens to specific molecular analyses. Included are coverages of mutational assays, instability testing, immunohistochemical assays, chromosomal studies, and gene expression analyses. The goal of our volume is to facilitate the performance of colorectal tumor biological experiments by investigators at various levels of training—from graduate students and postdoctoral fellows to principal investigators who desire to advance our understanding of colon cancer development.

Recent advances in the fields of molecular genetics, signal transduction, DNA repair, and genomic instability—especially as they relate to colorectal tumorigenesis—make this comprehensive coverage of molecular assays of this cancer particularly timely. The initial section of the volume describes gross microdissection of colon tumors and the establishment of cell lines and xenografted tumors. The next section describes chromosomal analyses, including comparative genomic hybridization and FISH assays. Mutational analyses of colon tumors and of blood samples to determine whether they have inherited a significant predisposition for colorectal cancer development follows. Microsatellite instability testing is also presented. Gene expression analyses including immunohistochemical assays, Western blotting, and microarray assays are in the final section to complete the volume.

Steven M. Powell, MD

Contents

Contributors

LAURI A. AALTONEN • *Department of Medical Genetics, University of Helsinki, Finland*

REID B. ADAMS • *Department of Surgery, University of Virginia Health System, Charlottesville, VA*

EGLE AVIZIENYTE • *Department of Medical Genetics, University of Helsinki, Finland*

LISA A. CERILLI • *Department of Pathology, University of Virginia Health System, Charlottesville, VA*

PERRY S. CHAN • *Molecular Genetics Laboratory, Dianon Systems Inc., Stratford, CT*

STEVEN M. COHN • *Department of Medicine/GI, University of Virginia Health System, Charlottesville, VA*

BAŞAK ÇORUH • *Department of Medicine/GI, University of Virginia Health System, Charlottesville, VA*

ROSANA COSME • *Department of Medicine/GI, University of Virginia Health System, Charlottesville, VA*

JULIE M. CUNNINGHAM • *Laboratory of Medicine and Pathology, Mayo Clinic, Rochester, MN*

SANDRINE DELBARY-GOSSART • *Department of Medicine/GI, University of Virginia Health System, Charlottesville, VA*

RAYMOND N. DUBOIS • *Division of Gastroenterology, Vanderbilt University Medical Center, Nashville, TN*

WA'EL EL-RIFAI • *Department of Medical Genetics, Haartman Institute and Helsinki University Central Hospital, University of Helsinki, Finland*

CHARIS ENG • *Department of Medical Genetics, University of Helsinki, Finland*

HENRY F. FRIERSON, JR. • *Department of Pathology, University of Virginia Health System, Charlottesville, VA*

STEVEN L. GERSEN • *Molecular Genetics Laboratory, Dianon Systems Inc., Stratford, CT*

WILLIAM M. GRADY • *Ireland Cancer Center, University Hospitals of Cleveland, Cleveland, OH*

KEVIN C. HALLING • *Molecular Genetics Laboratory, Mayo Clinic, Rochester, MN*

JEFFREY C. HARPER • *Department of Medicine/Surgery, University of Virginia Health System, Charlottesville, VA*

HONGMEI HE • *Ireland Cancer Center, University Hospitals of Cleveland, Cleveland, OH*

JIN JEN • *Department of Otolaryngology and Oncology, John Hopkins Medical School, Baltimore, MD*

HOSSAM M. KANDIL • *Division of Gastroenterology, Hepatology and Nutrition, University of Pittsburgh Medical Center, Pittsburgh, PA*

SAKARI KNUUTILA • *Department of Medical Genetics, Haartman Institute and Helsinki University Central Hospital, University of Helsinki, Finland*

ROGER QI LUO • *Department of Medicine/GI, University of Virginia Health System, Charlottesville, VA*

SANFORD MARKOWITZ • *Ireland Cancer Center, University Hospitals of Cleveland, Cleveland, OH*

STEPHEN J. MELTZER • *Department of Medicine/GI, Acrodigestive Interdisciplinary Program, Greenbaum Cancer Center, University of Maryland School of Medicine, VA Maryland HealthCare Systems, Baltimore, MD*

CHRISTOPHER A. MOSKALUK • *Departments of Pathology and Biochemistry and Molecular Genetics, University of Virginia Health System, Charlottesville, VA*

LOIS L. MYEROFF • *Ireland Cancer Center, University Hospitals of Cleveland, Cleveland, OH*

SVETLANA D. PACK • *Laboratory of Pathology, National Cancer Institute, NIH, Bethesda, MD*

YANN R. PARC • *Molecular Genetics Laboratory, Mayo Clinic, Rochester, MN*

THERESA T. PIZARRO • *Department of Medicine/GI, University of Virginia Health System, Charlottesville, VA*

STEVEN M. POWELL • *Department of Medicine/GI, University of Virginia Health System, Charlottesville, VA*

JAMES K. ROCHE • *Department of Medicine/GI, University of Virginia Health System, Charlottesville, VA*

PATRICK ROCHE • *Molecular Genetics Laboratory, Mayo Clinic, Rochester, MN*

STINA ROTH • *Department of Medical Genetics, Haartman Institute, University of Helsinki, Finland*

JOSHUA D. ROVIN • *Department of Surgery, University of Virginia Health System, Charlottesville, VA*

DARYL SHIBATA • *Department of Pathology, School of Medicine, University of Southern California, Los Angeles, CA*

MICHAL F. SMITH, JR. • *Department of Medicine/GI, University of Virginia Health System, Charlottesville, VA*

RHONDA F. SOUZA • *Department of Medicine/GI, University of Texas-Southwestern Medical Center at Dallas/Dallas VA Medical Center, Dallas, TX*

DAVID J. TESTER • *Laboratory of Medicine and Pathology, Mayo Clinic, Rochester, MN*

SAM THIAGALINGAM • *Department of Medicine/Genetics, Boston University School of Medicine, Boston, MA*

STEPHEN N. THIBODEAU • *Laboratory of Medicine and Pathology, Mayo Clinic, Rochester, MN*

KIMBERLY S. TUSTISON • *Department of Medicine/GI, University of Virginia Health System, Charlottesville, VA*

MARK T. WORTHINGTON • *Department of Medicine/GI, University of Virginia Health System, Charlottesville, VA*

JOANNE YU • *Department of Medicine/GI, University of Virginia Health System, Charlottesville, VA*

ZHENGPING ZHUANG • *Laboratory of Pathology, National Cancer Institute, Bethesda, MD*

1

Microdissection of Histologic Sections

Manual and Laser Capture Microdissection Techniques

Christopher A. Moskaluk

1. Introduction

The molecular analysis of human cancer is complicated by the difficulty in obtaining pure populations of tumor cells to study. One traditional method of obtaining a pure representation has been establishing cancer cell lines from primary tumors. However, this technique is time consuming and of low yield. Artifacts of cell culture include the selection of genetic alterations not present in primary tumors *(1,2)* and the alteration of gene expression as compared to primary tumors *(3)*. When molecular techniques move from experimental to diagnostic settings, the need for robust, reproducible and "real time" testing will probably therefore require the direct analysis of tissue samples.

Problems with the study of primary tissue samples include the heterogeneity of cell types and the range in the ratio of neoplastic cells relative to benign cells ("tumor cellularity"). All tissues, even malignant tumors, are composed of a mixture of cell types. No tumors are free of supporting stromal cells (fibroblasts, endothelial cells) and many tumors are invested with inflammatory cells and other residual benign tissue elements. Tumor cellularity and the degree of tumor necrosis not only varies between different neoplasms but can vary greatly between different areas in a single tumor mass. Molecular analyses of cancer in tissue samples may be hindered by insufficient number of viable target cells and a significant degree of contamination by nontarget cells. While it may be true that tests for specific genetic alterations may eventually make some histologic assessment superfluous *(4)*, proposed "gene expression profiling" studies (e.g., microarray assays) will require molecular analysis on pure representations of cancer cells *(5)*. Hence, histologic analysis of tumors will remain an

From: *Methods in Molecular Medicine, vol. 50: Colorectal Cancer: Methods and Protocols*
Edited by: S. M. Powell © Humana Press Inc., Totowa, NJ

important part of tissue procurement for molecular analysis and experimental correlation with molecular assays *(6)*.

To address these issues, various microdissection methodologies have been developed to obtain enriched and/or pure representations of target cells from histologic tissue sections. The methodologies can be separated into two basic strategies: selection of specific tissue elements for analysis, or the destruction of unwanted tissue elements. In the category of positive selection, the least complex methodology involves the manual dissection of tissue elements under direct microscopic visualization using scalpel blades, fine-gage needles, or drawn glass pipets *(7)*. The precision with which manual microdissection can be performed depends greatly on the architectural arrangement of the target tissue and the skill of the dissector. An extension of this method is the attachment of steel or glass needles to micromanipulator devices that allow for more fine control, enabling the dissection of individual cells *(8,9)*. The latter technique is quite laborious, which is a limitation to the procurement of large numbers of cells. Recent advances have brought the power of laser technology to microdissection, which allow both precise and rapid procurement of tissue elements. There are two prevalent laser-based techniques: laser capture microdissection (LCM) and laser microbeam microdissection with laser pressure catapulting (LMM-LPC). In LCM a transparent ethylene vinyl acetate thermoplastic film covers the tissue section, which is melted over areas of interest by an infrared laser thus embedding the target tissue *(10,11)*. When the film is removed from the histologic section the selected tissue remains on the film while unselected tissue remains in the tissue section (*see* **Figs. 1** and **2**). DNA, protein and RNA can all be subsequently isolated from the tissue attached to the film. In LMM-LPC, a pulsed ultraviolet nitrogen laser is used as a fine "optical scalpel" to cut out target tissue of interest *(12,13)*. The laser beam cuts

---

Fig. 1. *(opposite page)* Schematic diagram of laser capture microdissection. **(A)** The upper figure shows a side view of a histologic section and the microfuge tube cap which bears the thermoplastic ethylene vinyl acetate capture film (CapSure, Arcturus Engineering Inc.). The middle figure shows the CapSure cap in contact with the tissue and a burst of the infrared laser (not drawn to scale) traveling through the cap, film, and target tissue. The laser energy is absorbed by the thermoplastic film that melts and embeds the target tissue. The target tissue is not harmed in this process. The lower figure shows the result of a successful laser capture microdissection. The target tissue remains embedded in the thermoplastic film, and is lifted away from nontarget tissue in the histologic section. **(B)** The tissue-bearing cap is placed on a microfuge tube that contains a lysis buffer. After inversion of the tube and incubation, the desired biomolecules (DNA, RNA and/or protein) are released from the captured tissue into the solution.

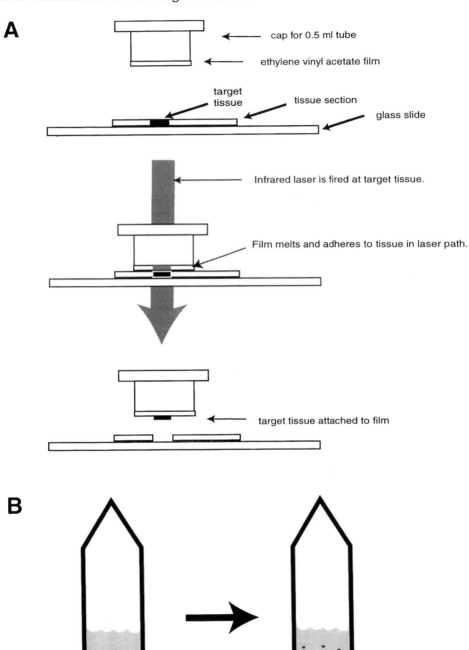

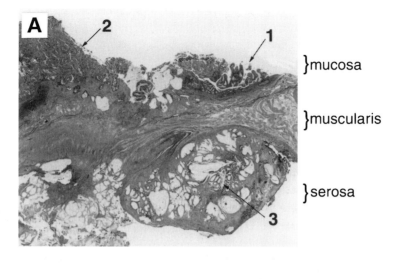

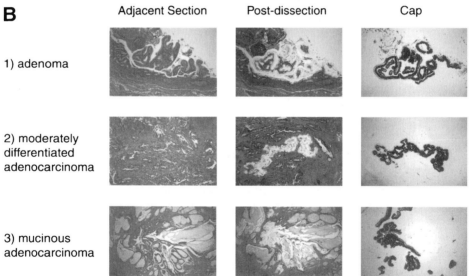

Fig. 2. Example laser capture microdissection of colon cancer. **(A)** Low power magnification of a histologic section of a human colon adenocarcinoma. Area 1 is an area of adenoma adjacent to the invasive carcinoma. Area 2 is an area of a typical moderately differentiated tubular adenocarcinoma in the region of the submucosa. Area 3 shows a more deeply invasive area of the carcinoma (in the serosa) with mucinous differentiation. Original magnification ×7. **(B)** In the left column, portions of a nondissected histologic section (same as in A) which is immediately adjacent to a histologic section used in laser capture microdissection are shown. The corresponding areas of the dissected

the tissue by "ablative photodecomposition" without heat generation or lateral damage to adjacent material *(14)*. The freed tissue is then catapulted from the surface of the histologic section into the cap of a microfuge tube by the force of a pulse of a high photon density laser microbeam. Both LCM and LMM-LPC have the precision to collect single cells, and the capacity to quickly collect thousands of targeted cells. Their drawback is the cost of the laser apparatuses, which range from $70,000 to $130,000.

The second strategy, removal or destruction of unwanted tissue, uses many of the same methodologies for positive selection. With manual techniques, it is sometimes easier to remove unwanted tissue from foci of targeted tissue, rather than to precisely dissect out the target tissue *(15)*. Laser photodecomposition can be used to destroy contaminating nontarget material *(16)*. DNA can also be destroyed by exposure to conventional ultraviolet light sources. The technique known as selective ultraviolet radiation fractionation (SURF) uses this principle *(17,18)*. Target tissue is covered with protective ink (either manually or with the aid of a micromanipulator), and then the histologic section is exposed to UV light. The integrity of the DNA in the target tissue is preserved and can be subsequently analyzed by polymerase chain reaction (PCR) assays. SURF has the advantages of being a rapid and relatively inexpensive technology, but has some of the limitations of other manual methods in terms of precision. It has also not been widely applied to analysis of RNA or protein content.

Presented here are two methods for microdissection that have yielded enriched populations of tumor cells used successfully in analysis of tumor-specific genetic alterations and gene expression. The first is a manual method which can be applied with a minimum of specialized equipment or expense. The second is laser capture microdissection, which requires the use of specialized equipment but offers increased precision. Manual microdissection is performed on hydrated tissue, and LCM is performed on dehydrated tissue. Hence, the latter method also offers greater protection to RNA and protein samples, which are more prone to degradation than DNA.

2. Materials
2.1. Histology

1. Series of containers suitable for slide baths.
2. Histology slide holders.
3. Xylene.

---

section are shown in the middle column. The tissue obtained from these areas by LCM is shown in the right column. The microdissected areas correspond to areas 1 (adenoma), 2 (tubular carcinoma) and 3 (mucinous carcinoma) shown in (A). Microdissection resulted in capture of neoplastic epithelium. Original magnification ×40.

4. 100% Ethanol.
5. 95% Ethanol.
6. 70% Ethanol.
7. Deionized water.
8. Harris hematoxylin (Sigma-Aldrich Co., St. Louis, MO).
9. Eosin Y solution, alcoholic (Sigma-Aldrich Co.).
10. Bluing solution (Richard-Allen medical, Richland, MI).
11. loTE buffer: 3 mM Tris-HCl (pH 7.5), 0.2 mM EDTA. Store at 4°C.
12. loTE/glycerol solution (100:2.5, v/v). Store at 4°C.

2.2. Manual Microdissection

1. Standard binocular light microscope with 4×, 10×, and 20× objectives and 10× oculars.
2. 30-gauge hypodermic needles.
3. 1 cc TB syringes.
4. #11 dissecting scalpel blades and scalpel handle.

2.3. Laser Capture Microdissection

1. Pixcell™ Laser Capture Microdissection System (Arcturus Engineering Inc., Mountain View, CA).
2. CapSure™ ethylene vinyl acetate film carriers (Arcturus Engineering Inc.).
3. 0.5 mL Eppendorf™ microfuge tubes.

2.4. DNA Isolation

1. 5% suspension (w/v) of Chelex 100 resin *(19)* (BioRad, Hercules, CA) in loTE buffer. Store at 4°C.
2. 10X TK buffer: 0.5 M Tris-HCl (pH 8.9), 20 mM EDTA, 10 mM NaCl, 5% Tween-20, 2 mg/mL proteinase K. Store at –20°C.

2.5. RNA Isolation (see Note 1)

1. Denaturing solution: 4 M guanidine isothiocyanate, 0.02 M sodium citrate, 0.5% sarcosyl. Store at room temperature.
2. 2 M sodium acetate (pH 4.0). Store at room temperature.
3. Chloroform:isoamyl alcohol (24:1). Store at room temperature.
4. Isopropanol. Store at room temperature.
5. Phenol equilibrated to pH 5.3–5.7 with 0.1 M succinic acid. Store at 4°C.
6. β-mercaptoethanol. Store at 4°C.
7. 2 mg/mL glycogen. Store at –20°C.

2.6. Protein Isolation

1. SDS sample buffer: 75 mM Tris-HCl (pH 8.3), 2% sodium dodecyl sulfate, 10% glycerol, 0.001% bromophenol blue, 100 mM dithiothreitol.
2. IEF sample buffer: 9 M urea, 4% NP40, 2% β-mercaptoethanol.

3. Methods

3.1. Preparation of Histologic Sections

Seven micron-thick sections are cut from formalin-fixed paraffin embedded tissue (FFPE) or frozen tissue using standard histologic techniques and placed on clean standard glass slides (*see* **Note 2**).

3.2. Staining of FFPE Histologic Sections for Manual Microdissection (DNA Isolation) (see Note 3)

1. Deparaffinization: place the sections in a xylene bath for 5 min. Repeat in a second xylene bath.
2. Removal of xylene and hydration: 100% ethanol bath for 2 min, 70% ethanol bath for 2 min, deionized water bath for 2 min.
3. Place in hematoxylin stain for 30 s (*see* **Note 4**).
4. Rinse in deionized water, repeat rinse.
5. Place in bluing solution for 15 s.
6. Dehydration: 70% ethanol bath for 30 s, 95% Ethanol bath for 30 s.
7. Place in eosin stain for 30 s.
8. Rinse in deionized water, repeat rinse.
9. Place in loTE 2.5% glycerol bath for 2 min (*see* **Note 5**).
10. Allow slides to air dry (*see* **Note 6**).

3.3. Staining of Frozen Sections for Manual Microdissection (DNA Isolation)

1. Fixation: 100% ethanol bath for 2 min.
2. Hydration: 70% ethanol bath for 30 s, deionized water bath for 30 s.
3. Continue from **step 3** in **Subheading 3.2.**

3.4. Staining of FFPE Histologic Sections for LCM (DNA Isolation)

1. Perform **steps 1–7** in **Subheading 3.2.**
2. After staining in eosin, rinse in a 95% ethanol bath, then repeat rinse in a second 95% ethanol bath.
3. 100% Ethanol bath for 1 min (use a clean ethanol bath, not the one used after xylene deparaffinization).
4. Xylene bath for 5 min (use a clean xylene bath, not the one used to deparaffinize sections).
5. Allow slides to air dry.

3.5. Staining of Frozen Histologic Sections for LCM (DNA Isolation)

1. Fixation: 100% ethanol bath for 2 min.
2. Hydration: 70% ethanol bath for 30 s, deionized water bath for 30 s.
3. **Steps 3–7** in **Subheading 3.2.**, followed by **steps 2–5** in **Subheading 3.4.**

3.6. Staining of Frozen Histologic Sections
for LCM (RNA and Protein Isolation) (see Note 7)

1. Ethanol-fixed frozen sections are dipped 15 times in RNase-free water using gloved hands or a slide holder.
2. 15 dips in hematoxylin stain.
3. The slide is dipped a few times in a deionized water bath to remove the majority of the stain, and is then dipped a few times in a fresh deionized water bath until the slide is clear of stain.
4. 15 dips in bluing reagent.
5. 15 dips in 70% ethanol.
6. 15 dips in 95% ethanol.
7. 15 dips in eosin stain.
8. 15 dips in 95% ethanol, then repeat in a fresh 95% ethanol bath.
9. 15 dips in 100% ethanol.
10. 5 min in xylene bath.
11. Air dry for at least 2 min or until the xylene is completely evaporated.

3.7. Manual Microdissection

1. Seat yourself squarely and comfortably in front of a standard light microscope (*see* **Note 8**).
2. Place the glass slide containing the tissue under the 4× objective and focus. Use either the 4×, 10×, or 20× objectives for the dissection, depending on the tissue target and your preferences.
3. Place a 30-gauge needle on the end of a 1 cc TB syringe, or if doing a broader dissection, place a fine tip scalpel blade at the end of a scalpel handle. When using the needle, tap the end of the needle against a hard surface to bend it into a small hook (you will see the hook only under the microscope).
4. Rest your hand on the microscope stage and bring your instrument to bear on the tissue. Perform as clean a dissection as possible by gently scraping the target tissue into a small heap (*see* **Note 9**). Keep a running estimate of the number of cells dissected.
5. Affix the dissected tissue to the end of your instrument, and place into a 1.5 mL microfuge tube. Disperse the tissue into the appropriate volume of buffer (*see* **Subheading 3.9.** for specific applications). If you are interrupted during the dissection, store tube at –20°C.

3.8. Laser Capture Microdissection (see Note 10)

1. Turn on the power to the laser control, the microscope and the video monitor components of the Pixcell LCM apparatus (Arcturus Engineering Inc.).
2. Place the slide to be dissected on the microscope stage over the 4× objective (tissue side up).
3. Adjust focus and light levels on the microscope so that the histologic image is seen clearly on the video monitor. Choose an appropriate microscope objective for the dissection and then refocus.

4. Position the histologic section so that the tissue of interest is on the monitor. Keep the stage controls set in their central position and move the slide around on the stage while doing this. Once the slide is positioned, activate the vacuum mechanism to hold the slide firmly in place on the stage.

5. Set the amplitude and laser pulse width on the laser control to the manufacturer's recommended settings initially (these values can be adjusted according to the requirements for the individual tissue section).

6. Place an ethylene vinyl acetate film-bearing microcentrifuge tube cap (CapSure, Arcturus Engineering Inc.) on the tissue section.

7. An aiming beam is projected onto the slide surface that allows pre-capture visualization. Lower the microscope light level until you can see the outline of the aiming beam on the video monitor. Position this target spot over the tissue area to be captured by moving the microscope stage (*see* **Note 11**).

8. Fire the laser beam. This administers a laser pulse of the power and duration selected on the laser control, which briefly melts the thermoplastic film allowing it to permeate the target tissue. Continue moving the microscope stage, positioning the aiming beam, and firing the laser until all the tissue of interest is captured (*see* **Note 12**).

9. After dissection, lift the CapSure cap off of the tissue, move the slide so that a blank area of glass is in the viewing area. Place the CapSure cap down on the blank area and inspect the captured tissue.

10. Place the CapSure cap on a 0.5 mL Eppendorf microcentrifuge tube. Label the tube, not the cap, with an indelible marker. The tube may contain extraction buffer for the specific applications outlined below.

3.9. DNA Isolation from Manual Microdissection

1. Prior to microdissection, place 15 µL of 5% Chelex resin per 100 cells expected to be dissected. If you decide to harvest more cells than the target number during the dissection, then add additional buffer after the dissection.

2. After the dissection, add 10X TK buffer to make tube contents 1X.

3. Vortex tube for 5 s, then spin briefly in a microcentrifuge to settle the contents.

4. Incubate in a 56°C waterbath overnight.

5. Vortex and centrifuge tube as above.

6. Add 1/10 the volume of 10X TK that was added initially.

7. Vortex 5 s, incubate at 56°C overnight.

8. Place in dry heating block set at 100°C for 10 min. Alternatively, incubate the tubes in a boiling water bath for 10 min (*see* **Note 13**).

9. Store at –20°C.

3.10. DNA Isolation from LCM

1. Place freshly diluted 1X TK buffer in a 0.5 mL Eppendorf microfuge tube at a ratio of 15 µL per 100 cells captured. Using the capping tool provided with the LCM apparatus, push the tissue-bearing CapSure cap to the prescribed distance into the tube on all sides. Invert the tube and shake.

2. Incubate the tube inverted in a 37°C incubator overnight.
3. Shake the tube then centrifuge briefly to settle the contents (you may have to cut the caps off of the tubes in order to centrifuge them).
4. Remove the CapSure cap, add 1% vol of 10X TK buffer, cap the tubes with a standard microfuge cap, then incubate for another day in a 56°C water bath.

3.11. RNA Isolation from Microdissection

1. Place the tissue-bearing CapSure cap onto a 0.5 mL Eppendorf microfuge tube (with its cap cut off) that contains 200 µL RNA denaturing buffer and 1.6 µL β-mercaptoethanol. Seat the cap using the cap fitting tool. Invert and vortex the tube several times over the course of 2 min to digest the tissue off the cap (*see* **Note 14**).
2. Centrifuge the tube briefly at top speed in a microcentrifuge to settle the contents. Remove the solution from the 0.5 mL tube and transfer it to a 1.5 mL microfuge tube.
3. Add 20 µL (0.1X vol) 2 *M* sodium acetate (pH 4.0), 220 µL (1X volume) water saturated phenol (bottom layer) and 60 µL (0.3X vol) chloroform-isoamyl alcohol.
4. Vortex vigorously, then centrifuge for 10 min at 12,000*g* (room temperature) to separate the aqueous and organic phases.
5. Transfer upper aqueous layer to a new tube.
6. Add 2 µL glycogen (2 mg/mL) and 200 µL isopropanol. Vortex vigorously.
7. Freeze solid in dry ice/ethanol bath. Alternatively, the tube may be left at −20°C overnight.
8. Centrifuge at 12,000*g* for 15 min at 4°C.
9. Remove the majority of the supernatant with a 1000 µL tip and then switch to a smaller pipet to remove the rest of the supernatant. This minimizes disruption of the RNA pellet.
10. Wash with 75% ethanol (4°C). Add the alcohol and centrifuge at 12,000*g* for 5 min at 4°C.
11. Remove the supernatant as explained above. All of the supernatant should be removed at this point.
12. Let the pellet air dry on ice to remove any residual fluid. Do not over dry the pellet, or it will be difficult to resuspend the RNA.
13. To RNA pellet add 15 µL RNase-free water, and 40 units RNase inhibitor (e.g., RNase block, Stratagene), 2 µL 10X DNase buffer (*see* enzyme supplier's recommendations) and 2 µL 10 U/µL RNase-free DNase1.
14. Incubate at 37°C for 2 h.
15. Centrifuge the tube briefly at top speed in a microcentrifuge to settle the contents. Add 30 mL DEPC water, 5 µL (0.1X volume), 2 *M* sodium acetate (pH 4.0), 55 µL (1X vol) water saturated phenol (bottom layer) and 16.5 µL (0.3X vol) chloroform-isoamyl alcohol.
16. Vortex vigorously then centrifuge at 12,000*g* for 10 min at room temperature.
17. Transfer upper layer to a new 1.5 mL microfuge tube.
18. Add 1 µL glycogen (2 mg/mL) and 50 µL isopropanol. Vortex vigorously.
19. Repeat **steps 7–12**.

3.12. Protein Isolation from Microdissection (see Note 7)

1. The sample buffer is chosen on the basis of the subsequent analysis: isoelectric focusing (IEF) or denaturing sodium dodecyl sulfate polyacrylamide gel electrophoresis (SDS-PAGE).
2. 10 μL of IEF sample buffer or 30 μL SDS sample buffer per 5000 cells are added to the microfuge tube containing the tissue. In the case of LCM, the tube is inverted so that buffer comes into contact with the tissue.
3. Vortex the tube vigorously for 1 min, or until the tissue is lysed (*see* **Note 14**).

4. Notes

1. Standard procedures for eliminating RNase from stock solution (treatment with diethylpyrocarbonate [DEPC]) should be followed. Alternatively, the reagents specified in this protocol can be purchased as part of the Micro RNA Isolation Kit from Stratagene Cloning Systems (La Jolla, CA).
2. Especially for LCM, it is important not to use treated glass slides (charged or coated) to increase tissue adhesion, which can interfere with transfer of tissue to the capture film. Store paraffin-embedded histologic sections in a dust-free box at room temperature. Store frozen histologic sections at –70°C.
3. DNA extraction can be performed from both FFPE and frozen tissue, although most of the DNA obtained from FFPE will be a few hundred basepairs or less in length. Five to 15 mL of the DNA extraction can be used in subsequent polymerase chain reaction (PCR) assays (33–100 cell equivalents).
4. Xylene and alcohol solutions should be changed regularly. The hematoxylin solution (which tends to coagulate) should be filtered through coarse filter paper prior to use each day. Bluing solution should be clear with no surface scum.
5. Longer incubation at this step will leach the eosin out of the tissue.
6. You may use a hair dryer set to the COOL setting to speed drying, but do not over dry the sections. Stain only as many sections as necessary. Stained sections should be stored at –20°C and can be reused as needed.
7. For protein and most RNA analysis, fresh frozen tissue is recommended, and the tissue needs to be frozen as quickly as possible following removal from the patient or animal to prevent degradation of these biomolecules. Place frozen sections in 95% ethanol kept on dry ice immediately after sectioning on a cryostat, and let fix for 5 min. It may be possible to obtain sufficient RNA from FFPE tissue to do reverse-transcriptase coupled PCR (RT-PCR) assays if the PCR product is less than 200 bp in length. At this juncture, it is recommended that protein analysis be carried out by LCM analysis, given the greater protection that the dehydrated tissue offers from proteolytic digestion.
8. Place a clean barrier on the adjacent desk if contamination with PCR product is a possibility. Place books, cushions, etc. under the elbow of your dissecting hand to give it stable support at the height required to reach the microscope stage.
9. During dissection, the tissue should be soft and pliable and not scatter due to static electricity. On the other hand, there shouldn't be a covering of liquid that causes the dissected tissue to float away. If upon storage or during a dissection

session the tissue becomes overly dried, it can be dipped momentarily into the loTE/glycerol buffer and allowed to dry.

10. Specific details on manipulation of the slide, caps and laser will depend on the specific model of the LCM apparatus. Consult the manufacturer's instruction manual. The NIH laser capture microdissection website (http://dir.nichd.nih.gov/lcm/lcm.htm) maintains updated protocols for biomolecule extraction and analysis from microdissected material.

11. If difficulty is encountered in balancing the light level for optimal visualization of both the tissue and the laser beam, mark the location of the laser beam on the video screen with pieces of tape, then readjust the light for optimal histologic resolution. The tape markers will have to be moved when switching between microscope objectives.

12. If tissue does not adhere to the thermoplastic film, increase the amplitude of the laser by five. If still not capturing, increase laser pulse width by five. If still not capturing, repeat the above two steps. If still not capturing, try dehydrating the tissue for longer periods in sequential 100% ethanol and xylene baths.

13. As an alternative to heat treatment of the tissue samples, the DNA extracts can be kept frozen until use in PCR. After assembling the PCR components (except for the thermostable DNA polymerase), the reactions can be incubated at 98°C for 5 min in the PCR machine, after which the DNA polymerase can be safely added.

14. Multiple LCM caps may be required to obtain the requisite number of cells for analysis. If this is the case, the microfuge tube can be briefly centrifuged to settle the fluid contents, and then another tissue-bearing cap can be placed on the tube and the lysis step repeated.

References

1. Okamoto, A., Demetrick, D. J., Spillare, E. A., Hagiwara, K., Hussain, S. P., Bennett, W. P., et al. (1994) Mutations and altered expression of p16INK4 in human cancer. *Proc. Natl. Acad. Sci. USA* **91,** 11,045–11,049.

2. Huang, L., Goodrow, T. L., Zhang, S. Y., Klein-Szanto, A. J., Chang, H., and Ruggeri, B. A. (1996) Deletion and mutation analyses of the p16/MTS-1 tumor suppressor gene in human ductal pancreatic cancer reveals a higher frequency of abnormalities in tumor-derived cell lines than in primary ductal adenocarcinomas. *Cancer Res.* **56,** 1137–1141.

3. Zhang, L., Zhou, W., Velculescu, V. E., Kern, S. E., Hruban, R. H., Hamilton, S. R., Vogelstein, B., and Kinzler, K. W. (1997) Gene expression profiles in normal and cancer cells. *Science* **276,** 1268–1272.

4. Cairns, P. and Sidransky, D. (1999) Molecular methods for the diagnosis of cancer. *Biochim. Biophys. Acta* **1423,** C11–C18.

5. Bowtell, D. D. L. (1998) Options available-from start to finish-for obtaining expression data by microarray. *Nature Genet.* **20,** 25–32.

6. Cole, K. A., Krizman, D. B., and Emmert-Buck, M. R. (1998) The genetics of cancer-a 3D model. *Nature Genet.* **20,** 38–41.

7. Zhuang, Z., Bertheau, P., Emmert-Buck, M. R., Liotta, L. A., Gnarra, J., Linehan, W. M., and Lubensky, I. A. (1995) A microdissection technique for archival DNA analysis of specific cell populations in lesions < 1 mm in size. *Am. J. Pathol.* **146,** 620–625.
8. Moskaluk, C. and Kern, S. (1997) Microdissection and PCR amplification of genomic DNA from histologic tissue sections. *Am. J. Pathol.* **150,** 1547–1552.
9. Lee, J. Y., Dong, S. M., Kim, S. Y., Yoo, N. J., Lee, S. H., and Park, W. S. (1998) A simple, precise and economical microdissection technique for analysis of genomic DNA from archival tissue sections. *Virchows Arch.* **433,** 305–309.
10. Simone, N. L., Bonner, R. F., Gillespie, J. W., Emmert-Buck, M. R., and Liotta, L. A. (1998) Laser-capture microdissection: opening the microscopic frontier to molecular analysis. *Trends Genet.* **14,** 272–276.
11. Emmert-Buck, M., Bonner, R., Smith, P., Chuaqui, R., Zhuang, Z., Goldstein, S., Weiss, R., and Liotta, L. (1996) Laser capture microdissection. *Science* **274,** 998–1001.
12. Schutze, K. and Lahr, G. (1998) Identification of expressed genes by laser mediated manipulation of single cells. *Nat. Biotechnol.* **16,** 737–742.
13. Schutze, K., Posl, H., and Lahr, G. (1998) Laser micromanipulation systems as universal tools in cellular and molecular biology and in medicine. *Cell Mol. Biol.* **44,** 735–746.
14. Srinivasan, R. (1986) Ablation of polymers and biological tissue by ultraviolet lasers. *Science* **234,** 559–565.
15. Deng, G., Lu, Y., Zlotnikov, G., Thor, A. D., and Smith, H. S. (1996) Loss of heterozygosity in normal tissue adjacent to breast carcinomas. *Science* **274,** 2057–2059.
16. Hadano, S., Watanabe, M., Yokoi, H., Kogi, M., Kondo, I., Tsuchiya, H., et al. (1991) Laser microdissection and single unique primer PCR allow generation of regional chromosome DNA clones from a single human chromosome. *Genomics* **11,** 364–373.
17. Shibata, D. (1993) Selective ultraviolet radiation fractionation and polymerase chain reaction analysis of genetic alterations. *Am. J. Pathol.* **143,** 1523–1526.
18. Shibata, D. (1998) The SURF technique: selective genetic analysis of microscopic tissue heterogeniety, in *PCR in Bioanalysis* (Meltzer, S. J., ed.), Humana, Totowa, NJ, pp. 39–47.
19. Walsh, P. S., Metzger, D. A., and Higuchi, R. (1991) Chelex 100 as a medium for simple extraction of DNA for PCR-based typing from forensic material. *Biotechniques* **10,** 506–513.

2

Isolation of a Purified Epithelial Cell Population from Human Colon

James K. Roche

1. Introduction

While *in situ* techniques have been valuable in identifying the presence and localization of cytoplasmic and membrane components in tissue *(1)*, there is often a need to study directly one or more cell types, free from its own microenvironment. For the human colon, isolation techniques to allow direct study have been described for mononuclear cells in the lamina propria, smooth muscle cells at or below the muscularis mucosae, and cells of the enteric nervous system, located between the subserosa and the lamina propria *(2–4)*. More recently, interest has risen to isolate populations of intestinal epithelial cells, for investigations of human colonic adenocarcinoma—which originates from colonic epithelia; as well as for study of the epithelial response to infection and inflammation. The technique for isolating epithelial cells from the human colon involves mechanical dissection to separate mucosa from the muscle layers which are discarded; and enzymatic digestion of collagen, followed by discontinuous gradient centrifugation in Percoll. The goal is to isolate >90% pure epithelial cells. Although the cells appear intact under the microscope, viability is variable from 50–80%. The yield depends on the size of the available tissue.

2. Materials

2.1. Buffers

1. Hanks balanced salt solution (1X) without Mg^{2+} and Ca^{2+} (store at room temperature).
2. Dulbecco's phosphate-buffered saline (1X) without Mg^{2+} ad Ca^{2+} (store at room temperature).

From: *Methods in Molecular Medicine, vol. 50: Colorectal Cancer: Methods and Protocols*
Edited by: S. M. Powell © Humana Press Inc., Totowa, NJ

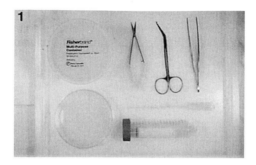

Fig. 1. Materials and instruments used for epithelial cell isolation. Moving clockwise from top left corner: surgical cutting board, small plastic container, surgical scissors, forceps, plastic transfer pipet, 50 mL centrifuge tube, and a Petri dish.

3. RPMI medium 1640 (1X), 0.1 μm filtered with L-glutamine (store at 4°C).
4. Percoll (sterile), 1000 mL, density 1.129 g/mL (store at 4°C).
5. 1 m*M* EDTA solution made in HBSS (store at 4°C).
6. 0.15% dithiothreitol solution made in HBSS (store at room temperature).
7. Trypan blue solution (*see* **Notes 1** and **2).**
8. HEPES buffer solution (1 *M*) (store at 4°C).

2.2. Chemicals

1. DNase enzyme (Worthington) (store at –20°C).
2. Dispase enzyme (Boehringer Mannheim) (store at 4°C).
3. Dithiothreitol DTT (Sigma) FW: 154.2.
4. Sodium chloride (Sigma) FW: 58.44.
5. Trypan blue (Kodak) FW: 960.81.
6. Thimerosal (Sigma) FW: 404.8.
7. EDTA disodium salt dihydrate (Sigma) FW: 372.2.

2.3. Equipment (see Note 3 and Fig. 1)

1. Fine tip transfer pipet (sterile).
2. Centrifuge tubes 50 mL.
3. One plastic surgical cutting board 12" × 12".
4. Forceps (small) (sterile).
5. Surgical scissors (sterile).
7. Flat bottom plastic disposable containers with tops.

3. Methods
3.1. Obtaining the Specimen

Obtain the surgical specimen. Select an appropriate area based on clinical diagnosis. Place tissue in 100 mL of ice-cold HBSS in a plastic disposable

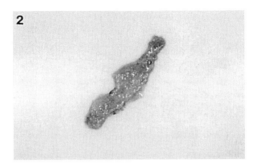

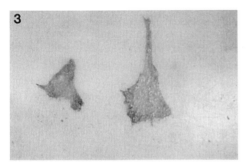 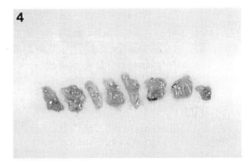

Fig. 2. Colonic specimen, shortly after surgical resection, opened longitudinally, with mucosal surface facing camera. To process this specimen, mucosa is stripped from the deeper muscle layers.

Fig. 3. Appearance of human colonic mucosa after it has been stripped from muscle and serosa. The next step is to cut the mucosa into 2 cm strips and then incubate with 0.15% Dithiothreitol/HBSS for 30 min to remove excess fat and other debris.

Fig. 4. Small pieces of colonic mucosa measuring 2 cm × 1 cm. The small sections will increase the surface area and allow more epithelial cells to be released from the tissue.

---

container and transport immediately to the laboratory. Begin the procedure as soon as the specimen is acquired. Long exposure of tissue to outside environment reduces cell yield (*see* **Note 4**).

3.2. Preparing and Dissecting the Mucosa

1. Remove the specimen from HBSS. Place tissue on a flat surface (dissecting board) covered with dry paper towels and remove fat, necrotic tissue and gross debris (*see* **Fig. 2**).
2. Place slightly stretched tissue flat on paper towels, mucosal side up. Using curved fine forceps, gently pinch and lift the mucosa at one edge of the specimen. Cut between the mucosal and the muscle layers with fine curved iris scissors, starting at the lifted edge of the specimen and if possible, longitudinally to the circular

folds. Put the mucosal strips in a 100 mm Petri dish containing HBSS. Cut the strips approx 4 cm in length and 1–2 mm in width. Be sure that no muscle is included underneath each mucosal strip. When in doubt, invert strip, inspect it visually and remove any muscle inadvertently included (*see* **Figs. 3** and **4**).

3.3. Removal of Residual Mucus and Epithelial Cells

1. After complete removal of the mucosa, rinse strip thoroughly in a Petri dish containing fresh HBSS and transfer them to a flat bottom plastic disposable container with 50 mL of HBSS, 0.15% dithiothreitol and a magnetic stirring bar (*see* **Note 5**). Place container on a stirring plate at room temperature, put lid on and set speed at approx $0.30g$ for 30 min to dissolve residual mucus and free additional debris. At the end of the stirring period, the solution will be slightly cloudy and small floating debris is usually observed.
2. Remove the mucosal strips and the stirring bar, rinse them in a Petri dish with fresh HBSS and transfer them to a new container with 100 mL of HBSS, 1 mM EDTA, pH 7.2. Stir at room temperature for 60 min to releases epithelial cells from the basal lamina. The solution will become cloudy as the epithelial cells detach from the lamina propria. Stirring must be gentle, yet vigorous enough to keep all tissue floating in suspension, and not simply to push the strip around at the bottom on the container.
3. Repeat the 60 min stirring period once or twice depending on the conditions of the specimen (*see* **Note 6**).
4. Collect EDTA solutions in 50 mL centrifuge tubes. Spin down $470g$ for 5 min and resuspend in 15 mL RPMI media.

3.4. Isolation and Purification of Intestinal Epithelial Cells Using Dispase and Percoll

1. Add 45 mg Dispase and 15 mg DNase to the combined epithelial cells (final enzyme concentrations 3 and 1 mg/mL, respectively) and incubate in a 37°C water bath for 30 min. Vortex for 10 s at 5 min intervals. Use the minimum force required to vortex to minimize damage to cells. Small intestinal specimens almost invariably require longer stirring periods than large bowel specimens due to the release of many more epithelial cells from a comparable surface area as a result of the presence of villi. Specimens with mucosal inflammation will require variable times, depending on the degree of inflammation and the extent and severity of damage to the epithelial cell layer.
2. Spin the cells at $200g$ for 5 min, carefully discard the supernatant and wash again in HBSS. Following wash, resuspend in 5 or 10 mL RPMI depending on the size of the pellet.
3. Prepare an aliquot of cells for trypan blue staining and microscopic examination (*see* **Note 2**). The preparation should be a mixture of epithelial cells, mononuclear cells, and red blood cells. The preparation should be 95–100% viable and mostly single cells, any clumps containing 3–4 cells at most.

4. A 50% Percoll solution is used to separate epithelial cells from mononuclear and red blood cells. For most preparations 2 gradients are sufficient, however 1 or 4 gradients can be used with small or large preps. Gradients are prepared by mixing 10 mL Percoll with 10 mL PBS in 50 mL centrifuge tubes. Adjust the cell suspension volume to 5 mL per gradient and overlay each gradient with 5 mL of cell suspension. Centrifuge the gradients at $470g$ for 20 min.

5. The epithelial cells will equilibrate at the top of the Percoll layer, while the mononuclear cells and red blood cells will pellet at the bottom of the tube. Collect the epithelial cell layer in a 50 mL centrifuge *excluding* as much of the gradient material below as possible (*see* **Note 7**). Most of the epithelial cells can be recovered in 10–15 mL, leaving at least 10 mL in the gradient tube. Do not include material form the conical portion of the tube!

6. Dilute the recovered epithelial cells with RPMI and centrifuge at $830g$ for 5 min. Resuspend the epithelial cells in RPMI, spin at $470g$ for 5 min, then transfer to a 15 mL tube.

7. Resuspend in a volume appropriate for counting, and prepare an aliquot for trypan blue staining. Count live epithelial cells, live mononuclear cells and dead cells.

8. Final step: what to do with cells?
   a. Freeze cells at –80°C (*see* **Note 8**).
   b. Use cells in functional assay.

4. Notes

1. Please handle with caution! Thimerosal in powder form is toxic by inhalation, after contact with skin, and when swallowed. It is irritating to eyes, respiratory system, and skin. It is also a possible mutagen with target organs being kidneys and nerves. Wear suitable protective clothing, gloves, and eye/face protection when dealing with thimerosal as a powder. When thimerosal is dissolved, gloves are still recommended.

2. Counting solution: 45 µL (4.5% NaCl, 0.2% thimerosal).
   180 µL (0.2% trypan blue, 0.2% thimerosal).

3. Any equipment labeled "Sterile" means autoclaved individually wrapped to assure sterility.

4. When dealing with any human tissue, please use the utmost care to assure the safety of yourself and your lab. Dispose of anything that comes into contact with human tissue in your contaminated materials box. Isopropyl alcohol (70%) sterilizes everything.

5. Most of the solutions such as EDTA, 0.15% dithiothreitol, and trypan blue solutions can be made ahead of time.

6. A minimum of 2 EDTA incubations ensures higher epithelial cell counts.

7. When collecting the cells from the Percoll, use a fine tip plastic transfer pipet. When pipeting the cells in the centrifuge tubes, try not to make any bubbles. Bubbles may harm the epithelial cells.

8. At the end of the isolation, centrifuge the cells into a pellet and discard supernatant. Using a pipetman, place the cells in the cryogenic tube excluding as much of

the media as possible. Fast freeze the cells by placing the tubes in a small volume of liquid nitrogen. Label tubes with cell type, cell number, diagnosis, patient name/number, and so on.

References

1. Planchon, S., Fiocchi, C., Takafuji, V., and Roche, J. K. (1999) Transforming growth factor-β1 preserves epithelial barrier function: identification of receptors, biochemical intermediates, and cytokine antagonists. *J. Cell Physiol.* **181,** 55–66.
2. Youngman, K. R., Simon, P. L., West, G. A., Cominelli, F., Rachmilewitz, D., Klein, J. S., and Fiocchi, C. (1993) Localization of intestinal interleukin 1 activity and protein and gene expression to lamina propria cells. *Gastroenterology* **104,** 749–758.
3. Strong, S. A., Pizarro, T. T., Klein, J. S., Cominelli, F., and Fiocchi, C. (1998) Proinflammatory cytokines differentially modulate their own expression in human intestinal mucosal mesenchymal cells. *Gastroenterology* **114,** 1244–1256.
4. Graham, M. F., Diealmann, R. F., Elson, C. O., Ditar, K. N., and Ehrlich, H. F. (1984) Isolation and culture of human intestinal smooth muscle cells. *Proc. Soc. Exp. Biol. Med.* **176,** 503–507.

3

Xenografting Human Colon Cancers

Jeffrey C. Harper, Reid B. Adams, and Steven M. Powell

1. Introduction

Xenografting of human tumors has been used to produce samples which are enriched for neoplasia and optimal for subsequent molecular analyses. Molecular studies of xenograft tumors generated from both human colon and pancreatic adenocarcinomas have led to the discovery of important genetic alterations underlying these malignancies (e.g., Smad4, Smad2) *(1,2)*. Moreover, analysis of pancreatic xenografts helped facilitate the discovery of BCRA2 through identification of homozygous deletions *(3)*. Furthermore, xenografted tumors have facilitated the discovery of distinctive allelic loss patterns in pancreatic and stomach adenocarcinomas *(4,5)*. Comparative genomic hybridization analysis of xenografted human gastric cancers has demonstrated consistent DNA copy number changes, including both gains and losses of chromosomal regions *(6)*.

Previous studies have demonstrated that genetic changes found in these xenografted tumors are stable and correlate well with the corresponding primary tumor genetic alterations *(4,7)*. Additional genetic alterations which might occur during propagation of these human tissues in immunodeficient mice appear to occur only rarely. Thus, xenograft tumors generated from human stomach carcinomas provide optimal specimens to identify clear, unambiguous changes which occur during tumorigenesis.

2. Materials

1. Forceps, curved dissection and blunt end (Fisher Scientific, Pittsburgh, PA).
2. Scissors, eye dissection grade (Fisher Scientific).
3. 70% Ethanol pads and spray bottle.
4. Towels (sterile field) and gauze.
5. Safety razor blades (Fisher Scientific).

From: *Methods in Molecular Medicine, vol. 50: Colorectal Cancer: Methods and Protocols*
Edited by: S. M. Powell © Humana Press Inc., Totowa, NJ

6. Plastic Petri dishes (100 × 15 mm) (Fisher Scientific).
7. Anesthetizing chamber.
8. Metophane (Mallinckrodt Veterinary, Inc.).
9. Autoclip wound closing system (Fisher Scientific).
10. RPMI with FBS and Penn Strep (Gibco-BRL, Gaithersburg, MD).
11. Matrigel (Becton Dickinson Labware, Bedford, MA).
12. Sterile hood.
13. Liquid nitrogen.
14. −80°C Freezer.
15. Autoclave.
16. Cryovials (5 mL) (Fisher Scientific).
17. 1.7 mL snap cap centrifuge tubes (Fisher Scientific).
18. Mice: immune deficient mice are used (nu/nu from Harlan or SCID from Charles River, 3 to 9 wk old) (*see* **Notes 1** and **2**).

3. Methods.
3.1. Implantation (see Notes 3–8)

1. Fresh tissue from surgically resected tumors are obtained for implantation. Immediately the tumor tissue is placed in ~5 mL of RPMI/FBS/Pen Strep. After implantation any remaining tumor tissue is placed in a cryovial and snap frozen in liquid nitrogen. Then, this tissue is stored in the −80°C freezer.
2. Sterilize by autoclaving all surgical instruments. Sanitize the sterile hood with 70% ethanol and spray all items placed in the hood.
3. Prepare the tumor tissue for implantation by placing a viable piece in a Petri dish in a pool of RPMI. Using a razor and forceps chop twelve 3–4 mm sub samples. Place three pieces in a sterile 1.7 mL snap cap centrifuge tube containing 50 µL Matrigel. Prepare a mouse by placing it in a anesthetizing chamber that has had Metofane poured on gauze. Do not let the Metofane liquid come in contact with the mouse. Observe the mouse's respiration and muscular movement. When the breathing is slowed, remove the mouse and place it on a surgical towel. Regulate the depth of anesthesia.
4. Mouse surgery is started by wiping the skin area to be cut with a 70% ethanol pad, typically over the shoulders and hips. Using the forceps pull up a fold of skin and make a ~1 cm incision. Insert the blunt end forceps and form a pocket under the skin (~2 cm deep). Using the same forceps, remove the tumor and Matrigel from the centrifuge tube and place in the formed pocket. Close the wound with the forceps and staple it with the Autoclip system. Repeat on the next site for implantation. Place the mouse in a clean sterile cage. Check the mouse after 15 min. It should be active.

3.2. Harvesting the Xenograft Tumors

1. Xenografts may be harvested when an obvious subdermal growth is noticed. Typically at least 1 cm × 2 cm. Longer growth periods may result in larger tumors; however, necrosis may be a concern.

2. A mouse with a xenograft growth is anesthetized as before. The growth area is sanitized with a 70% ethanol pad. The skin adjacent to the growth is pulled up with forceps and cut with scissors. Observation of the blood supply to the growth is made. This is referred to as the pedicle. The pedicle and a small amount of xenograft is left in the mouse to allow for future harvests. All remaining tumor is removed. The harvest is then divided in a Petri dish according to the various analysis to be performed (i.e., RNA extraction, cell suspension initiation). The remaining tissue is snap frozen in a cryovial in liquid nitrogen and stored in the –80°C freezer.

4. Notes

1. Two to five mice per case have been used for implantations to increase the likelihood of tumor growth.
2. Sterile surgical materials and conditions and technique. These mice are immunodeficient, thus utmost care needs to be taken to prevent infections from developing in these animals.
3. RPMI is made as follows: 500 mL 1X RPMI, 10 mL penicillin/streptomycin, 5 mL glutamine, 2.979 g HEPES (25 mM HEPES) mixed and filtered to sterilize.
4. Snap freezing is done by immersing a sample in bath of liquid nitrogen for approximately 2 min.
5. Minimize the time from the removal of the sample from RPMI media and the implantation once arterial supply of nutrients to tissue is gone.
6. Matrigel immersed tissue should be in the gel for 10–15 min before implantation. During implantation most of the Matrigel should also be transferred to the mouse.
7. The depth of anesthesia of the mouse is regulated by placing a small container (i.e., 1.7 mL centrifuge tube) with gauze saturated with Metofane over the mouse's nose at various intervals.
8. Four to six implantation sites between two mice were routinely performed for each resection.

References

1. Hahn, S. A., Schutte, M., Hoque, A. T., Moskaluk, C. A., da Costa, L. T., Rozenblum, E., et al. (1996) DPC4, a candidate tumor suppressor gene at human chromosome 18q21.1. *Science* **271**, p. 350–353.
2. Thiagalingam, S., Lengauer, C., Leach, F. S., Schutte, M., Hahn, S. A., Overhauser, J., et al. (1996) Evaluation of candidate tumour suppressor genes on chromosome 18 in colorectal cancers. *Nature Genet.* **13**, 343–346.
3. Schutte, M., da Costa, L. T., Hahn, S. A., Moskaluk, C., Hoque, A. T., Rozenblum, E., et al. (1995) Identification by representational difference analysis of a homozygous deletion in pancreatic carcinoma that lies within the BCRA2 region. *Proc. Natl. Acad. Sci. USA* **92**, 5950–5954.
4. Hahn, S. A., Seymour, A. B., Hoque, A. T., Schutte, M., da Costa, L. T., Redston, M. S., et al. (1995) Allelotype of pancreatic adenocarcinoma using xenograft enrichment. *Cancer Res.* **55**, 4670–4675.

5. Yustein, A. S., Harper, J. C., Petroni, G. R., Cummings, O. W., Moskaluk, C. A., and Powell, S. M. (1999) Allelotype of gastric adenocarcinoma. *Cancer Res.* **59,** 1437–1441.
6. El-Rifai, W., Harper, J. C., Cumings, O. W., Hyytinen, E. R., Frierson, H. F., Jr., Knuutila, S., and Powell, S. M. (1998) Consistent genetic alterations in xenografts of proximal stomach and gastro-esophageal junction adenocarcinomas. *Cancer Res.* **58,** 34–37.
7. McQueen, H., Wyllie, A., Piris, J., Foster, E., and Bird, C. (1991) Stability of critical genetic lesions in human colorectal carcinoma xenografts. *Br. J. Cancer* **63,** 94.

4

Comparative Genomic Hybridization Technique

Wa'el El-Rifai and Sakari Knuutila

1. Introduction

Screening for chromosomal changes in solid tumors was long hindered by methodological problems encountered in standard cytogenetic analysis. Comparative genomic hybridization (CGH), a technique that emerged in 1992 (1) has proved to be a powerful tool for molecular cytogenetic analysis of neoplasms. The main prerequisite of the technique is DNA isolated from tumor samples. As no cell culture of tumor material is required, the technique has been successfully used to study fresh and frozen tissue samples, as well as archival formalin-fixed paraffin-embedded tissue samples. CGH allows to screen entire tumor genomes for gains and losses of DNA copy number, enabling consequent mapping of aberrations to chromosomal subregions. The technique is based on fluorescence *in situ* hybridization. Tumor and reference DNA are differentially labeled with fluorochromes (green and red, respectively) and mixed in equal amounts. The mixture is cohybridized competitively to a normal metaphase slide prepared from a lymphocyte cell culture of a normal healthy individual. After hybridization and washes, the chromosomes are counterstained with DAPI (blue) and slides are mounted with an antifading medium. Using a fluorescence microscope, a DNA copy number increase becomes visible by the heightened intensity of green hybridized tumor DNA, whereas a decrease is visible in red. Detailed analysis is performed using a sensitive monochrome charge-coupled device (CCD) camera mounted on a fluorescence microscope and automated image analysis software. Green, red, and blue images are obtained for each metaphase. Using CGH analysis software, the chromosomes are classified based on the DAPI-banding pattern and the relative intensities of the green and red colors along each chromosome are calculated (*see* **Fig. 1**). The sensitivity of the technique in detecting DNA copy

From: *Methods in Molecular Medicine, vol. 50: Colorectal Cancer: Methods and Protocols*
Edited by: S. M. Powell © Humana Press Inc., Totowa, NJ

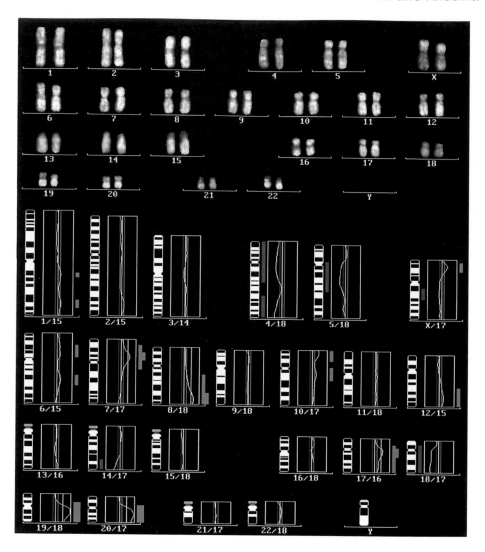

Fig. 1. CGH karyotype (**upper**) and profile of DNA copy number changes in a gastric carcinoma tumor (**lower**). In the lower panel, the red line represents a threshold of 0.85 for detection of losses while the green line(s) represent a threshold of 1.17 for gains, respectively. Gains and losses are drawn as green and red bars, respectively. High-level amplifications are shown as wide green bars. Image was analyzed using ISIS digital image analysis (Metasystems).

number gains is about 2 Mb and approx 10 Mb for DNA copy number losses. High-level amplifications of smaller sequences can be detected if the amplicon size multiplied by the number of amplification is ~2 Mb. However, CGH can not reveal balanced structural chromosomal rearrangements, such as translocations and inversions. Several methodological papers to improve CGH and overcome hybridization artifacts have been published *(2–5)*.

Since the introduction of CGH, more than 300 publications have appeared providing important genetic information related to the development and progression of several tumors. Several novel amplicons and losses have thus been identified in a large number of solid tumors that otherwise had remained poorly characterized by standard cytogenetics *(6,7)*. For tumors of the gastrointestinal tract (GIT), novel genetic changes were identified by CGH. Gastric adenocarcinomas have shown recurrent amplicons on chromosome arms 7p, 17q, and 20q *(8,9)*. Barrett's tumors of the esophagus demonstrated a unique deletion in 14q31–q32 not seen in gastric or gastroesophageal junction carcinomas *(10)*. In colorectal tumors, in addition to gains in chromosome arms 17q and 20q, chromosomes 1 and 13 and chromosome arm 7p were frequently gained *(11,12)*. Despite the similarities of the genetic changes observed in gastric carcinomas and colorectal carcinomas, gains in chromosome 13 were not a frequent finding in gastric carcinomas *(8,9,13)*. Gastric carcinomas from patients with hereditary nonpolyposis colorectal cancer had less genetic changes than sporadic gastric carcinomas *(14)*. In addition to adenocarcinomas, studies of both benign and malignant stromal tumors of the GIT showed a novel consistent deletion at 14q22 that had rarely been reported in any other tumors of the GIT. Moreover, such a unique deletion was not seen in histopathologically related leiomyomas and leiomyosarcomas *(15)*.

CGH has been able to reveal chromosomal areas that contain amplified cellular oncogenes. The androgen receptor gene was shown to be amplified in prostate cancers, the *BCL2* gene in lymphomas, and the *KRAS2* gene in nonsmall cell lung cancer tumors. CGH has shown copy number amplification in chromosomal regions containing these genes. Similarly, losses have helped to trace candidate tumor suppressor genes. Losses detected at 19p in the intestinal hamartomatous polyps in Peutz–Jeghers syndrome *(16)* have enabled to trace a novel cancer gene, *STK1/LKB1 (17)*.

2. Materials

2.1. DNA Isolation

1. Tumor: paraffin-embedded tissue, frozen tissue, blood or bone marrow sample. Reference: normal tissue sample or blood sample from a normal healthy individual.
2. Xylene (Riedel-de Haën, GmbH, Germany) for paraffin-embedded tissue and absolute ethanol solution.
3. Proteinase K: 1 mg/mL solution (Merck, GmbH, Darmstadt, Germany).
4. RNase: ribonuclease 10 mg/mL (Sigma, St. Louis, MO).
5. Lysis buffer: 50 mM Tris-HCl, pH 8.5, 1 mM Na$_2$EDTA, 0.5% Tween.
6. 10% SDS.

7. 6 *M* NaCl (saturated).
8. TE buffer: 10 m*M* Tris-HCl, 0.2 m*M* Na$_2$EDTA, pH 7.5.

2.2. Preparation of Slides

1. Fixed cells from lymphocyte cell culture.
2. Steamer or hot water bath.
3. Glass slides cleaned in 70% ethanol.
4. Fixative, methanol: acetic acid 3:1.

2.3. Labeling of DNA

1. Sterile water.
2. Prepare N buffer from unlabeled deoxynucleotide triphosphates (10 m*M* dNTPs; Gibco-BRL, Gaithersburg, MD) by adding 20 µL of dATP, 20 µL dGTP, 6 µL dTTP, 6 µL dCTP, 6.8 µL mercaptoethanol (14.7 *M*), 10 µL BSA (10 mg/mL, Gibco-BRL), 50 µL 1 *M* MgCl$_2$, and 500 µL Tris-HCl (1 *M*, pH 7.6) to 381 µL sterile water for a total volume of 1 mL. Mix and store at –20°C.
3. Prepare a mixture of fluorescein isothiocyanate (FITC)-dCTP and FITC-dUTP (1:1) (DuPont, Boston, MA) for labeling the tumor DNA and a similar mixture of Texas red (TR) for labeling the reference DNA.
4. DNA polymerase I/DNase I: DNA polymerase I (10 U/µL, Promega, Madison, WI) and DNase I (0.5 U/µL, Gibco-BRL).
5. Genomic DNA from a tumor sample and a normal tissue sample.

2.4. Hybridization and Washings

1. Water bath and incubator.
2. Cot-1 DNA (1 µg/µL: Gibco-BRL), and 3 *M* Na Acetate (pH 7.0).
3. 70% formamide/2X SSC (1X SSC: 0.15 *M* NaCl–15 m*M* sodium citrate, pH 7.0).
4. PN buffer: 0.1 *M* NaH$_2$PO$_4$-0.1 *M* Na$_2$HPO$_4$-0.1% NP40 (pH 8.0). Prepare as follows: Solution (A) 13.8 g NaH$_2$PO$_4$ and adjust volume to 1000 mL using H$_2$O. Solution (B) 89 g Na$_2$HPO$_4$ and adjust volume to 5000 mL using H$_2$O. Adjust pH of solution B to pH 8.0 using solution A and add 5 mL of Nonidet P-40 (NP-40) to your buffer.
5. Hybridization buffer: 50% formamide, 10% dextran sulfate, 2X SSC.
6. Proteinase K buffer: 20 m*M* Tris-HCl, pH 7.6, 2 m*M* CaCl$_2$, pH 7.5 (2 mL 1 *M* Tris-HCl+ 2 mL 0.1 *M* CaCl$_2$ + 98 mL H$_2$O).
7. An antifading medium with 4',6-diamidino-2-phenylindole-dihydrochloride (Vectashield-DAPI ™; Vector Laboratories Inc, Burlingame, CA).
8. 50% formamide/2X SSC (pH 7.0).
9. 2X SSC.
10. 0.1X SSC.

3. Methods

3.1. DNA Isolation (see Note 1)

Salting out procedure is recommended for DNA extraction, especially for paraffin-embedded tissue sections. The procedure is simple and nontoxic, and the DNA obtained yields better CGH hybridization for paraffin-embedded tissue sections than does the standard phenol chloroform method. The same procedure can also be used for DNA extraction from frozen tissue sections and blood samples.

3.1.1. Preparation of Tissue Sections and Deparaffinization

1. Prepare 30–60 sections, each of 3–6 micron thickness in a 15-mL polypropylene tube.
2. For deparaffinization, add 8–10 mL Xylene for 10 min at 55°C.
3. Centrifuge for 5 min at 550*g* and discard supernatant.
4. Repeat **steps 2–3** two more times.
5. Dehydrate with 8–10 mL absolute ethanol for 10 min at 55°C.
6. Centrifuge for 5 min at 550*g* and discard supernatant.
7. Repeat **steps 5–6** two more times.
8. Dry at 37°C or 55°C for 2–4 h.
9. Add 1 mL lysis buffer and incubate overnight at 55°C.

3.1.2. Cell Digestion

The cell lysates are digested as follows:

1. Add 300 µL proteinase K solution and mix well.
2. Incubate at 55°C overnight.

It is recommended to check the suspension after 12–24 h and add more proteinase K, if it is not clear. This step is preferably completed within 72 h. Proteinase K can be re-added every 6–12 h. Longer incubation will result in degraded DNA.

3.1.3. RNase Treatment

Add 10 µL of 10% SDS + 10–20 µL RNase to the suspension and incubate for 1–3 h at 37°C.

3.1.4. Precipitation of Proteins and Collection of DNA

1. Add 300 µL of 6 *M* NaCl and vortex vigorously for 2 min.
2. Centrifuge at 550*g* 30 min at room temperature or +4°C to precipitate the proteins.
3. Carefully, transfer the supernatant containing the DNA to another polypropylene tube.
4. Repeat **steps 1–4** one to two times.
5. Add two volumes of cold absolute ethanol and keep at –20°C overnight.
6. Centrifuge 30–60 min at 550*g*. Discard the alcohol.
7. Let the DNA pellet dry at 55°C for 20 min.
8. Add 50–100 µL TE and incubate at 55°C for at least 4 h. Dissolving the DNA may require 1–2 d incubation with intermittent mixing.
9. Measure the DNA and run the samples on ethidium bromide/1.4% agarose gel electrophoresis to estimate the DNA fragments' length.

3.2. Preparation of Metaphase Slides (see Note 2)

1. Adjust the humidity to 70–80% and the temperature to 25°C in a hood.
2. From a distance of 30 cm, drop one to two drops from your fixed cell suspension onto the slide.
3. Keep the slide 5 min inside the humid hood before taking it out.
4. Check your metaphases with a phase-contrast microscope and accept only slides with black spread metaphases.
5. Allow the slides to age at room temperature (25–30°C) for 1–2 wk.
6. Aged slides can be successfully used for another 2 wk.

3.3. Labeling of DNA (see Notes 3 and 4)

Standard nick translation reaction is used for labeling DNAs.

1. For labeling 1 µg of DNA, the following ingredients are mixed in one 1.5 mL Eppendorf tube and the volume of the reaction is adjusted to 50 µL using sterile water. 1 µg DNA, 5 µL N buffer, 1.5 µL Fluorochrome mix, 8–12 µL DNA polymerase I/DNaseI, 1.2 µL DNA polymerase I.
2. Incubate at +15°C for 40–75 min. The DNA polymerase I/DNase I volume and the reaction time are adjusted in order to obtain DNA fragments ranging from 600 to 2000 bp.
3. Stop the reaction by heating the Eppendorf tube at 70°C for 10 min.
4. Add 400 ng (800 ng for paraffin-embedded tumors) of each of both labeled DNAs (tumor and reference of the same sex), 20 µg of unlabeled Cot-1 DNA, 10 µL of 3 M Na acetate and 700 µL absolute ethanol. Mix and keep for at least 2 h at –20°C to precipitate the DNA probe.
5. In a microcentrifuge at 4°C, spin the probe for 30 min at 10,000g. Discard supernatant and allow the DNA pellet to dry at 37°C for 20–30 min.
6. The DNA probe is dissolved in 10 µL of hybridization buffer for at least 2 h at 37°C.

3.4. CGH Procedure

For optimum CGH hybridization, use slides aged for 10–20 d at room temperature.

3.4.1. Pretreatment and Denaturation (see Note 5)

1. Refix the slides in methanol:acetic 3:1 overnight at +4°C.
2. Incubate the slides in 2X SSC at 42°C for 40 min, then wash in distilled water.
3. Dehydrate the slides in ethanol solution (70%, 85%, and absolute) for 5 min each.
4. Denaturate, the maximum of four slides at one time, in prewarmed (65–70°C) 70% formamide/2X SSC for 2 min.
5. Quickly, remove slides and dehydrate them in a sequence of ice-cold 70%, 85%, and 100% ethanol, for 2 min each, followed by air drying.
6. Add 10 µL of proteinase K into a prewarmed (37°C) coplin jar containing 100 mL of proteinase K buffer and incubate the slides for 5–10 min.

7. Dehydrate slides in a sequence of 70%, 85%, and 100% ice-cold ethanol for 2 min each and air dry.
8. Denaturate probe at 75°C for 5 min in a water bath or heat block and immediately shake on ice.

3.4.2. Hybridization

1. Apply 10 μL of probe on a slide, add a 18 × 18 mm cover slip, and seal with rubber cement.
2. Incubate at 37°C in a moist chamber for 48–72 h.

3.4.3. Washings

1. Remove rubber seal and cover slips.
2. Incubate slides in a prewarmed (45°C) coplin jar containing 50% formamide/2X SSC for 10 min. Repeat two times more.
3. Incubate slides in a prewarmed (45°C) coplin jar containing 2X SSC for 10 min. Repeat once more.
4. Incubate slides in a prewarmed (45°C) coplin jar containing 0.1X SSC for 10 min.
5. At room temperature, incubate slides in a sequence of coplin jars containing 2X SSC, PN buffer, and distilled water, each for 10 min.
6. Air dry slides.
7. Mount the slides with 10 μL VectaShield-DAPI medium and add cover slips.

3.4.4. Image Analysis (see **Notes 6** and **7**)

Images are captured using a cooled charge-coupled device (CCD) camera mounted on a fluorescence microscope equipped with appropriate filters to detect FITC, TR, and DAPI. We use an epifluorescence microscope (Zeiss) and the ISIS digital image analysis system (Metasystems GmbH, Altlussheim, Germany) based on an integrated high-sensitivity monochrome CCD camera and automated CGH analysis software. Three-color images (red for reference DNA, green for tumor DNA, and blue for counterstaining) are acquired from 8–10 metaphases per sample. Only metaphases of good quality with strong uniform hybridization are included in the analysis. Chromosomes not suitable for CGH analysis are excluded (i.e., chromosomes heavily bent, overlapping, or with overlying artifacts). Chromosomal regions are interpreted as over-represented, when the corresponding ratio exceeds 1.17 (gains) or 1.5 (high-level amplification), and as underrepresented (losses), when the ratio is less than 0.85.

4. Notes

1. The salting out method yields a better DNA quality from paraffin-embedded tissue sections than does standard phenol chloroform and is used routinely in our laboratory.

2. Black metaphases give smooth and strong hybridization, whereas grey and light-grey metaphases tend to give poor granular hybridization. If the slide is too dense, add a few drops of methanol:acetic fixative to your cell suspension. If metaphase spreading is poor, increase humidity. Avoid excessive exposure of the slides to humidity as it results in light-gray metaphases not suitable for CGH.

3. Direct fluorochrome-conjugated DNA gives a stronger and smoother hybridization. A fluorochrome mixture of dCTP and dUTP nucleotides ensures efficient labeling of more DNA sequences and reduces hybridization artifacts. For DNA from paraffin-embedded tissue section, the time of nick translation reaction is two-thirds of the time used for the reference DNA.

4. If DNA concentration is below 150 ng/μL, add 2.5 μL of 10 mM MgCl$_2$ in the nick translation reaction. Diluted DNA samples contain excess TE (Tris-EDTA) which chelates Mg^{2+} necessary for the enzymes to function during nick translation.

5. Fuzzy chromosomes with poor banding are an indication of high denaturation temperature and/or prolonged time. Try reducing either or both of them. Fresh slides are more sensitive to denaturation.

6. There are several CGH-analysis software packages available. The thresholds should be calculated based on control results. A negative control (FITC-labeled normal DNA vs TR-labeled normal DNA) and a quality control should be included In each CGH experiment. In the quality control, FITC-labeled DNA from a tumor with known DNA copy number changes is hybridized against TR-labeled normal DNA.

7. Some software packages offer an option to use a 99% confidence interval to confirm the CGH results. Briefly, intra-experiment standard deviations for all positions in the CGH ratio profiles are calculated from the variation of the ratio values of all homologous chromosomes within the experiment. Confidence intervals for the ratio profiles are then computed by combining them with an empirical inter-experiment standard deviation and by estimating error probabilities based on the t-distribution.

References

1. Kallioniemi, A., Kallioniemi, O.-P., Sudan, D., Rutovitz, D., Gray, J., Waldman, F., and Pinkel, D. (1992) Comparative genomic hybridization for molecular cytogenetic analysis of solid tumors. *Science* **258,** 818–821.
2. Kallioniemi, O. P., Kallioniemi, A., Piper, J., Isola, J., Waldman, F. M., Gray, J. W., and Pinkel, D. (1994) Optimizing comparative genomic hybridization for analysis of DNA sequence copy number changes in solid tumors. *Genes Chromosom. Cancer* **10,** 231–243.
3. Larramendy, M. L., El-Rifai, W., and Knuutila, S. (1998) Comparison of fluorescein isothiocyanate- and Texas red-conjugated nucleotides for direct labeling in comparative genomic hybridization. *Cytometry* **31,** 174–179.
4. du Manoir, S., Schrock, E., Bentz, M., Speicher, M. R., Joos, S., Ried, T., Lichter, P., and Cremer, T. (1995) Quantitative analysis of comparative genomic hybridization. *Cytometry* **19,** 27–41.
5. El-Rifai, W., Larramendy, M. L., Björkqvist, A.-M., Hemmer, S., and Knuutila, S. (1997) Optimization of comparative genomic hybridization using

fluorochrome conjugated to dCTP and dUTP nucleotides. *Lab. Invest.* **77,** 699–700.

6. Knuutila, S., Björkqvist, A.-M., Autio, K., Tarkkanen, M., Wolf, M., Monni, O., et al. (1998) DNA copy number amplifications in human neoplasms. Review of comparative genomic hybridization studies. *Am. J. Pathol.* **152,** 1107–1123.
7. Knuutila, S., Aalto, Y., Autio, K., Björkqvist, A.-M., El-Rifai, W., Hemmer, S., et al. (1999) DNA copy number losses in human neoplasms. *Am. J. Pathol.* **155,** 683–694.
8. Kokkola, A., Monni, O., Puolakkainen, P., Larramendy, M. L., Victorzon, M., Nordling, S., et al. (1997) 17q12-21 amplicon, a novel recurrent genetic change in intestinal type of gastric carcinoma: a comparative genomic hybridization study. *Genes Chromosom. Cancer* **20,** 38–43.
9. El-Rifai, W., Harper, J. C., Cummings, O. W., Hyytinen, E. R., Frierson, H. F., Jr., Knuutila, S., and Powell, S. M. (1998) Consistent genetic alterations in xenografts of proximal stomach and gastro-esophageal junction adenocarcinomas. *Cancer Res.* **58,** 34–37.
10. van Dekken, H., Geelen, E., Dinjens, W. N., Wijnhoven, B. P., Tilanus, H. W., Tanke, H. J., and Rosenberg, C. (1999) Comparative genomic hybridization of cancer of the gastroesophageal junction: deletion of 14q31-32.1 discriminates between esophageal (Barrett's) and gastric cardia adenocarcinomas. *Cancer Res.* **59,** 748–52.
11. Ried, T., Knutzen, R., Steinbeck, R., Blegen, H., Schrock, E., Heselmeyer, K., et al. (1996) Comparative genomic hybridization reveals a specific pattern of chromosomal gains and losses during the genesis of colorectal tumors. *Genes Chromosom. Cancer* **15,** 234–245.
12. Al-Mulla, F., Keith, W. N., Pickford, I. R., Going, J. J., and Birnie, G. D. (1999) Comparative genomic hybridization analysis of primary colorectal carcinomas and their synchronous metastases. *Genes Chromosom. Cancer* **24,** 306–314.
13. Sakakura, C., Mori, T., Sakabe, T., Ariyama, Y., Shinomiya, T., Date, K., et al. (1999) Gains, losses, and amplifications of genomic materials in primary gastric cancers analyzed by comparative genomic hybridization. *Genes Chromosom. Cancer* **24,** 299–305.
14. Larramendy, M. L., El-Rifai, W., Kokkola, A., Puolakkainen, P., Monni, O., Salovaara, R., et al. (1998) Comparative genomic hybridization reveals differences in DNA copy number changes between sporadic gastric carcinoma and gastric carcinomas from patients with hereditary nonpolyposis colorectal cancer. *Cancer Genet. Cytogenet.* **106,** 62–65.
15. El-Rifai, W., Sarlomo-Rikala, M., Knuutila, S., and Miettinen, M. (1998) DNA copy number changes in development and progression in leiomyosarcoma of soft tissues. *Am. J. Pathol.* **153,** 985–990.
16. Hemminki, A., Tomlinson, I., Markie, D., Jarvinen, H., Sistonen, P., Bjorkqvist, A. M., et al. (1997) Localization of a susceptibility locus for Peutz-Jeghers syndrome to 19p using comparative genomic hybridization and targeted linkage analysis. *Nature Genet.* **15,** 87–90.
17. Hemminki, A., Markie, D., Tomlinson, I., Avizienyte, E., Roth, S., Loukola, A., et al. (1998) A serine/threonine kinase gene defective in Peutz-Jeghers syndrome. *Nature* **391,** 184–187.

5

Fluorescence *In Situ* Hybridization

Application in Cancer Research and Clinical Diagnostics

Svetlana D. Pack and Zhengping Zhuang

1. Introduction
1.1 Fluorescence In Situ *Hybridization*

An opportunity to look inside of the individual cell for the direct visualization *in situ* of "what happened?" is the most wonderful feature offered by fluorescence *in situ* hybridization (FISH). DNA *in situ* hybridization is a technique that allows the visualization of defined sequences of nucleic acids within the individual cells. The method is based on the site specific annealing (hybridization) of single-stranded labeled DNA fragments (probes) to denatured, homologous sequences (targets) on cytological preparations, like metaphase chromosomes, interphase nuclei, or naked chromatin fibers. Visualization of hybridization sites becomes possible after detection steps by using a wide spectrum of the fluorescent dyes available.

Much has been achieved during the last decade in the human genome analysis due to the development of nonradioactive methods of DNA *in situ* hybridization. General usefulness of FISH for physical mapping *(1–2)* was greatly enhanced by improved DNA resolution. Interphase cytogenetics has become an useful diagnostic tool in cancer cytogenetics *(3–11)*. The high resolution of FISH analysis allows for a sensitive visualization of gene alterations. This has implications for the diagnosis of constitutional microdeletion syndromes (**Fig. 1A**), translocations in a variety of human diseases *(12–18)* as well as the identification of deletions of tumor suppressor genes and amplification of oncogenes in different types of human malignancies *(19–25)* (**Fig. 1B**). Fiber FISH technique allows to produce decondensed stretched interphase chromatin for orientation and ordering cosmids, PACs, BACs, and YACs while gener-

From: *Methods in Molecular Medicine, vol. 50: Colorectal Cancer: Methods and Protocols*
Edited by: S. M. Powell © Humana Press Inc., Totowa, NJ

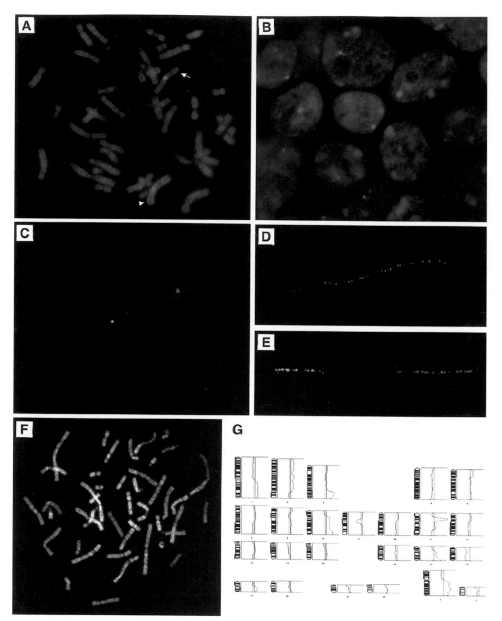

Fig. 1. Representative FISH data demonstrating: **(A)** Constitutional VHL gene deletion (chromosome 3p25) detected in VHL patient's blood lymphocytes using the cDNA probe g7 (rhodamine signal). A centromeric alpha-satellite probe specific for chromosome 3 (FITC signal) was used as a control. Chromosomes are counterstained with DAPI. **(B)** Allelic deletion of the MEN1 locus (chromosome 11q13) in pituitary adenoma tumor cells. Dual-color FISH was performed on tumor touch preparation

ating contigs in particular region of interest, definition and approximate sizing of gaps and overlaps (**Fig. 1C–E**). These new high-resolution FISH technologies have widespread applications for long-range genome mapping.

Comparative Genomic Hybridization (CGH) is one of the applications of FISH. The method has been developed to detect an integral pattern of the genetic changes in the tumor genome including aneuploidies, extended chromosomal deletions (losses), presence of extra chromosomal fragments (gains) and amplifications (*26–27*) (**Fig. 1F,G**). The genomic DNA from tumor cells is the only requirement for the analysis. The principle of the method is the competitive hybridization of the tumor and referent normal DNAs labeled differently (used as a probe) to the metaphase chromosomes from the normal donor (used as a template). A specially designed software for CGH analysis allows to measure the ratio of hybridization efficiency tumor:normal DNA along the axis of each individual chromosome. This method is extremely valuable as the first approach to study genetically unknown cancer syndromes or unknown tumor entity, especially associated with the hereditary condition. By using CGH on a series of tumors it is possible to identify specific chromosomal rearrangements characteristic for this tumor type. Consistent chromosomal loss will indicate region of localization of the putative tumor-supressor genes. Consistent areas of gain or amplification would show location of the putative oncogenes involved in tumor initiation and progression. In one experiment it is possible to unravel all chromosomal losses and gains occurred in tumor genome.

In order to detect translocation another FISH technique can be applied, Spectral Karyotyping (SKY) (*28*). A combination of chromosomal painting probes labeled with different fluorochromes covering all 23 pairs of human chromosomes (or 20 pairs of the mouse chromosomes) is now commercially available

---

using the MEN1 locus specific cosmid 10B11 (red signal) and chromosome-specific alpha–satellite for chromosome 11 (green FITC signal). FISH detects an aneusomy for chromosome 11. (**C**) Three-color FISH for high resolution mapping. Physical ordering and estimation of the distances between three BAC clones (orange-red-green) in the contig from Carney Complex critical region (chromosome 2p16) using depleted chromatin fibers as a template. (**D, E**) Fiber FISH using BAC clones from Carney Complex critical region, overlapped (D), and approx 80 kb apart from each other (E). (**F, G**) CGH analysis of squamous cell type esophageal carcinoma. (F) Normal metaphase spread after simultaneous hybridization of the tumor (FITC fluorescence) and normal referent (rhodamine fluorescence) DNAs. Chromosomal regions with loss appear red whereas areas of gain have extra green fluorescence. (D) The CGH image profile for the same tumor, computed as a mean value for ten metaphase spreads. The parallel vertical lines represent tumor:reference rations. The bold median line represents ratio of 1.0, and red and green line indicate ratio of 0.9 and 1.1, respectively. Red represents losses and green represents gains and amplification.

(Applied Spectral Imaging, Carlsbad, CA; Vysis, Inc., Downers Grove, IL). Requirement for this experiment is metaphase spreads obtained from the tumor cells.

How does FISH contribute to the study of neoplastic process and what are the main current advantages of the method?

1.2. The Method and How It Works

1.2.1. The Main Problem

Tumor specimens available for the study are usually pathologic lesions removed surgically from patients and represent heterogeneous composition of different cell types including normal epithelial, stromal, and endothelial cells. Thus, homogenized tissue samples will reflect an average content of cell population and in most cases mask genetic alterations present in tumor cells while using the most accurate DNA analysis. A combination of microdissection of small histological sections and polymerase chain reaction (PCR) on small cell populations helps to avoid this problem, but not always. There are some types of tumor cells which are difficult to distinguish from normal ones, or the area with tumor cells on the slide is too small to clearly identify. In both cases there is a chance to ignore affected cells and misread the result of LOH testing. FISH is a very helpful and powerful alternative.

1. The method is simple and provides the desired result the next day.
2. The result is not an average evaluation of the entire cell population but individual cell scoring. This is critically important for heterogeneous tumor samples.
3. Polymorphism of genetic markers in the area of interest is not a necessary condition of success.
4. There is no need in cell cultivation that is problematic for certain types of tumor cells and also time consuming. Possibility to use frozen tissue specimens, frozen sections, slides after Diff-Quick provides an access to the entire archival collection of patient specimens available.

1.2.2. Procedure

FISH is a mulitstep procedure, which includes:

1. Preparation of specimen (fixation, digestion, dehydration).
2. Probe preparation (labeling, precipitation).
3. Denaturation.
4. Hybridization.
5. Washing.
6. Detection.
7. Microscope analysis.

The most crucial part for the successful FISH experiment is a quality of slide preparation. In our experiments fresh tumor tissue was found to be the best for touch preps as well as frozen tissue samples. Both provide well separated nicely-shaped interphase cells without multilayer tissue fragments. Frozen tissue sections usually give less satisfying results. Even 5 microns section contains more than one layer of cells and is too thick for FISH analysis without confocal microscopy. Sometimes it is helpful to make touch preps from frozen section after thawing and adding a drop of water on the section. It provides better cell separation. We then allow slides to dry 10–15 min and fix cells in ethanol series—70%, 85%, 100%.

The next important step is protein digestion and cytoplasm removal, which facilitate better probe accessibility and fluorescence background reduction. For this purpose we use pepsin treatment for 3–10 min with the following washes in PBS buffer. After dehydration in ethanol slides are ready for denaturation.

The probe and the target DNA are denatured thermally. Formamide is added to reduce the melting temperature of the double stranded DNA. If genomic DNA probes are used, an additional pre-annealing step with an excess of unlabeled total genomic DNA or the Cot1-fraction of human DNA prior to the hybridization is required to block repetitive sequences *(29)*. The denaturation of the specimen is more critical than the denaturation of the probe DNA. The golden middle line is probe penetration should be optimal with a maximum preservation of specimen morphology. Temperature control is very important. We recommend not to exceed 72°C for one slide by adding 1°C per additional slide.

DNA preparation usually follows standard procedures. Qiagen kit is a satisfying option for the probe DNA extraction. We also recommend to do phenol:chlorophorm extraction one or two times. The DNA probe labeling for FISH is generally performed by Nick-translation, random priming, or PCR proved to be the simplest and most reliable labeling protocols. During the labeling reaction modified nucleotide analogs are incorporated. They are linked to haptens, e.g., biotin, digoxigenin. Recently, nucleotide analogs became available, that are directly conjugated to fluorochromes such as Spectrum Orange-dUTP, Spectrum Green-dUTP, Spectrum Red-dUTP, FITC-dUTP, and so on.

The hybridization reaction is usually carried out at 37°C overnight (for about 16 h). Shorter hybridization time (1–2 h) is sufficient for probes that detect repetitive sequence motifs. If entire genomes are hybridized, e.g., using CGH, prolonged hybridization time (2–3 nights) is necessary.

The detection reaction is performed indirectly with fluorochromes linked to avidin or antibodies against the reporter molecules. If probes were labeled directly using modified nucleotides that are conjugated with fluorochromes, detection steps are not required. Numerous fluorochromes are available including fluorochromes emitting in the blue (AMCA, Cascade blue), in the green (FITC, rhodamine-110), and in the red (rhodamine, TRITC, Texas Red,

Cy-3). More recently, fluorochromes that emit in the infrared, such as Cy-5, became commercially available.

FISH signals are visualized by epifluorescence microscopy. New generations of specific filter sets allow to precisely separate the fluorochromes *(30–31)*. Double and triple band pass filters *(32)* provide an opportunity to simultaneously visualize and analyze two or three fluorochromes. This was an important development, particularly, with respect to the needs of routine diagnostic laboratories. Digital imaging devices with a high photon detection efficiency and a high dynamic range, charge coupled device (CCD) cameras increase the sensitivity significantly and provide the basis to quantify fluorescence images *(33)*. A sensitivity of modern CCD cameras in a broad spectral range allows to add fluorochromes emitting in the infrared spectrum, such as Cy-5 in fluorescence detection systems. For the analysis of the three-dimensional specimens, like tissue sections, interphase nuclei, preference should be given to the confocal laser scanning microscopy *(34)*.

2. Materials
2.1. Reagents
2.1.1. Reagents for Tissue Culture

1. RPMI-1640 (Gibco-BRL).
2. Penicillin-streptomycin, 100X (Gibco-BRL).
3. L-glutamin, 100X (Gibco-BRL).
4. Fetal bovine serum (Gibco-BRL).
5. Phytohemagglutinin (PHA) (Murex Biotech Ltd , Dartford, England, cat. no. HA15).
6. Ethidium bromide, 10 mg/mL, (Gibco-BRL, cat. no. 5585UA).
7. Colcemid, 10 mg/mL (Boehringer Mannheim, cat. no. 295892).
8. Methanol (JT Baker, cat. no. 9093-03).
9. Glacial acetic acid (Malinckrodt, cat. no. UN2789).

2.1.2. Reagents for Slide Processing

1. 20X SSC (prepare 2X SSC, 0.1X SSC, 4X SSC/0.1% Tween-20), store at room temperature up to 1 mo.
2. 70%, 85%, 100% Ethanol (–20°C) (VWR, cat. no. MK70194).
3. Deionized sterile water.
4. Pepsin, 10% stock solution (Sigma, cat. no. P 6887, 5 g). Dissolve 100 mg/mL in sterile water, keep on ice, make 50 µL aliquots, store at –20°C.
5. HCl (Sigma, cat. no. 251-2, 50 mL, 2 *N*).
6. Formamide deionized (American Bioanalytical, cat. no. AB-600, 500 mL).
7. Tween 20 (Sigma, cat. no. P5927).
8. Dextran sulfate (Sigma, cat. no. D7037, 50 g).

2.1.3. Labeling Reagents

1. Nick translation kit (Boehringer Mannheim, cat. no. 976776).
2. Digoxigenin-11-dUTP (Boehringer Mannheim, cat. no. 1093088, 25 nmol, 25 μL).
3. Biotin-16-dUTP (Boehringer Mannheim, cat. no. 1093070, 50 nmol, 50 μL).
4. DNA, COT-1, Human (Boehringer Mannheim, cat. no. 1581074, 500 μg).
5. DNA, Herring sperm (Gibco-BRL, cat. no. 15634-017, 10 mg/mL, 1 mL).

2.1.4. Detection Reagents

1. Anti-digoxigenin-rhodamine, F(ab)2-fragment (Boehringer Mannheim, cat. no. 1207 750, 200 μg), stock solution: 200 μg/1 mL sterile water, prepare in the darkness, aliquote 60 μL, store at –20°C in foil. Working solution 1 μg/mL.
2. Fluorescein avidin D (Vector Laboratories, cat. no. A-2001, 5 mg/mL, 5 mg) prepare aliquotes 15 μL, store at –20°C in foil. Working solution 5 μg/mL.
3. DAPI, 4'6'-diamino 2-phenylindole (Serva, cat. no. 18860, 10 mg), stock solution: 2.5 mg/mL. Dissolve 10 mg DAPI/4 mL sterile water, aliquot 100 μL, store at –20°C in the dark. Working solution: 250 ng/mL in Vectashield Mounting Medium.
4. Vectashield Mounting Medium (Vector Laboratories, cat. no. H1000, 10 mL).
5. Albumin bovine, Fraction V (ICN Biomedicals Inc., cat. no. 160069).

2.2. Reagents Preparation

2.2.1. DAY 1

1. Ethanol series: prepare 70, 85, 100% ethanol (500 mL each). Store at –20°C.
2. 0.01 M HCl: Add 0.4 mL 1 M HCl to 39.6 mL distilled water. Place coplin jar in 37°C water bath.
3. Phosphate-buffered saline (1X PBS): prepare a 1X PBS solution. Store at room temperature (RT).
4. 1X PBS/MgCl$_2$: add 50 mL of 1 M MgCl$_2$ to 950 mL of 1X PBS.
5. Denaturation solution (70% formamide/2X SSC): mix 28 mL formamide/8 mL distilled water/4 mL. 20X SSC in a coplin jar.
6. Hybridization solution (hybrisol): 50% formamide/2X SSC/10% dextran sulfate. Prepare 10 mL, make aliquots 1 mL, keep at –20°C.

Detection Solutions

1. Detection buffer (DB): 4X SSC/0.1% Tween-20/1% BSA. Mix well 10 mL 20X SSC/40 mL distilled water. 50 μL Tween-20/0.5 g BSA in a 50 mL tube. Leave overnight at 37°C to completely dissolve BSA. Centrifuge for 5 min at 3000 rpm to remove particulates.
2. Antidigoxigenin rhodamine detection solution (1 μg/mL): add 50 μL of the anti-dig-rhodamine stock solution (200 mg/mL) to 10 mL DB. Mix well. Store in a dark bottle (or in a foil) at 4°C up to 6 mo.
3. Avidin–FITC detection solution (5 mg/mL): add 10 μL of the avidin-FITC stock solution (50 mg/mL) to 10 mL DB. Mix well. Storage is the same as above.

4. Double-color detection solution: mix 50 μL of the anti-dig-rhodamine stock solution (200 μg/mL) and 10 μL of the avidin-FITC stock solution (5 mg/mL) in 10 mL DB. Storage is the same as above.
5. DAPI (250 ng/mL). Make gradual dilutions:
    a. (1:100) 5 μL of DAPI (2.5 mg/mL) stock solution dissolve in 495 μL of Vectashield Mounting Medium (DAPI II, 25 μg/mL).
    b. (1:100) 100 μL of DAPI II dissolve in 9 mL 900 μL of Vectashield Mounting Medium (DAPI III, 250 ng/mL). Store at –20°C in a dark.

2.2.2. DAY 2: Washing Solutions

1. 2X SSC: mix 100 mL 20X SSC with 900 mL distilled water. Keep at RT.
2. 50% Formamide/2X SSC: mix 20 mL formamide/16 mL distilled water/4 mL 20X SSC. Prepare 3 (40 mL) coplin jars. Heat to 45°C in a water bath. Discard after use.
3. 0.1X SSC: mix 5 mL 20X SSC with 995 mL distilled water. Keep at RT.
4. 4X SSC/0.1% Tween-20: 200 mL 20X SSC/1 mL Tween-20/dH$_2$O to 1 L volume. Keep at RT.

3. Methods
3.1. Preparation of Tumor Tissue Specimens for FISH

1. Make touch preps using fresh tissue sample, frozen tissue sample or frozen tissue section. Gently apply small piece of tissue or wet frozen tissue section on a dry clean slide. Check under the microscope. Allow slides to dry (*see* **Note 1**).
2. Fixation in ethanol series of 70, 85, 100% (10 min each). Then air dry.

3.1.1. Pepsin Treatment

1. Immerse slides at 37°C in coplin jar for 5–10 min with pepsin solution (add 20 μL pepsin stock solution to 40 mL prewarmed 0.01 *M* HCl at 37°C). Control digestion under the microscope (*see* **Note 2**).
2. Wash 2 × 5 min in 1X PBS, at room temperature with shaking.
3. Wash 1 × 5 min in 1X PBS/MgCl$_2$.
4. Dehydrate slides in 70, 85, 100% ethanol for 2 min each.
5. Air dry slides.

3.2. Preparation of Metaphase Chromosomes from the Normal Peripheral Blood Lymphocytes and Lymphoblastoid Cells (EBV Transformed) for CGH

3.2.1. Blood Cell Culture

1. To grow the lymphocytes from the whole blood mix in tissue culture flask 25cm^2:
    a. 10 mL RPMI-1640, with penicillin/streptomycin and L-glutamin and 15% FBS.
    b. 0.1 mL PHA (phytohemagglutinin).
    c. 20 drops of blood (use tissue culture flask 25cm^2).

2. Culture for 72 or 96 h at 37°C (shake flasks once a day).
3. Add 5 mL of fresh media with supplements 1 d before harvesting.

3.2.2. B-Cells Culture

1. Grow cells in 10 mL RPMI-1640, with penicillin/streptomycin and L-glutamin and 15% FBS.
2. Split the culture 2 d before harvesting.
3. Change the media again next day, leave overnight (*see* **Note 3**).

3.2.3. Harvesting

1. Add ethidium bromide (8 μg/mL) for one hour. Use 100 μL of stock solution (0.8 mg/mL) per 10 mL media.
2. After 1 h add colcemid (10 μg/mL) 100 μL to 10 mL flask and mix well by shaking or pipeting.
3. Transfer to 15 mL tube immediately.
4. Incubate at 37°C for 15 min.
5. Centrifuge for 5min at 1000 rpm.
6. Remove supernatant.
7. Add 5 mL of prewarmed (37°C) 0.075 *M* KCl/each tube drop by drop while tapping tubes.
8. Resuspend thoroughly using Pasteur pipet.
9. Add more 0.075 *M* KCl to total 10 mL.
10. Incubate at 37°C water bath for 17 min.
11. Add 1 mL of freshly prepared fixative (3:1; Methanol Glacial acetic acid) to each tube and slowly invert the tube 2 or 3 times.
12. Centrifuge as in **step 5**.
13. Remove supernatant and tap well.
14. Add freshly prepared fixative (2 mL per tube) drop by drop while tapping tubes.
15. Add more fixative to total 10 mL/tube.
16. Leave on ice 20–30 min.
17. Resuspend very well with the Pasteur pipet.
18. Centrifuge as in **step 5**.
19. Change fixative 10 mL.
20. Resuspend again.
21. Repeat **steps 18** and **19** more than three times until cells become white.
22. If slides will be made the next day, fill up with freshly prepared fixative, tighten caps and store at 4°C.
23. Change fixative three times before making slides.
24. Drop suspension onto clean slides (dip slides in ethanol/ether (50:50) and wipe with Kim wipes) (*see* **Note 4**).

3.3. Preparation of Extended Chromatin Fibers

This a modification of the method of Thomas Haaf and David Ward *(35)*.

1. Wash normal lymphoblastoid cells (or cells of interest) in PBS twice.
2. Apply three separate drops of cell suspension (100,000 cells) on top of clean dry slide (wipe slide after exposure in 100% ethanol). Try to make spots of cell monolayer about 5 mm in diameter. Wait until spots dry (5–10 min).
3. Cell lysis. As soon as drops dried immerse slides vertically in a coplin jar with high concentration salt–detergent solution (2 M NaCl, 25 mM Tris-HCl, 1% Triton X-100) for 15 min.
4. Carefully remove slide from the lysis solution holding slide in a vertical position. Viscous chromatin streams will float down the slide.
5. Allow slides to dry overnight.
6. Fixation in a coplin jar containing 70% ethanol or cold fresh Methanol:Glacial Acetic acid (3:1) for 30 min (*see* **Note 5**).
7. Proceed through the ethanol series of 80, 90, 100% for dehydration (5 min each). Air dry.
8. Slides can be kept in a coplin jar with 100% ethanol at –20°C sealed with parafilm for several months.

3.4. Probe Preparation

3.4.1. Labeling

PCR machine is perfect to perform a nick-translation reaction as well. Best to use the DNA concentration 0.5-1 µg/µL. Label 2 µg of DNA. If nick-translation kit from Boehringer Mannheim is used,

1. Make dNTP mix first: A:G:C:T + Dig-11-dUTP (or biotin-16-dUTP)=1:1:1:2/3 + 1/3.
2. Mix in Eppendof tube:

   x µL (2 µg) DNA probe
   10 µL dNTP mix
   2 µL 10X buffer
   x µL dH$_2$O
   2 µL Enzyme mix
   20 µL Total
3. Incubate at 15°C for 2 h 15 min. Keep on ice.
4. The size of the labeled DNA fragments should be checked on 1% agarose gel using 100bp marker. Use 2 µL from 20 µL of labeled mix. A smear should be in a range 100–400 bp. For CGH total human genomic DNA fragments should be below 1000 bp in size (*see* **Note 6**).
5. Heat at 65°C for 10min to inactivate the enzymes.
6. Keep at –20°C for prolonged storage.

3.4.2. Precipitation

1. For the genomic DNA probes add 50-fold excess (w/w) of human Cot-1DNA and 100X (w/w) of Herring Sperm DNA per probe amount, 1/10 v/v Na acetate (3%) and 2.5X v/v of total volume of 100% ethanol. Example:

18 µL DNA (~2 µg)
10 µL herring sperm DNA (100X)
50 µL human Cot 1 DNA (50X)
22 µL DW (up to 100 µL)
10 µL Na Acetate 3% (1/10 v)
275 µL ethanol 100% (2.5X) v/v

There is no need in Cot-1 if cDNA is used as a probe.

2. Precipitate at –70°C for 30 min or at –20°C for 2–3 h.
3. Centrifuge at 12,000 rpm, at 4°C for 10 min. Remove the supernatant.
4. Add 500 µL of 70% alcohol.
5. Centrifuge for 5 more min.
6. Carefully remove the supernatant, do not lose the pellet.
7. Leave open tube to dry until the pellet becomes clear (10–15 min at RT).
8. Add 50% Hybrisol solution (80 µL for a final concentration 25 ng/µL for single probe use, 40 µL for a final concentration of 50 ng/µL for two-color FISH, 24 µL for a final concentration of 80 ng/µL for three-color experiment).
9. Dissolve the probe at 37°C in a thermomixer (or water-bath) for 2–3 h, vortexing every 20 min.
10. For hybridization use 250 ng per half slide (10 µL).
11. Store the rest of the probe at –20°C for several months.

3.4.3. Denaturation

3.4.3.1. SLIDE DENATURATION

1. Denature slide for 2 min in a coplin jar with 70% formamide/2X SSC prewarmed to 72°C. Exact time is important! Add 1°C per extra slide.
2. Dehydrate through a cold ethanol series (70%, 85%, 100%), 2 min each, and air dry.

3.4.3.2. PROBE DENATURATION

1. Denature probe in 78°C water bath for 10 min.
2. Incubate at 37°C for pre-annealing for 30 min (genomic probe). Skip this step for the cDNA probe.
3. Prewarm slides to 37°C.
4. Apply 10 µL of the probe DNA per half slide (total DNA amount should be 250 ng for genomic clones; 500 ng–1 µg of each tumor and normal genomic DNAs for CGH), cover slip with 22 × 22mm cover glass, seal with rubber cement.

3.4.4. Hybridization

Incubate overnight at 37°C in a moist chamber. For CGH continue hybridization for 3 nights.

3.4.5. Washing

1. Remove rubber cement with a forceps. Soak slides in 2X SSC solution at RT. Quickly remove coverslips. Do not dry the slides. All washes are done at 45°C preferably in a shaking water bath.

2. Wash in 50% formamide/2X SSC, twice for 7 min.
3. 1X SSC twice for 5 min.
4. 0.1X SSC twice for 5 min (*see* **Note 7**).
5. 4X SSC/0.1% Tween-20, 5 min at RT.

During the following steps slides should be kept wet and protected from light!

3.4.6. Detection

1. Drain excess of fluid.
2. Apply 60 µL of the detecton solution, coverslip.
3. Incubate 40 min at 37°C in a moist chamber in the dark.

3.4.7. Washes 2

1. Remove coverslip and immediately transfer slide into solution.
2. 4X SSC/0.1% Tween-20, 3 × 2 min at 45°C with shaking.
3. 4X SSC/0.1% Tween-20, 1 min at room temperature.

3.4.8. Counterstaining

1. Drain excess of fluid.
2. Drop 9 µL of DAPI (250 ng/µL) on each half of the slide and coverslip with 24 × 50 mm coverslip.
3. Slides are ready for analysis. Store slides in a light protected folder for several months at –20°C (*see* **Note 8**).

3.5. Fluorescence Microscopy

1. Fluorescence microscopes from several leading brands like Zeiss, Leica, Olimpus, Nikon are widely used in different research, diagnostic laboratories around the world for different FISH applications.
2. Digital imaging devices (CCD cameras) are necessary components for a successful high resolution FISH imaging. Photometrics, Sony, Hamamatsu manufacture very sensitive and reliable CCD cameras.
3. For double, three-color FISH experiments triple-band pass filter should be used to visualize simultaneously specific probes and counterstained chromosomes, nuclei or chromatin fibers. FITC, rhodamine, DAPI filters are necessary for a gray-scale image acquisitions.
4. There are different kinds of software currently available for FISH analysis, e.g., from Applied Imaging, Imagenetics, Scanalytics. IP Lab Spectrum (Scanalytics, Fairfax, VA) is a good option for multi-color FISH image analysis.

3.6. Solutions

1. dNTP mix: dATP: dCTP :dGTP: dTTP, (0.5 mM:05 mM:0.5 mM:0.05 mM), store aliquots at –20°C.
2. 10X NT-buffer: 0.5 M Tris-HCl, pH 8.0, 50 mM MgCl$_2$, 0.5 mg/mL BSA, store aliquots a –20°C.

3. β-Mercaptoethanol (0.1 *M*): 34.7 μL of 99% solution (14.4 *M*), 5 mL of ddH$_2$O, store aliquots at –20°C.
4. DNase I stock solution (1 mg/mL) (Boehringer Mannheim GmbH, cat. no. 104 159, 100 mg 2000 U/mg). Dissolve in 0.15 *M* NaCl /50% glycerol. Store aliquots at –20°C. Working solution (1 μg/mL), 1:1000 stock solution diluted in cold ddH$_2$O.
5. DNA polymerase (Kornberg-fragment, *E. coli*) (Boehringer Mannheim, cat. no. 104 485, 500 U).

3.7. Nick-Translation

1. To label 2 μg DNA mix:

    x μL DNA (2μg)
    10 μL dNTP mix
    10 μL 10xNT-buffer
    10 μL 0.1 *M* β-mercaptoethanol
    4 μL bio-16-dUTP or dig-11-dUTP, 1 m*M*
    x μL ddH$_2$O
    0.5–3 μL DNAse
    2 μL polymerase (*E. coli*, Kornberg-fragment)
    100 μL total

2. Incubate at 15°C for 2 h.
3. Check the fragment's size on agarose gel. The DNA fragment smear should be in a range of 100–400 bp for genomic clones and 100–1000 bp for CGH.
4. If DNA-fragments are too large, add more DNase and incubate at 15°C for 20–30 min.
5. Incubate at 65°C for 10 min to stop the nick-translation.
6. Store labeled DNA at –20°C.
7. If after detection excess of the background is seen on the slides, this step can be repeated at 60°C. Excess of the background only on the chromosomes is due to insufficient suppression of the repetitive sequences and can be eliminated by the increasing of the amount of Cot-1 DNA added to a probe (to 100X).
7. Failure of hybridization might be due to DNA purity problem. Two times phenol-chloroform extraction of the original probe DNA can help to improve the result.

4. Notes

1. If not immediately used, slides should be kept frozen at –20°C. Storage at RT over two weeks may result in week hybridization intensity.
2. Digestion should be monitored under the microscope every 5 min. Underdigested slides will have trim of the cytoplasm around cell nuclei and later give autofluorescence background. Digestion should proceed until nicely shaped clean nuclei show up. Overdigested specimens will display poor nuclei morphology, destructed chromatin. That slides should be discarded.
3. Change of the cell culture media each of 2 d before harvesting results in high mitotic index.

4. Optimum conditions for metaphase slide preparation should be determined first. If chromosomes overlap or retain the cytoplasm some modification can be used. Immerse clean slides in a jar with the cold distilled water. Drain excess water and drop cell suspension on the slide. Warm up the slide in a humid environment (on top of a jar with close to boiling water) for few seconds. This may improve chromosome spreading.

5. Monitor this step under the microscope. Sometimes after fixation in 70% ethanol straight chromatin fibers loose their shape. In that case slides after lysis buffer should be left to dry for several more days and then fixed in ethanol 70% or methanol acetic acid (3:1).

6. In order to control the size of the labeled fragments a "self-made" kit can be prepared and used. After 2 h of nick-translation, if the fragment is too large, an extra amount of the DNase can be added to a labeling mix to proceed reaction for 30 min more until the optimum lengths of the DNA fragments is reached.

References

1. Pack, S. D., Tanigami, A., Sato, T., Ledbetter, D., and Fukuda, M. N. (1997) Assignment of trophoblast/endometrial epithelium cell adhesion molecule trophinin gene Tro to human chromosome bands Xp11. 21-11. 22 by *in situ* hybridization *Cytogenet. Cell Genet.* **79(1–2),** 123–124.

2. Pack, S. D., Pak, E., Tanigami, A., Ledbetter, D. H., and Fukuda, M. N. (1999) Assignment of bystin gene BYSL to human chromosome band 6p21. 1 by *in situ* hybridization *Cytogenet. Cell Genet.* **83,** 76–77

3. Nederlof, P., van der Flier, S., Raap, A. K., Tanke, H. J., van der Ploeg, M., Kornips, F., and Geraedts, J. P. M. (1989) Detection of chromosome aberrations in interphase tumor nuclei by non-radioactive *in situ* hybridization. *Cancer Genet. Cytogenet.* **42,** 87–98.

4. Tkachuk, D. C., Pinkel, D., Kuo, W.-L., Weier, H.-U., and Gray, J. W. (1991) Clinical applications of fluorescence *in situ* hybridization. *Genet. Anal. Techn. Appl.* **8,** 67–74.

5. Ried, T., Lengauer, C., Cremer, T., Wiegant, J., Raap, A. K., van der Ploeg, M., Groitl, P., and Lipp, M. (1992) Specific metaphase and interphase detection of the breakpoint region in 8q24 of Burkitt lymphoma cells by triple-color fluorescence in situ hybridization. *Genes Chrom. Cancer* **4,** 69–74.

6. Lengauer, C., Green, E. D., and Cremer, T. (1992) Fluorescence in situ hybridization of YAC clones after Alu-PCR amplification. *Genomics* **13,** 826–828.

7. Ried, T., Lengauer, C., Lipp, M., Fischer, C., Cremer, T., and Ward, D. C. (1993) Evaluation of the utility of interphase cytogenetics to detect residual cells with a malignant genotype in mixed cell populations: a Burkitt lymphoma model. *DNA Cell Biol.* **12,** 637–643.

8. Demetrick, D. J. (1996) The use of archival frozen tumor tissue imprint specimens for fluorescence *in situ* hybridization. *Modern Pathol.* **9(2),** 133–136.

9. Pack, S., Vortmeyer, A., Pak, E., Liotta, L., and Zhuang, Z. (1997) Detection of single metastatic cells in lymph node tissue by fluorescent *in-situ* hybridization. *Lancet* **350,** 264–265.

10. Pack, S. D., Turner, M. L., Zhuang, Z., Vortmeyer, A. O., Boni, R, Scarulis, M., Marx, S. J., and Darling, T. N. (1998) Cutanious tumors in patients with multiple endocrine neoplasia type I show allelic deletion of the MEN1 gene *J. Invest. Dermatol.* **110,** 438–441.
11. Pack, S., Boni, R., Vortmeyer, A., Pak, E., and Zhuang, Z. (1998) Detection of gene deletion in single metastatic tumor cells in the exicion margin of a primary cutanious melanoma by fluorescent *in situ* hybridization. *J. Natl. Cancer Inst.* **90(10),** 782–783.
12. Kuwano, A., Ledbetter, S. A., Dobins, W. B., Emanuel, B. S., and Ledbetter, D. H. (1991) Detection of deletions and cryptic translocations in Miller-Dieker syndrome by *in situ* hybridization. *Am. J. Hum. Genet.* **49(4),** 707–714.
13. Hirota, H., Matsuoka, R., Kimura, M., Imamura, S., Joho, K., Ando, M., Takao, A., and Momma, K. (1996) Molecular cytogenetic diagnosis of Williams syndrome. *Am. J. Med. Genet.* **64(3),** 473–477.
14. Shaffer, L. G., Kennedy, G. M., Spikes, A. S., and Lupski J. R. (1997) Diagnosis of CMT1A duplications and HNPP deletions by interphase FISH: implications for testing in the cytogenetics laboratory. *Am. J. Med. Genet.* **69(3),** 325–331.
15. Krantz, I. D., Rand, E. B., Genin, A., Hunt, P., Jones, M., Louis, A. A., et al. (1997) Deletions of 20p12 in Allagille syndrome: frequency and molecular characterization. *Am. J. Med. Genet.* **70(1),** 80–86.
16. Kumar, S., Pack, S. D, Kumar, D., Walker, R., Quezado, M., Zhuang, Z., et al. (1999) Detection of EWS-FLI-1 fusion in Ewing's sarcoma/peripheral primitive neuroectodermal tumor by fluorescence in-situ hybridization using formalin-fixed paraffin-embedded tissue. *Human Pathol.* **30(3),** 324–330.
17. Chan, C. C., Pack, S. D., Pak, E., Tsokos, M., and Zhuang, Z. (1999) Translocation of chromosomes 11 and 22 in choroidal metastatic Ewing's Sarcoma detected by fluorescence in-situ hybridization. *Am. J. Opthalmol.* **127(2),** 226–228.
18. Pack, S. D., Zbar, B., Pak, E., Ault, D. O., Humphrey, J., Pham, T., et al. (1999) Germline deletions in VHL syndrome detected by fluorescence *in situ* hybridization (FISH). *Cancer Res.* **59(2),** 5560–5563.
19. Stilgenbauer, S., Döhner, H., Bulgary-Mörschel, M., Weitz, S., Bentz, M., and Lichter, P. (1993) Retinoblastoma gene deletion in chronic lymphoid leukemias: a combined metaphase and interphase cytogenetic study. *Blood* **81,** 2118–2124.
20. Vortmeyer, A., Choo, D., Pack, S., Oldfield, E., and Zhuang, Z. (1997, July 2) VHL gene alterations associated with endolymphatic sac tumors. *J. Natl. Cancer Inst.* **89(13),** 970–972.
21. Zhuang, Z., Vortmeyer, A. O., Pack, S., Huang, S., Pham, T., Wang, C., et al. (1997) Somatic mutations of the MEN1 tumor suppressor gene in sporadic gastrinomas and insulinomas. *Cancer Res.* **57(21),** 4682–4686.
22. Zhuang, Z., Ezzat, S., Vortmeyer, A. O., Weil, R., Oldfield, E. H., et al. (1997) Mutations of the MEN1 tumor suppressor gene in pituitary tumors. *Cancer Res.* **57(24),** 5446–5451.
23. Lubensky, I. A., Pack, S., Ault, D., Vortmeyer, A. O., Libutti, S. K., Choyke, P. L., et al. (1998) Multiple neuroendocrine tumors of the pancreas in von Hippel-

Lindau Disease Patients: Histopathologic and Molecular Genetic Analysis. *Am. J. Pathol.* **153(1),** 1378–1384.

24. Zhuang, Z., Park, W-S., Pack, S. D., Schmidt, L., Vortmeyer, A. O., Pak, E., et al. (1998) Trisomy 7 harboring non-random duplication of the mutant c-met proto-oncogene allele in hereditary papillary renal carcinomas. *Nat. Genet.* **20,** 66–69.

25. Thibleton, C., Pack, S., Sakai, A., Beaty, M., Pak, E., Vortmeyer, A. O., et al. (1999) Allelic loss of 11q13 as detected by MEN1- FISH is not associated with mutation of the MEN1 gene in lymphoid neoplasms *Leukemia* **13(1),** 85–91.

26. Kallioniemi, A., Kallioniemi, O.-P, Sudar, D., Rutovitz, D., Gray, J. W., Waldman, F., and Pinkel, D. (1992) Comparative genomic hybrization for molecular cytogenetic analysis of solid tumors. *Science* **258,** 818–821.

27. Pack, S. D., Karkera, J. D., Zhuang, Z., Pak, E., Hwu, P., Balan, K. W., et al. (1999) Molecular cytogenetic fingerprinting of esophageal squamous cell carcinoma by comparative genomic hybridization (CGH) reveals consistent pattern of chromosomal alterations. *Genes Chrom. Cancer* **25,** 160–168.

28. Schrock, E., du Manoir, S., Veldman, T., Schoell, B., Wienberg, J., Ferguson-Smith, M. A., et al. (1996) Multicolor spectral karyotyping of human chromosomes. *Science* **273(5274),** 494–497.

29. Cremer, T., Lichter, P., Borden, J., Ward, D. C., and Manuelidis, L. (1988) Detection of chromosome aberrations in metaphase and interphase tumor cells by in situ hybridization using chromosome specific library probes. *Hum. Genet.* **80,** 235–246.

30. Ploem, J. S. and Tanke, H. J. (1987) Introduction to fluorescence microscopy, in *RMS microscopy handbooks series,* No. 10, Oxford Science Publications.

31. Marcus, D. A. (1988) High-performance optical filters for fluorescence analysis. *Cell Motil. Cytoskelet.* **10,** 62–70.

32. Johnson, C. V., McNeil, J. A., Carter, K. C., and Lawrence, J. B. (1991) A simple, rapid technique for precise mapping of multiple sequences in two colors using a single optical filter set. *Genet. Anal. Techn. Appl.* **8,** 24–35.

33. Hiraoka, Y., Sedat, J. W., and Agard, D. A. (1987) The use of a charge-coupled device for quantitative optical microscopy of biological structures. *Science* **238,** 36–41.

34. Cremer, C. and Cremer, T. (1978) Considerations on a laser-scanning microscope with high resolution and depth of field. *Microscopia Acta* **81,** 31–44.

35. Haaf, T. and Ward, D. C. (1994) Structural analysis of alpha-satellite DNA and centromere proteins using extended chromatin and chromosomes. *Hum. Mol. Gen.* **3(5),** 697–709.

6

Microsatellite Analysis to Assess Chromosome 18q Status in Colorectal Cancer

Jin Jen

1. Introduction

Loss of the long arm of chromosome 18 (18q) is one of the most common genetic changes in colorectal cancer. This chapter describes the method to determine chromosome 18q status using microsatellite markers. Specifically, tumor and normal tissue are separated by microdissection of routine formalin-fixed paraffin embedded tissues obtained from surgical resection. Total genomic DNA are isolated and subjected to polymerase chain reaction (PCR) using polymorphic microsatellite markers located on the long arm of chromosome 18 *(1)*.

Microsatellite markers are short tandem repeat DNA sequences located throughout the genome *(2)*. Their lengths are highly variable in the population and are readily assayed by PCR using small amounts of DNA *(3,4)*. The normal cells of an individual carry two alleles, one inherited from each parent. When analyzed by denaturing gel electrophoresis, these alleles are usually detected as two amplified products of nearly equal intensity varying in size by one or more tandem repeats. In tumor tissues, however, chromosomal losses occur which can be detected by a change in the relative intensity of the two PCR products. A schematic outline of this procedure is shown in **Fig. 1**.

2. Materials
2.1. Tissue Source

Hematoxylin and eosin stained (H&E) primary tumor slides (6 mm thickness) made from fresh or paraffin embedded tissues.

From: *Methods in Molecular Medicine, vol. 50: Colorectal Cancer: Methods and Protocols*
Edited by: S. M. Powell © Humana Press Inc., Totowa, NJ

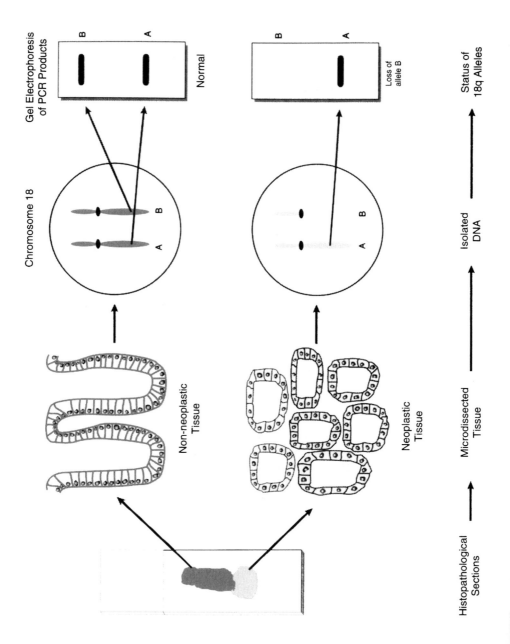

Gel Electrophoresis of PCR Products

Chromosome 18

Non-neoplastic Tissue

Neoplastic Tissue

Normal

B

A

Loss of allele B

B

A

Histopathological Sections

Microdissected Tissue

Isolated DNA

Status of 18q Alleles

2.2. Tissue Dissection

1. Razor blades, xylenes (J. T. Baker), black fine-point Sharpie pen, and Kim wipes.
2. Standard and dissecting microscopes.
3. Ventilated hood, 55°C heating block, a small boiling water bath.
4. 1.5 mL microcentrifuge tubes, racks, and a microcentrifuge.

2.3. DNA Extraction

All reagents are from Sigma unless otherwise specified.

1. TE-9: 500 mM Tris 9.0, 20 mM EDTA, 10 mM NaCl.
2. 10X SDS/Proteinase K: 5 mg/mL proteinase K (Boehringer and Mannheim), 10% sodium dodecyl sulfate.
3. LoTE: 3 mM Tris-HCL, pH 7.5, 0.3 mM EDTA.
4. PC-8: mixed 1:1 with aqua-phenol (Appligene), pH 8.0 and chloroform (J. T. Baker).
5. 100% and 70% ethanol, sterile water (Gibco-BRL), 7.5 M ammonium acetate and glycogen (Boehringer and Mannheim).

2.4. Sequence of the Primers for Microsatellite Amplification

All primers diluted to 100 ng/µL with sterile water (*see* **Notes 1** and **2**).

1. D18S55: 5'-GGGAAGTCAAATGCAAAATC-3' and
   5'-AGCTTCTGAGTAATCTTATGCTGTG-3'.
2. S18S58: 5'-GCTCCCGGCTGGTTTT-3' and
   5'-GCAGGAAATCGCAGGAACTT-3'.
3. D18S61: 5'-ATTTCTAAGAGGACTCCCAAACT-3' and
   5'-ATATTTTGAAACTCAGGAGCAT-3'.
4. D18S64: 5'-AACTAGAGACAGGCAGAA-3' and
   5'-ATCAGGAAATCGGCACTG-3'.
5. D18S69: 5'-CTCTTTCTCTGACTCTGACC-3' and
   5'-GACTTTCTAAGTTCTTGCCAG-3'.

Fig. 1. *(opposite page)* Strategy for determining the allelic status of the long arm of chromosome 18. Neoplastic tissue and non-neoplastic control tissue were separated by microdissection of routine histopathological sections from resection specimens. Total genomic DNA was isolated from each tissue sample. The polymerase chain reaction (PCR) was used to amplify polymorphic microsatellite markers capable of distinguishing between the maternal and the paternal copies of chromosome 18. Allelic loss (alleles are designated as A and B on chromosome 18) was observed as absence or a relative reduction of the PCR product corresponding to the loss of chromosomal arm. From **ref. 1**, with permission. Copyright 1994, Massachusetts Medical Society.

2.5. End Labeling of PCR Primers

1. T4 kinase, polynucleotide buffer (New England Biolabs), ^{32}P-γ-ATP (Amersham).
2. Chromospin-30 column (Clontech, CA).
3. Clinical centrifuge (Beckman).

2.6. PCR Amplification of Microsatellite Markers

1. 10X PCR buffer: 166 mM (NH$_4$)$_2$SO$_4$, 670 mM Tris-HCl, pH 8.8, 67 mM MgCl$_2$, and 100 mM β-mercaptalethanol.
2. dNTP mix (25 mM each made from 100 mM stock, Phamarcia).
3. DMSO, Taq polymerase, and mineral oil.
4. 96-well PCR plate (Hybaid), adhesive Plate Seal taps for 96 well plate (Research Product International), and PCR thermocycler (Hybaid).

2.7. Gel Electrophoresis

1. Formamide containing acrylamide gel mix: 7% acrylamide with 19:1 *bis*-acrylamide, 32% formamide, 5.6 M urea, and 1X TBE (90 mM Tris borate, 2 mM EDTA, pH 8.0).
2. 10% ammonium persulfate, TEMED (Bio-Rad).
3. Sequencing apparatus and power supply (Stratagene, CA).

2.8. Fluorography

1. Large blocking paper (GBM002, Schleicher and Schuell).
2. –80°C freezer.
3. Kodak X-Omat film and a film processor.

3. Methods

3.1. Tissue Microdissection and Processing

1. For each case to be analyzed use 2–5 H&E stained slides. Examine each slide under a standard microscope to determine the size, the relative position, and the histology of the tumor. Identify regions with the highest tumor components. Use a black Sharpie pen to demarcate the tumor if needed.
2. Place the slide under a low-powered dissecting microscope, use a clean Sharpie pen to dot cover the exact tumor area(s) to be dissected. Sometimes, more than one tumor area may be desired for microdissection (*see* **Notes 3** and **4**).
3. Do the same for each slide. In general, 2–5 slides are sufficient for at least 10 independent PCR reactions. However, 10 or more slides may be desired for very small tumors (less than 2 mm^2 in size).
4. In a ventilated hood, pipet transfer ~2 μL xylenes on to the corner of a new razor blade. Use this blade corner to carefully scrape off the Sharpie-covered tumor area(s). Use the same pipet tip to help transfer the tissue from the blade into a 1.5 mL microfuge tube containing 400 μL xylenes. Label the tube with case number and the letter "T" for tumor. Cap the tube immediately to avoid cross contamination.

5. Place the scraped slide under dissecting microscope and use a new blade to remove the remaining tumor cells from the slide until it is tumor free.
6. Use a Kim wipe to clean the tip of the Sharpie pen and dot cover the remaining nonneoplastic region of the slide.
7. Repeat **step 4** to obtain the normal tissue sample for control. Place tissue in a separate 1.5 mL xylenes containing tube and cap. Label the tube with "N" for normal.

3.2. DNA Extraction

1. Leave the tissue in xylenes for at least 15 min. Vortex the tubes containing the microdissected tissues for 15 s or until thoroughly mixed. The solution should be black in appearance with a tint of pink from eosin stain.
2. Place the tubes in a microfuge and spin at >10,000 rpm for 5 min.
3. Remove the xylenes from the tube using a pipetman and take care not to touch the pellet at the bottom (some removal of the fine black particles is acceptable because they are mostly the ink from the Sharpie pen).
4. Place the tube containing the pellet in a 58°C heating block for 15 min until the tissue pellet becomes dry and flaky in appearance.
5. Add 360 μL TE-9 and 40 μL 10X SDS/Proteinase K to each sample. Vortex to resuspend the pellet and incubate at 58°C for 16 to 20 h.
6. Vortex the tubes containing digested tissue samples and place them in a boiling water bath for 5 min and then let the samples stand at room temperature for at least 15 min (*see* **Note 5**).
7. Spin samples briefly in a microcentrifuge to bring down condensation and add 400 mL phenol/chloroform to each tube.
8. Cap the tube and vortex thoroughly. Spin for 5 min at top speed in a microcentrifuge and transfer the aqueous top phase to a fresh 1.5 mL tube. The interphase should be black in appearance and aqueous phase may be slightly pink.
9. Add another 400 μL phenol/chloroform to the extracted sample and repeat **step 8**.
10. Transfer the aqueous phase to another fresh tube and add 150 μL 7.5 *M* ammonium acetate, 3 μL glycogen, and 1 mL 100% ethanol to the sample.
11. Vortex to mix and spin the samples at 12,000 rpm for 10 min.
12. Drain out the ethanol and add 400 μL 70% ethanol. Invert the tube a few times to mix and spin for 2 min. Drain out the ethanol and repeat wash one more time (*see* **Note 6**).
13. After draining out the ethanol, spin the tube one more time and pipet out the remaining ethanol.
14. Air dries the pellet in the hood for 2 min and resuspend in 30 μL LoTE. Store at 4°C until use.

3.3. ^{32}P Labeling of the Oligo Primers

1. For every marker, label any one of the PCR primers using a 1.5 mL screw-top tube and add the following (*see* **Note 7**):

   1 μL   DNA (100 ng)
   2 μL   10X polynucleotide kinase buffer (NEB)

     14 µL   H$_2$O
      2 µL ^{32}P-γ-ATP (6000 mCi/ mM, 150 µCi/µL)
      1 µL   T$_4$ Kinase (10 U/µL, New England Biolabs)
Total: 20 µL   37°C 30 min

2. Prepare a ChromaSpin-30 column following the manufacturer's instruction.
3. Place the spin-dried column on top of a new screw top tube and place the setup in a 15 mL conical tube.
4. Add 30 µL Lo-TE to the kinase reaction mix and load the entire 50 µL on to the column at the center of the packed resin.
5. Spin the column for 15 min and the labeled primers should now be recovered in the collection tube.
6. Measure the total volume of recovery, which is usually greater than 40 µL. Add sterile water to bring the final volume to 100 µL.

3.4. PCR Amplification

1. Make a PCR master mix that is 2× more than the actual number of samples needed. Mix everything except *Taq* and labeled primer.

  1x =   1 µL   10X PCR buffer
         4 µL   H$_2$O
     0.5 µL   dNTP (25 mM each)
         1 µL   DMSO
     0.5 µL   Unlabeled primer (100 ng/µL)
         1 µL   Labeled primer

       1 U *Taq*/10 µL reaction

2. To a 96-well plate, aliquot 2 µL DNA template to each well (*see* **Note 8**).
3. Just before use, add Taq polymerase to the master mix and add ^{32}P-labeled primer behind a shield. Mix briefly and spin the reaction mixture for 30 s to collect the sample to the bottom of the tube.
4. Add 8 µL of the completed master mix to each well and top with 1 drop of mineral oil.
5. Cover the plate with PlateSeal Tape and PCR using block control option.
6. PCR for 1 cycle at 95°C for 2 min and then 30 cycles at 95°C for 30 s, 50°C for 1 min, and 70°C for 1 min followed by one cycle at 70°C for 5 min.
7. At the completion of PCR, add 15 µL stop buffer directly into the wells. Heat the plate in a PCR thermocycler at 95°C for 10 min then place immediately on ice. Load 5 µL/sample on formamide containing 7% polyacrylamide gel.

3.5. Gel Electrophoresis and Fluorography

1. Make the 7% gel mix and set up polyacrylamide gel apparatus as for sequencing *(5,6)* (*see* **Note 9**). Prerun the gel at 2000 V for 15 min. Rinse out the wells and load 5 µL of the sample per well.
2. Arrange so that the tumor and the normal control for each case are loaded immediately adjacent to each other.

3. Run gel under settings at 2000 to 2200 V for about 2 h until the first dye is just at the bottom of the gel (*see* **Note 10**).
4. Stop the run and take apart the glass plates (*see* **Note 11**).
5. Place a sheet of pre-cut GBM 002 paper onto the gel and lift to transfer the gel to the filter.
6. Cover the gel with plastic wrap and place on top of another sheet of GBM002 paper.
7. Immediately place the gel in a cassette with X-ray film closest to the gel.
8. Expose the film at –80°C for 4 to 24 h.
9. Develop and process the film for analysis of allelic status at chromosome 18q (*see* **Note 12**).
10. A loss of chromosome 18q is considered when the analyzed allele is heterozygous and the relative intensity of the two alleles in the tumor DNA differs from that of the normal control by a factor of at least 1.5 *(7)* (*see* **Note 13**).

4. Notes

1. The five microsatellite markers were selected based on their location on the chromosome and their easily distinguishable allele pattern. In general, D18S61 and D18S58 markers alone will be able to determine the chromosome status in 80% of the cases. The other markers are needed only when the data from the first two markers is inconclusive.
2. Although commercially available, the PCR primers for these markers are designed to generate PCR products that are smaller in size to ensure the success of each PCR reaction.
3. It is most important to carefully microdissect the tumor from the nonneoplastic component on the slide. Make every effort to select for regions that have the highest percentage of tumor cells. A highly enrich tumor sample is essential for the unambiguous interpretation of the chromosome 18q status.
4. The black Sharpie ink is used to mark the tumor regions as well as allowing the tissue to settle down to the bottom of the xylenes solution. However, do so gently so that the tissue will not be scraped or peeled off by the tip of the Sharpie pen.
5. After boiling, it is important to let the tubes stand for at least 15 min at room temperature before spinning as spinning earlier will deform the tube and cause leaking during phenol/chloroform extraction.
6. When washing the DNA with 70% ethanol, pay attention to the location of the pellets as they are only loosely attached to the tube at this point and can be easily lost resulting in a poor DNA yield.
7. It is recommended that one only use ^{32}P isotope within 2 wk of the calibration date. A good labeling reaction typically generates probes with a specific activity of greater than 10^8 cpm/μg DNA. Typically, 10^6 cpm should be used for each 10 μL PCR reaction. More probes can be used when specific activity of the probe is low.
8. When setting up PCR reaction in a 96-well plate, dot each well with a marker as you go so you will not get lost. Also look up from the bottom of the plate after adding DNA to be sure that there is DNA sample in each well.

9. Only purchase formamide from Sigma as other brands may not work. The gel mix should be kept at 4°C and used within one month.
10. The recommended total run time of the gel is approximate. For markers D18S64 and D18S69, shorter time may be needed.
11. The acrylamide gel can also be fixed with 5% methanol/acetic acid and dried to allow better resolution but doing so is more labor intensive and time consuming.
12. Fluorescent labeled probes can also be used in the same way for the analysis described. In this case, automatic sequencing capacity will be required.
13. For colorectal cancer, novel alleles representing the replication error phenotype (RER) phenotype occur at more than 2 of the 5 markers in ~15% of the cases. We have previous showed that these tumors usually retain chromosome 18q and are thus considered as having retention of chromosome 18q *(1)*.

Acknowledgments

This work was supported in part by the Hopkins GI SPORE grant CA-62924. The author would like to thank Mr. Robert Yuchem for photographic assistance.

Reference

1. Jen, J., Kim, H., Piantadosi, S., Liu, Z.-F., Levitt, R. C., Sistonen, P., Kinzler, K. W., Vogelstein, B., and Hamilton, S. R. (1994) Allelic loss of chromosome 18q and prognosis in colorectal cancer. *New Engl. J. Med.* **331,** 213–221.
2. Beckman, J. S. and Weber, J. L. (1992) Survey of human and rat microsatellites. *Genomics* **12,** 627–631.
3. NIH/CEPH collaborative mapping group. (1992) A comprehensive genetic linkage map of the human genome. *Nature* **258,** 67–86.
4. Saiki, R. K., Gelfand, D. H., Stoffel, S., et al. (1988) Primer-directed enzymatic amplification of DNA with a thermostable DNA polymerase. *Science* **239,** 487–491.
5. Sambrook, J., Fritsch, E. F., and Maniatis, T. (1989) *Molecular Cloning—A Laboratory Manual.* Cold Spring Harbor Laboratory, Cold Spring Harbor, NY, pp. 13.45–13.57.
6. Litt, M., Hauge, X., and Sharma, V. (1993) Shadow bands seen when typing polymorphic dinucleotide repeats: some causes and cures. *Biotechniques* **15,** 280–284.
7. Louis, D. N., Deimling, A., and Seizinger, B. R. (1992) A $(CA)_n$ dinucleotide repeat assay for evaluating loss of allelic heterozygosity in small and archival human brain tumor specimens. *Am. J. Pathol.* **141,** 777–782.

7

The SURF Technique

Selective Genetic Analysis of Microscopic Tissue Heterogeneity

Darryl Shibata

1. Introduction
1.1. Selective Ultraviolet Radiation Fractionation

Selective ultraviolet radiation fractionation (SURF) is a simple technique for the isolation of histologically defined microscopic tissue regions *(1,2)*. Very small numbers (100–400) of cells can be rapidly isolated with relatively crude equipment. The isolated cells can be analyzed genetically by PCR, thereby allowing a direct comparison between microscopic phenotype with genotype. The ability to compare genotype between different tissue areas provides opportunities to analyze many disease processes, including the heterogeneity expected of multistep tumor progression.

1.2. Tissue Microdissection Techniques

Tissues are complex mixtures of different cell types. This heterogeneity can hinder analysis if the cells of interest are only a minority of all cells. Conversely, the high sensitivity of many molecular techniques may allow detection of rare sequences that are absent from most cells. Tissue analysis can be improved by first refining the target such that only the desired cells are examined. Toward this goal, various investigators have used physical microdissection techniques to isolate specific cells (for example **refs. 3–5**, and many others).

An alternative to physical isolation are *in situ* hybridization techniques. Unfortunately, the sensitivity of *in situ* techniques are limited and not generally useful for mutation analysis of single-copy genes. *In situ* amplification techniques have been useful for the analysis of viral infections *(6,7)*.

From: *Methods in Molecular Medicine, vol. 50: Colorectal Cancer: Methods and Protocols*
Edited by: S. M. Powell © Humana Press Inc., Totowa, NJ

1.3. Advantages of SURF

Tissue microdissection can be tedious and requires great skill. The operator must be able to cut the desired region away from the undesired cells and the underlying microscope slide. He/she must also lift the isolated tissue and place it into the appropriate isolation tube. Multiple dissections require great care to prevent crosscontamination.

An alternative to the direct isolation of desired cells is the elimination of undesired cells. This approach has multiple technical advantages. First, the elimination of the unwanted cells greatly reduces the chance of contamination. Second, this approach is more amenable to technical innovation. For example, an elegant method to eliminate undesired DNA utilized a computer-controlled laser *(8)*. Essentially, a laser destroys everything on a microscopic slide except the small areas of interest. The SURF approach is less complicated and mimics the masking techniques used for the mass production of consumer electronic microcircuits. Electronic integrated chips are small and complex, and direct physical dissection would be extremely inefficient. Instead, a photographic mask or picture of the desired pattern is projected onto a photosensitive material. The optical pattern is converted into a physical pattern with the exposed areas eliminated whereas the protected areas remain. Extremely fine structures can be constructed because of the high resolution of light.

Microscopic tissue sections are "photosensitive" because the DNA present in the slides can be destroyed by ultraviolet light. Therefore, analogous to electronic circuits, masking techniques can be used to protect the cells of interest and ultraviolet light can be used to eliminate the DNA present in all other undesired cells. The resolution can be theoretically greater than conventional microscopy since ultraviolet light has a shorter wavelength than visible light. Hence, we have the technique of SURF (**Fig. 1**).

SURF requires some practice and modification of existing tools. One primary requirement is the ability to recognize histologic features. As such, the technique is ideal for pathologists although most individuals can achieve competence after several days or weeks of study. SURF places the emphasis on which areas to analyze because the subsequent isolation is greatly simplified. Of note: real surfing is much harder than SURF.

Before PCR, genetic analysis required large amounts of fresh tissue since hybridization probes required weeks to detect 1–10 µg of DNA. Now, over a decade after the PCR revolution, large amounts of DNA are still extracted from bulk tissues even though PCR allows the genetic analysis of small numbers of molecules. Depending on the situation, it is both unnecessary and unwise to perform genetic studies on bulk extracted DNA, unless it can be safely assumed that tissue heterogeneity is either not present or unimportant.

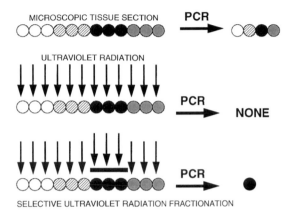

MICROSCOPIC TISSUE SECTION   **PCR**

ULTRAVIOLET RADIATION

PCR   **NONE**

PCR

SELECTIVE ULTRAVIOLET RADIATION FRACTIONATION

Fig. 1. Principles of SURF.

2. Materials
2.1. Preparations for SURF

1. Formalin-fixed, paraffin embedded tissues (*see* **Note 1**).
2. Plastic slides (*see* **Note 2**).
3. Stainless steel metal tray.
4. 90°C oven.
5. Hematoxylin and eosin stains (*see* **Table 1**).
6. "Sharpie" (Sanford Corporation, Bellwood, IL) marking pen.

2.2. SURF

1. Microdotter (*see* **Note 3**).
2. Ink from a Sharpie marking pen (*see* **Note 4**).
3. Inverted microscope (*see* **Note 5**) with photodocumentation system.

2.3. After SURF

1. Short-wave (254- or 302-nm) ulltraviolet transilluminator.
2. Photocopier.
3. Sterile scissors and forceps.
4. Sterile microfuge tubes (500 µL).
5. DNA extraction solution: 100 mM Tris-HCl, 2 mM EDTA, pH 8.0.
6. 20 mg/mL Proteinase K.
7. 42 to 56°C water bath.

3. Methods
3.1. Preparations for SURF

1. Select an appropriate formalin-fixed, paraffin-embedded tissue (*see* **Note 1**).

2. Place a single 5-µ thin tissue section on a plastic slide (*see* **Note 2**) using standard histology techniques. The plastic slides should be handled by their edges only.
3. A Sharpie marking pen is used to label the slides.
4. The slides (tissue-face-up) are place on a flat metal tray over small water drops. The water drops provide surface tension to prevent curling of the slides.
5. The slides are heated on the metal plate in a 90°C oven for 5–8 min. This baking melts the paraffin and firmly adheres the tissue to the slide. The slides should remain flat.
6. The slides are stained with conventional histologic hematoxylin and eosin reagents (**Table 1**). For some tissues that tend to fall off, each step may be shortened because only light staining is necessary.
7. The stained slides can be stored at room temperature. Coverslips are not used because they result in the loss of histologic detail. However, histologic features are usually adequate to distinguish between cells of different phenotypes.

3.2. SURF

1. The stained plastic slides are taped (transparent tape) onto glass slides so they can be moved by the microscope stage.
2. Areas of interest are identified by histologic microscopic criteria.
3. Ink dots are placed either manually or using a modified microdotter attached to a micromanipulator (*see* **Note 3** and **Fig. 2**). The dots are placed directly on the tissue. A "good" dot is thick enough to totally prevent the passage of light. Multiple small dots are placed to cover 100–400 cells (**Fig. 3**). Fewer cells can be covered but a larger number of cells prevents false allelic dropout and allows the use of less-robust PCR assays.
4. Photography allows the documentation of the tissues covered with each dot (*see* **Note 6**).
5. Approximately 10–20 areas per slide can be protected ("dotted") in 10–30 min.

3.3. After SURF

1. After the ink dots dry, the plastic sections, still attached to the glass slides, are placed face-down on a photocopier and then copied. Ideally the tissues are magnified by 200%. The photocopies allow a precise documentation of the location of each dot. Each dot is given an identifying number or letter. Note that at this point, only the back of the plastic slide must be protected against contamination because the front will be sterilized by UV radiation.
2. The plastic slides are removed from the glass slide and then placed directly (tissue-side-down) on a short-wave UV transilluminator. Both 254-nm and 302-nm wavelengths work fine. The time of illumination varies with the transilluminator and must be increased as the transilluminator ages (from 90 min for a new transilluminator to 3–4 h with an older one). The protection by the dots is almost complete so excess UV exposure does not appear to be a problem.
3. The slides are moved around every 20–30 min to ensure uniform exposure.
4. Afterwards, the plastic with attached allots are cut out with sterile scissors (2–4 mm squares) and placed directly into 0.5-mL microfuge tubes. In this way, there can be little doubt that the desired cells are indeed placed into the tube.

Table 1
Staining of Plastic Slides

Reagent	Interval	Purpose
Clear-Rite 3[a]	3 min	Deparaffinize
Ethanol 100%	6 dips	Wash
Ethanol 95%	6 dips	Wash
Water	6 dips	Wash
Hematoxylin	4 dips	Stain
Water	6 dips	Wash
0.5% Ammonium hydroxide	2 dips	Darken stain
Water	2 dips	Wash
Eosin	3 dips	Stain
Ethanol 95%	6 dips	Wash
Ethanol 100%	6 dips	Wash
Shake and air-dry	2 min	Dry

[a]Clear-Rite 3 (Richard-Allen Medical, Richland, MI). Each dip is approx 2–4 s.

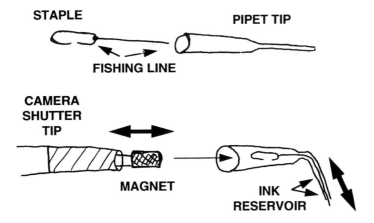

Fig. 2. A simple apparatus for placing protective dots. The bend in the pipet tip is induced with an autoclave. A micromanipulator is attached at the camera shutter tip to allow the precise placement of the dotter above the microscope slide.

5. The DNA is extracted (33 μL of 100 mM Tris-HCl, 2 mM EDTA, pH 8.0, with 0.7 μL of 20 mg/mL Proteinase K) overnight at 42°C or 4 h at 56°C.
6. The tubes are boiled for 5–7 min, vortexed, centrifuged, and stored at –20°C.
7. The dots should be scraped off with a pipet tip if they have not already fallen off to ensure complete extraction. If desired, the entire fraction including the ink dot and plastic can be subjected to PCR. Typically 8–10 μL

DOTS PLACED ON A SQUAMOUS CELL LUNG CANCER

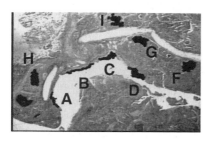

MICROSCOPIC PHENOTYPE
A) METAPLASIA
B) DYSPLASIA
C) DYSPLASIA
D) CARCINOMA IN SITU
F) CARCINOMA IN SITU
G) CARCINOMA IN SITU
H) DEEPER CANCER
I) DEPPER CANCER

BEFORE DOTS   **AFTER DOTS**

AIRWAY

BASEMENT   EPITHELIAL
MEMBRANE   SURFACE

p53 MUTATION ANALYSIS

WATER BLANK
NORMAL
COMPOSITE
NO DOT
CONTROLS

WILD TYPE

MUTANT

A B C D E F G H I J K

Fig. 3. Example of SURF on a squamous cell lung cancer *(13)*. The p53 point mutation was detected using radiolabeled allelic specific hybridization probes in a dot blot format. The p53 mutation was present in metaplastic, dysplastic and throughout the tumor tissue, but was absent from normal tissue (L). Loss of heterozygosity is not evident in this example.

are used in a 50 µL PCR so that multiple loci can be analyzed from the same dissected cells. PCR of many different targets (*see* **Note 7**) with appropriate controls is possible (*see* **Note 8**).

4. Notes

1. SURF is best performed on conventional formalin-fixed, paraffin-embedded tissue. Tissues are sometimes preserved with other fixatives. Fixatives that prevent subsequent PCR analysis are "B-5", Zenkers, Carnoy's, and Bouin's (*9*). Optimal fixatives are 10% buffered formalin (used almost universally for human tissues) and ethanol-based fixatives. Prolonged fixation (>5 d) in formalin degrades the DNA and the usual overnight fixation typically yields amplification in >90% of cases. Very old blocks paraffin blocks can be used (*10*).

2. Plastic slides have the optical properties of glass but the attached tissue and plastic can be cut by scissors. Specific isolation of tissue is greatly facilitated by this approach and the investigator can be confident that the desired tissues are indeed present in the desired tubes. Plastic slides are currently not commercially available. In art stores, "acetate" sheets can be purchased. The thickness should be about "10 mil" or 0.1 cm. These sheets are also called "desk protectors" in stationary stores. The sheets should be purchased flat and not extensively rolled.

   Using gloves, the sheets are cut into "microscope" slides with sterile scissors. These slides are dipped into a 0.1% poly-L-lysine adhesive solution (Catalog Number P 8920, Sigma Diagnostics, St. Louis, MO) for 5 min and air-dried. Conventional slide carriers that hold slides vertically (long dimension-up) appear to work best when dipping or staining plastic slides. The coated slides are stored at room temperature.

3. Dots can be place manually using a fine point Sharpie pen. However, a micromanipulator greatly facilitates placing the dots on the desired areas. The current setup in my laboratory consists of an inverted microscope and a video camera and recorder. The "dotter" is a custom designed camera shutter cord mounted on a simple micromanipulator (**Fig. 2**). The parts are:
   a. Stapled staple with 1 lb fishing line (monofilament) tied around it.
   b. Autoclaved gel loader pipet tip bent at about 60°.
   c. Flexible camera shutter cord with a small magnet at the tip.

   The tips (**Notes 1** and **2**) are autoclaved for 1 h in aluminum foil. The bend is induced when the tips are placed in the aluminum foil and becomes "permanent" after autoclaving. The sterile tips are placed on the camera shutter cord and the magnet provides a direct control link.

   After assembly, modifications to the pipette tip can be made with a sterile scissors. A Sharpie pen is broken open and its wick (covered with plastic) is squeezed to place a drop of ink onto a clean glass slide. The ink is usually too thin and is usually aged for 5–15 min, until the correct consistency is reached (depends on temperature and humidity, with differences present between pens). The dotter tip is placed into the ink pool and 0.2–0.4 cm (length) of ink is drawn up, by capillary action. With the dotter about 0.2 to 0.3 cm above the slide, the shutter is depressed to move the fishing line out of the ink reservoir and onto the slide (**Fig. 2**). The fishing line is flexible so that it is usually impossible to dislodge the tissue from the slide. Therefore, a single dotter can be used to dot multiple regions. The shape and consistency of the dots will change with time as the ink slowly dries (about 30–50 min).

4. Various UV protective ink umbrellas have been tried without success (many inks contain substances that inhibit subsequent PCR). The ink in Sharpie marking pens works well because it blocks UV radiation, produces sharp dots, and does not inhibit PCR.

5. An inverted microscope allows the direct visualization of the dotting process because one can observe the approach of the microdotter or ink pen towards the tissue section.

6. It is essential to document the site and phenotype of each dot. This can be done several ways. First, each dot is assigned an identification number. A photograph is taken before and after each dot to document the exact number and types of cells covered by the ink dot. A video camera with a digital frame grabber (made by various companies) is most convenient since many pictures are required for each slide. Second, the phenotype of each dot (normal, dysplastic, cancer, and so forth) is written down (**Fig. 3**).

7. Radioactive techniques and a large number of PCR cycles (36–48) are usually needed since the number of starting molecules is low. The PCR products from the fractions are analyzed by conventional techniques including dot-blot hybridization, restriction enzyme digestion, SSCP, direct sequencing, and electrophoresis (such as microsatellite size analysis) *(11,12)*. Loss of heterozygosity studies are also possible but require careful attention to PCR conditions since many PCR cycles are necessary to detect the low numbers of starting molecules.

   Virtually any target can be analyzed with SURF and PCR. The biggest concern is the size of the PCR product. It must be short enough (<200 bp with <160 bp better) to be preserved in the fixed tissue but long enough (5100 bp) to be readily inactivated by UV radiation.

8. The following controls should be used: No dot control: An adjacent square of similar but unprotected tissue should also be isolated and analyzed by PCR. It should demonstrate no PCR products. If PCR products are detected with this negative control, a longer PCR target or greater exposure to the UV radiation is necessary. Duplicates: Each tissue section should be SURFed at least twice to verify the distribution of each mutation. Positive controls: If difficulty is encountered in getting detectable PCR products, the tissue not exposed to UV radiation should be amplified to verify that its DNA is intact. A shorter PCR target usually corrects this problem unless the tissue has been fixed in B-5, Bouin's, or Zenkers.

Acknowledgments

The author thanks the many talented students and technicians who have gone SURFing in my laboratory, including Zhi-Hua Li, Jenny Tsao, Qioping Shu, Susan Leong, and Bridgette Duggan, Antonio Hernandez, and Adrian Ireland.

References

1. Shibata, D., Hawes, D., Li, Z. H., Hernandez, A., Spruck, C. H., and Nichols, P. W. (1992) Specific genetic analysis of microscopic tissue after selective

ultraviolet radiation fractionation and the polymerase chain reaction. *Am. Pathol.* **141,** 539–543.

2. Shibata, D. (1993) Selective ultraviolet radiation fractionation and polymerase chain reaction analysis of genetic alterations. *Am. J. Pathol.* **143,** 1523–1526.

3. Meltzer, S. J., Yin, J., Huang, Y., McDaniel, T. K., Newkirk, C., Iseri, O., et al. (1991) Reduction to homozygosity involving p53 in esophageal cancers demonstrated by the polymerase chain reaction. *Proc. Natl. Acad. Sci. USA* **88,** 4976–4980.

4. Bianchi, A. B., Navone, N. M., and Conti, C. J. (1991) Detection of loss of heterozygosity in formalin-fixed paraffin-embedded tumor specimens by the polymerase chain reaction. *Am. J. Pathol.* **138,** 279–284.

5. Volgelstein. B., Fearon, E. R., Hamilton, S. R., Kern, S. E., Preisinger, A. C., Leppert, M., et al. (1988) Genetic alterations during colorectal-tumor development. *N. Engl. J. Med.* **319,** 1525–1532.

6. Haase, A. T., Retzel, E. F., and Staskur, K. A. (1990) Amplification and detection of lentiviral DNA inside cells. *Proc. Natl. Acad. Sci. USA* **87,** 4971–4975.

7. Nuovo, G. J., MacConnell, P., Forde, A., and Delvenne, D. P. (1991) Detection of human papillomavirus DNA in formalin-fixed tissues by *in situ* hybridization after amplification by polymerase chain reaction. *Am. J. Pathol.* **139,** 847–854.

8. Hadano, S., Watanabe, M., Yokai, H., Kogi, M., Kondo, I., Tsuchiya, H., Kanazawa, I., Wakasa, K., and Ikeda, J. E. (1991) Laser microdissection and single unique primer PCR allow generation of regional chromosome DNA clones from a single human chromosome. *Genomics* **11,** 364–673.

9. Greer, C. E., Peterson, S. L., Kiviat, N. B., and Manos, O. M. (1991) PCR amplification from paraffin-embedded tissues. *Am. J. Clin. Pathol.* **95,** 117–124.

10. Shibata, D., Martin, W. J., and Arnheim, N. (1988) Analysis of DNA sequences in forty-year-old paraffin-embedded thin-tissue sections: a bridge between molecular biology and classical histology. *Cancer Res.* **48,** 4564–4566.

11. Shibata, D., Schaeffer, J., Li, Z. H., Capella, G., and Perucho, M. (1993) Genetic heterogeneity of the c-K-ras locus in colorectal adenomas but not adenocarcinomas. *J. Natl. Cancer Inst.* **85,** 1058–1063.

12. Shibata, D., Peinadoa, M. A., Ionov, Y., Malkhosyan, S., and Perucho, M. (1991) Genomic instability in simple repeat sequences is a very early somatic event in colorectal tumorigenesis that persists after transformation. *Nature Genetics* **6,** 273–281.

13. Zheng, J., Shu, Q., Li, Z. H., Tsao, J. L., Weiss, L. M., and Shibata, D. (1994) Patterns of p53 mutations in squamous cell carcinoma of the lung: early acquisition at a relatively early age. *Am. J. Pathol.* **145,** 1444–1449.

8

Microsatellite Instability Testing

Yann R. Parc and Kevin C. Halling

1. Introduction

Microsatellites are tandem repeats of simple sequences that occur abundantly and are randomly interspersed throughout the human genome. They typically consist of 10–50 copies of 1–6 bp motifs, and are characterized by a high degree of polymorphism. Despite the variability observed among individuals, microsatellite are replicated faithfully at each cell division in normal germline and somatic cells (1).

In 1993, three research groups described a novel type of genomic instability, which has been called microsatellite instability (MSI) or replication error (RER), in a subset of sporadic colorectal cancers and in most tumors from patients with HNPCC (2–4). Microsatellite instability is a change of any length (due to either insertion or deletion of repeating units) in a microsatellite within a tumor when compared to normal tissue.

In CRC, three MSI phenotypes have been described (5,6). The MSI-H phenotype is characterized by MSI at >30–40% of the loci examined, the MSI-L phenotype by MSI at <30–40% of the loci examined and the MSS phenotype by an absence of MSI at any of the loci examined. In sporadic CRC the MSI-H phenotype is associated with distinct clinicopathologic features (e.g., proximal tumor site, high grade, diploidy, favorable survival) (3,5,6). The MSI-L and MSS phenotypes, on the other hand, are not associated with distinct clinicopathologic features (5).

The MSI-H phenotype is the result of defective DNA mismatch repair. Inactivating mutations of one of at least five different DNA MMR genes (hMLH1, hMSH2, PMS1, PMS2, and hMSH6/GTPBP) are the cause of the MSI-H phenotype in HNPCC-associated tumors (7–11). Hypermethylation of

From: Methods in Molecular Medicine, vol. 50: Colorectal Cancer: Methods and Protocols
Edited by: S. M. Powell © Humana Press Inc., Totowa, NJ

the *hMLH1* promoter is the etiology of the MSI-H phenotype in over 90% of sporadic CRC *(12–14)*.

MSI has been reported in a variety of other malignancies *(15)*. However, among sporadic tumors, the MSI-H phenotype appears to be most common in cancers of the stomach, endometrium and upper urinary tract *(16)*. Interestingly, these are also the same types of tumors that frequently occur in HNPCC patients *(17)*.

MSI analysis can be used to: 1) identify tumors with defective MMR (i.e., the tumors with the MSI-H phenotype), 2) as a screening test for the identification of colorectal cancer patients that may have HNPCC *(18–21)*, and 3) to identify colorectal cancer patients that may have a favorable prognosis (i.e., the MSI-H tumors) *(3,22–25)*. Additionally, the identification of the MSI-H phenotype in CRC may have treatment implications beyond prognostication since some studies suggest that tumors with the MSI-H phenotype are resistant to chemotherapeutic agents such as cisplatin and N-Methyl-N'-nitro-N-nitrosoguanidine *(26–28)*.

In this chapter we describe methods that we use in our laboratory to assess tumors for MSI. Additional information on technical guidelines for the detection of MSI can be found in the report of a recent National Cancer Institute workshop on microsatellite instability *(21)*.

2. Materials

2.1. DNA Extraction

1. Paraffin-embedded normal and tumor tissue sections (10 microns thick).
2. Scalpels (Bard-Parkers®, Franklin Lakes, NJ).
3. Microfuge tube (2.0 mL) (Sarstedt, Nümbrecht, Germany).
4. QIAamp tissue kit (Qiagen Inc, Santa Clarita, CA).

2.2. Polymerase Chain Reaction

1. Ampli*Taq*® Gold with GeneAmp® kit (Perkin Elmer, Branchburg, NJ).
2. Ampli*Taq* DNA polymerase with GeneAmp kit (Perkin Elmer).
3. GeneAmp dNTPs (Perkin Elmer, Branchburg, NJ).
4. 5X PCR buffer: 100 µL of dATP, dGTP, and dTTP, 20 mL dCTP, 500 µL of 10X PCR buffer (provided with the AmpliTaq polymerase kit), 180 µL deionized and filtered water.
5. α-^{32}P-dCTP, 111 Tbq/mmol, 3000 Ci/mmol (New England Nuclear, Boston, MA).
6. Primers (Integrated DNA Technologies, Inc., Coralville, IA) (*see* **Table 1** and **Note 1**).

2.3. Gel Electrophoresis and Autoradiography

1. Acrylamide/Bis 19:1 (5% C) powder "30g" (Bio-Rad Laboratories, Hercules, CA).
2. 10X TBE stock (National Diagnostics, Atlanta, GA).

Table 1
Primer Sequences

	5' Primer	3'Primer
ACTC	5'-TTCCATACCTGGGAACGAGT-3'	5'-TTGACCTGAATGCACTGTGA-3'
TP53	5'-AGGGATACTATTCAGCCCGAGGTG-3'	5'-ACTGCCACTCCTTGCCCCATTC-3'
D18S34	5'-CAGAAAATTCTCTCTGGCTA-3'	5'-CTCATGTTCCTGGCAAGAAT-3'
D18S61	5'-ATATTTTGAAACTCAGGAGCAT-3'	5'-ATTTCTAAGAGTCCCAAACT-3'
D18S49	5'-GTTTATTGTTGTAGGGTGTGCTCCT-3'	5'-GTTTGCTTCCTTCTGGAATATCTCC-3'
D5S346	5'-ACTCACTCTAGTGATAAATCG-3'	5'-AGCAGATAAGACAGTATTACTAGTT-3'
BAT 26	5'-TGACTACTTTGACTTCAGCC-3'	5'-AACCATTCAACATTTTAACCC-3'
MFD 15	5'-GTTTGCAAGAATCAAATAGACAAT-3'	5'-GTTTGCTGGCCATATATATATTTAAACC-3'
D2S123	5'-GTTTAAACAGGATGCCTGCCTTTA-3'	5'-GTTTGGACTTTCCACCTATGGGAC-3'
BAT 25	5'-GTTTCGCCTCCAAGAATGTAAGT-3'	5'-GTTTCTGCATTTTAACTATGGCTC-3'

GTTT is a non-annealing 5' "tail" that increases the specificity of the PCR.

3. Urea (Fisher Biotech, Fair Lawn, NJ).
4. Corning® filter systems and bottle top filters (Corning Incorporated, Corning, NY).
5. Ammonium persulfate (Sigma Chemical Co., St. Louis, MO).
6. TEMED (Boerhinger Mannheim Corp., Indianapolis, IN).
7. Sequencing gel electrophoresis apparatus, Model S2 (Gibco-BRL, Gaithersburg, MD).
8. Glass plates (pair) (provided with sequencing apparatus).
9. Spacers and combs (provided with sequencing apparatus).
10. 0.5 M EDTA, pH 8.0 (Bio Whittaker, Walkersville, MD).
11. 10% Ammonium persulfate: 1 g of ammonium persulfate in 10 mL of water. Stable for 6 mo if stored at 4°C.
12. Formamide (Oncor, Gaithersburg, MD).
13. Bromophenol blue (Sigma Chemical).
14. Xylene cyanole FF (Sigma Chemical).
15. Filter paper (35 × 45 cm) (Bio-Rad Laboratories).
16. Bio-Max MR film (Kodak, Rochester, NY).
17. Autoradiography cassettes, X-Omatic cassette (Kodak).
18. Loading buffer: 47.5 mL of formamide, 2 mL of 0.5 M EDTA (pH 8.0), 0.025 g of bromophenol blue, 0.025 g of xylene cyanole FF, bring to 50 mL with deionized and filtered water. Stable for 1 year at –20°C.

3. Methods

3.1. DNA Extraction

1. Cut one 5 μ and several 10 μ sections from the paraffin-embedded normal and tumor tissue blocks with a microtome (*see* **Note 2**). Sections from a single block may suffice for DNA extraction if the tissue in that block contains both normal and tumor tissue. The number of slides required for DNA extraction depends on how large the foci of normal and tumor tissue are (*see* **Note 3**). We recommend that at least one cm² of normal and tumor tissue be used.
2. Stain the 5 μm but not the 10 μm slide with hematoxylin and eosin (H&E) (*see* **Note 4**).
3. A pathologist should then circle (on the H&E stained slide with a fine point flare pen) foci of normal and tumor tissue that will be used for DNA extraction. The pathologist should try to identify areas that contain ≥70% tumor cells (*see* **Note 5**).
4. Using the H&E slide as a template, circle the corresponding areas of "normal" and "tumor" on the bottom side of the unstained slides (*see* **Note 5**).
5. Using separate scalpel blades, scrape the encircled "normal" and "tumor" tissue from the unstained slides into a 2.0 mL microfuge tube.
6. DNA extraction is then performed as described in the procedure provided with the QIAamp DNA extraction kit (*see* **Note 6**).
7. Store the DNA at 4°C until further use. The DNA concentration will generally be approx 25 ng/μL in our experience. However, we do not standardly determine the concentrations of the samples.

3.2. Polymerase Chain Reaction

1. All of the reagents required for PCR except for dNTPs are contained in the GeneAmp kits.
2. A typical PCR mixture contains the following:

> 2 mL DNA (extracted) (~50 ng)
> 0.8 mL forward primer (20 μ*M*) (16 pmol)
> 0.8 mL reverse primer (20 μ*M*) (16 pmol)
> 2.4 mL 2 m*M* MgCl$_2$
> 2.0 mL Ampli*Taq* (0.5 units/μL) (1 unit)
> 4.0 mL 5X PCR buffer
> H$_2$O to 20 μL

3. It may be necessary to vary the concentrations of the various reaction components to optimize the PCR results (*see* **Note 7**). However, PCR conditions that have been found to be optimal for the microsatellites that we use in our laboratory are shown in **Table 2**.
4. The PCR generally consists of 35 cycles of 30 s at 95°C, 30 s at the annealing temperature that might vary from 55°C to 65°C, and 30 s at 72°C.
5. This is followed by an extension step of 10 min at 72°C. The cycling parameters used for each primer pair are shown in **Table 3**.
6. If Ampli*Taq* Gold GeneAmp is used, an activating step of 10 min at 95°C should be performed before the 35 amplification cycles.
7. The PCR products can be stored at –20°C or immediately subjected to electrophoretic analysis. It is recommended that the PCR products be analyzed within 1 wk, since additional storage leads to weaker and less distinct signals.

3.3. Gel Preparation, Electrophoresis and Autoradiography

1. Prepare 1 L of stock acrylamide solution in the following fashion.
2. Add 48 mL of ultra-pure water to two 30 g Acrylamide/Bis 19:1 (5% C) powder containers. Dissolve the acrylamide with a stir bar.
3. In a 1 L beaker, add 100 mL of 10X TBE buffer to 420 g of urea.
4. When the acrylamide mix has dissolved, add it to the beaker containing the urea/TBE mix.
5. Bring to 1 L with deionized and filtered water.
6. Wrap the container with aluminum foil to protect the acrylamide from photodegradation.
7. Dissolve the urea by mixing with a stir bar. This typically takes 1/2–1 h.
8. Vacuum-filter the solution through a Corning filter systems and Bottle Top filters to remove impurities.
9. Store at 4°C in the dark. The acrylamide mix should be stable for 6 mo under these conditions.
10. Prepare a gel "sandwich" according to standard techniques.
11. Allow 60 mL of the acrylamide gel solution to come to room temperature in a 250 mL vacuum flask.
12. Degas the solution for 10 min under vacuum.

Table 2
PCR Composition for the Different Markers[a]

	ACTC	TP53	D18S34	D18S61	D18S49	D5S346	BAT 26	MFD 25	D2S123	BAT 25
H_2O	11.2	11.7	10.5	12	12.075	9.2	9.6	9.6	9.6	9.6
5X buffer with MgCl$_2$				4						
5X buffer without MgCl$_2$	4	4	4		4	4	4	4	4	4
MgCl$_2$ 25 mM	0.8	1.6	1.6	0.8	0.8	2.8	2.4	2.4	2.4	2.4
Primer A 20 pmol/µL	0.8	0.2	0.8	0.8	0.4	0.8	0.8	0.8	0.8	0.8
Primer B 20 pmol/µL	0.8	0.2	0.8	0.8	0.4	0.8	0.8	0.8	0.8	0.8
Taq polymerase	0.2*	0.1*	0.1*	0.2*	0.125*	0.2♣	0.2♣	0.2♣	0.2♣	0.2♣
α-P^{32} (dCTP)	0.2	0.2	0.2	0.2	0.2	0.2	0.2	0.2	0.2	0.2
DNA	2	2	2	2	2	2	2	2	2	2

[a]Volume are expressed in µL. *Regular Taq polymerase, ♣ Taq Gold polymerase.

Table 3
PCR Thermal Cycler Parameters and Gel Run Times for the Different Markers

	ACTC	TP53	D18S34	D18S61	D18S49	D5S346	BAT 26	MFD 25	D2S123	BAT 25
Activating step						95°C/10'	95°C/10'	95°C/10'	95°C/10'	95°C/10'
Annealing temp	60°C	60°C	60°C	60°C	62°C	58°C	58°C	58°C	58°C	58°C
Product size	68–96	103–135	89–119	157–179	102–118	96–122	100	150	197–227	100
Gel run time (h)	1.5	2	2	2.5	2	2	2	2.5	3	2

13. Add 400 μL of 10% ammonium persulfate and 10.2 μL of TEMED and mix by swirling.
14. Pour the mixture between the gel sandwich plates.
15. Insert the blunt end of a sharkstooth comb approx 7 mm deep into the top of the gel sandwich.
16. Allow the gel to polymerize for 1 h.
17. Remove the comb and wash the loading space with running buffer (1X TBE).
18. Place the teeth of the sharkstooth comb barely into the surface of the gel.
19. Pre-electrophorese for 30 min at 70 V.
20. Prepare samples for electrophoresis by diluting 1 μL of the PCR products with 19 μL of loading buffer.
21. Denature PCR products at 95°C for 2 min and quickly place on ice to prevent renaturation.
22. Load the normal and tumor tissue PCR products for each patient in adjacent wells (*see* **Note 8**).
23. The running time varies according to the product size (**Table 3**), but 70 V should be applied in all cases.
24. When the electrophoresis is complete, remove the upper plate of the gel sandwich and place a Bio-Rad filter paper on the gel.
25. Dry the gel on a vacuum gel dryer at 80°C for 1 h.
26. Expose a film to the gel in a cassette for 12 h (*see* **Note 9**).
27. Develop the film.

3.4. Interpretation

Compare the banding pattern of the PCR products from the normal and tumor tissue of the patient to determine if the tumor exhibits MSI, loss of heterozygosity (LOH) or no change at that marker. Two patterns of MSI have been noted in our laboratory that we call pattern 1 and pattern 2 alterations. Pattern 1 alterations appear as marked alterations in repeat length (often heterogenous in nature and appearing as a ladder), whereas pattern 2 alterations are minor changes in repeat length (typically two bp) (*see* **Note 10**). Representative examples of pattern 1 and 2 MSI alterations and LOH are shown in **Fig. 1**. Both patterns can be observed in MSI-L and MSI-H tumors, however, pattern 1 predominates in the MSI-H group, and pattern 2 predominates in the MSI-L group *(3,5,15)*.

4. Notes

1. Primers. For formalin-fixed paraffin-embedded tissue, primers should be designed such that the PCR product size is <200 bp in length. It is difficult to obtain PCR product for larger amplicons when DNA is extracted from paraffin-embedded material. Longer PCR amplicons, however, can be amplified from frozen fresh tissue. If paired normal DNA cannot be obtained, BAT26 can be used as a single marker to assess a tumor for the MSI-H phenotype due to quasi-monomorphic nature of this mononucleotide repeat *(29)*.

N   T   N   T   N   T

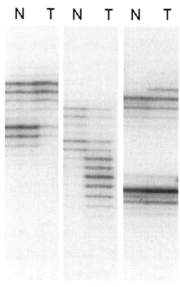

LOH   Pattern 1 Pattern 2

Fig. 1. Examples of LOH and microsatellite instability (pattern 1 and 2) at the p53 locus. N; normal DNA, T; tumor DNA.

2. The microtome blade should be changed or shifted to a new section of the blade between different patient samples. This prevents PCR contamination between samples.
3. It may be necessary to use several unstained slides to obtain enough tissue for DNA extraction if the foci of normal or tumor tissue are small.
4. Do not stain the slides that will be used for DNA extraction. Staining appears to inhibit the quality of the PCR.
5. A tumor cell content of 70% has been recommended for LOH analysis. However, a lower tumor cell content (as low as 30–40%) will still allow for the identification of tumor MSI. The size of the foci circled by the pathologist will frequently be a compromise between quantity and quality. The goal is to maximize the amount of tissue circled while maintaining a high tumor content.
6. The QIAamp kit has provided excellent results for DNA extraction.
7. Thermal cycling parameters and reagent concentrations may be modified to optimize the PCR. The most important parameters that can be modified to increase the quality of the reaction are the $MgCl_2$ concentration and the annealing temperature. AmpliTaq Gold polymerase sometimes but not always increases the quality of the reaction. Additionally, a non-hybridizing GTTT(T) sequence can be added to the 5' end of the primers to increase the specificity of the PCR *(30)*.
8. Load control samples at regular intervals as lane markers in the event that some or all of the test samples fail to provide good signals.

9. If the signals observed after a 12-h room temperature exposure are weak, expose the gel at –70°C for 12 h. Perform autoradiography on a s film for 36 h. Occasional instances of MSI will be detected with this longer exposure but not with the shorter 12-h exposure.

10. Pattern 1 is almost always easily recognized. However, pattern 2 can sometimes be difficult to recognize and can be overinterpreted. It is important not to mistake bands not present in the normal as definitive evidence of MSI if the intensity of the signals in the normal lane are significantly weaker than in the tumor lane.

References

1. Weber, J. L. and Wong, C. (1993) Mutation of human short tandem repeats. *Human Mol. Genet.* **2,** 1123–1128.

2. Ionov, Y., Peinado, M. A., Malkhosyan, S., Shibata, D., and Perucho, M. (1993) Ubiquitous somatic mutations in simple repeated sequences reveal a new mechanism for colonic carcinogenesis. *Nature* **363,** 558–561.

3. Thibodeau, S. N., Bren, G., and Schaid, D. (1993) Microsatellite instability in cancer of the proximal colon. *Science* **260,** 816–819.

4. Aaltonen, L. A., Peltomaki, P., Leach, F. S., Sistonen, P., Pylkkanen, L., Mecklin, J. P., et al. (1993) Clues to the pathogenesis of familial colorectal cancer. *Science* **260,** 812–816.

5. Thibodeau, S. N., French, A. J., Cunningham, J. M., Tester, D., Burgart, L. J., Roche, P. C., et al. (1998) Microsatellite instability in colorectal cancer: different mutator phenotypes and the principlal involvment of hMLH1. *Cancer Res.* **58,** 1713–1718.

6. Lengauer, C., Kinzler, K. W., and Vogelstein, B. *(1997)* DNA methylation and genetic instability in colorectal cancer cells. *Proc. Natl. Acad. Sci. USA* **94,** 2545–2550.

7. Fishel, R., Lescoe, M. K., Rao, M. R., Copeland, N. G., Jenkins, N. A., Garber, J., et al. (1993) The human mutator gene homolog MSH2 and its association with hereditary nonpolyposis colon cancer. *Cell* **75,** 1027–1038.

8. Leach, F. S., Nicolaides, N. C., Papadopoulos, N., Liu, B., Jen, J., Parsons, R., et al. (1993) Mutations of a mutS homolog in hereditary nonpolyposis colorectal cancer. *Cell* **75,** 1215–1225.

9. Bronner, C. E., Baker, S. M., Morrison, P. T., Warren, G., Smith, L. G., Lescoe, M. K., et al. (1994) Mutation in the DNA mismatch repair gene homologue hMLH1 is associated with hereditary non-polyposis colon cancer. *Nature* **368,** 258–261.

10. Nicolaides, N. C., Papadopoulos, N., Liu, B., Wei, Y. F., Carter, K. C., Ruben, S. M., et al. (1994) Mutations of two PMS homologues in hereditary nonpolyposis colon cancer. *Nature* **371,** 75–80.

11. Papadopoulos, N., Nicolaides, N. C., Wei, Y. F., Ruben, S. M., Carter, K. C., Rosen, C. A., et al. (1994) Mutation of a mutL homolog in hereditary colon cancer. *Science* **263,** 1625–1629.

12. Kane, M. F., Loda, M., Gaida, G. M., Lipman, J., Mishra, R., Goldman, H., et al. (1997) Methylation of the hMLH1 promoter correlates with lack of expression of

hMLH1 in sporadic colon tumors and mismatch repair-defective human tumor cell lines. *Cancer Res.* **57,** 808–811.

13. Herman, J. G., Umar, A., Polyak, K., Graff, J. R., Ahuja, N., Issa, J. P., Markowitz, S., et al. (1998) Incidence and functional consequences of hMLH1 promoter hypermethylation in colorectal carcinoma. *Proc. Natl. Acad. Sci. USA* 6870–6875.

14. Cunningham, J. M., Christensen, E. R., Tester, D. J., Kim, C.-Y., Roche, P. C., Burgart, L. J., and Thibodeau, S. N. (1998) Hypermethylation of the hMLH1 promoter in colon cancer with microsatellite instability. *Cancer Res.* **58,** 3455–3460.

15. Honchel, R., Halling, K. C., and Thibodeau, S. N. (1995) Genomic instability in neoplasia. *Semin. Cell Biol.* **6,** 45–52.

16. Peltomaki, P., Lothe, R. A., Aaltonen, L. A., Pylkkanen, L., Nystrom-Lahti, M., Seruca, R., et al. (1993) Microsatellite instability is associated with tumors that characterize the hereditary non-polyposis colorectal carcinoma syndrome. *Cancer Res.* **53,** 5853–5855.

17. Lynch, H. T., Smyrk, T., and Lynch, J. (1997) An update of HNPCC (Lynch syndrome). *Cancer Genet. Cytogenet.* **93,** 84–99.

18. Moslein, G., Tester, D. J., Lindor, N. M., Honchel, R., Cunningham, J. M., French, A. J., et al. (1996) Microsatellite instability and mutation analysis of hMSH2 and hMLH1 in patients with sporadic, familial and hereditary colorectal cancer. *Hum. Mol. Genet.* **5,** 1245–1252.

19. Beck, N. E., Tomlinson, I. P., Homfray, T., Hodgson, S. V., Harocopos, C. J., and Bodmer, W. F. (1997) Genetic testing is important in families with a history suggestive of hereditary non-polyposis colorectal cancer even if the Amsterdam criteria are not fulfilled. *Br. J. Surg.* **84,** 233–237.

20. Dietmaier, W., Wallinger, S., Bocker, T., Kullmann, F., Fishel, R., and Ruschoff, J. (1997) Diagnostic microsatellite instability: definition and correlation with mismatch repair protein expression. *Cancer Res.* **57,** 4749–4756.

21. Boland, C. R., Thibodeau, S. N., Hamilton, S. R., Sidransky, D., Eshelman, J. R., Burt, R. W., et al. (1998) A National Cancer Institute workshop on microsatellite instability for cancer detection and familial predisposition: development of international criteria for the determination of microsatellite instability in colorectal cancer. *Cancer Res.* **58,** 5248–5257.

22. Löthe, R. A., Peltomäki, P., Meling, G. I., Aaltonen, L. A., Nyström-Lahti, M., Pylkkänen, L., et al. (1993) Genomic instability in colorectal cancer: relationship to clinicopathological variables and family history. *Cancer Res.* **53,** 5849–5852.

23. Bubb, V. J., Curtis, L. J., Cunningham, C., Dunlop, M. G., Carothers, A. D., Morris, R. G., et al. (1996) Microsatellite instability and the role of hMSH2 in sporadic colorectal cancer. *Oncogene* **12,** 2641–2649.

24. Cawkwell, L., Li, D., Lewis, F. A., Martin, I., Dixon, M. F., and Quirke, P. (1995) Microsatellite instability in colorectal cancer: improved assessment using fluorescent polymerase chain reaction. *Gastroenterology* **109,** 465–471.

25. Lukish, J. R., Muro, K., DeNobile, J., Katz, R., Williams, J., Cruess, D. F., et al. (1998) Prognostic significance of DNA replication errors in young patients with colorectal cancer. *Ann. Surg.* **227,** 51–56.

26. Aebi, S., Kurdi-Haidar, B., Gordon, R., Cenni, B., Zheng, H., Fink, D., Christen, R. D., et al. (1996) Loss of DNA mismatch repair in acquired resistance to cisplatin. *Cancer Res.* **56,** 3087–3090.

27. Fink, D., Nebel, S., Aebi, S., Zheng, H., Cenni, B., Nehmé, A., et al. (1996) The role of DNA mismatch repair in platinum drug resistance. *Cancer Res.* **56,** 4881–4886.

28. Fink, D., Zheng, H., Nebel, S., Norris, P. S., Aebi, S., Lin, T.-P., et al. (1997) *In vitro* and *in vivo* resistance to cisplatin in cells that have lost DNA mismatch repair. *Cancer Res.* **57,** 1841–1845.

29. Zhou, X. P., Hoang, J. M., Li, Y. J., Seruca, r., Carneiro, F., Sobrinho-Simoes, M., et al. (1998) Determination of the replication error phenotype in human tumors without the requirement for matching normal DNA by analysis of mononucleotide repeat microsatellites. *Genes Chrom. Cancer* **21,** 101–177.

30. Brownstein, M. J., Carpten, J. D., and Smith, J. R. (1996) Modulation of nontemplated nucleotide addition by Taq DNA polymerase: primer modifications that facilitate genotyping. *Biotechniques* **20,** 1004–1006.

9

Immunohistochemical Analysis for *hMLH1* and *hMSH2* Expression in Colorectal Cancer

Kevin C. Halling and Patrick C. Roche

1. Introduction

Defective DNA mismatch repair (MMR) occurs in the majority of tumors from patients with hereditary non-polyposis colorectal cancer (HNPCC) and approx 15% of sporadic colorectal cancer (CRC) *(1,2)*. In HNPCC-associated tumors, defective MMR is most often due to inactivating mutations of the DNA MMR genes *hMLH1* and *hMSH2 (3,4)*. Defective MMR in sporadic CRC, on the other hand, is generally due to hypermethylation of the *hMLH1* promoter *(5–7)*. As might be expected, inactivating mutations of *hMSH2* and *hMLH1* lead to a loss of *hMSH2* or *hMLH1* expression respectively and hypermethylation of the *hMLH1* promoter to a loss of *hMLH1* expression *(5–8)*. One of the hallmarks of defective DNA MMR is a type of genetic instability known as microsatellite instability (MSI). Tumors with defective DNA MMR generally exhibit MSI at the majority of the loci examined (MSI-H phenotype) *(8,9)*.

Immunohistochemical analysis for *hMLH1* and *hMSH2* is useful for: 1) assessing colorectal tumors for defective MMR; 2) screening CRC patients for HNPCC; and 3) identifying the defective MMR gene in tumors with a MSI-H phenotype. The last mentioned utility is helpful since it identifies the gene that needs to be sequenced to find the causative mutation (or promoter hypermethylation). Immunohistochemical analysis for *hMLH1* and *hMSH2* may eventually also be used to guide CRC patient treatment since: 1) tumors with defective MMR appear to have a better prognosis than tumors that do not, and 2) tumors with defective MMR appear to be resistant to chemotherapeutic agents such as cisplatin and *N*-Methyl-*N'*-nitro-*N*-nitrosoguanidine *(2,10–16)*.

In this chapter we describe the methods that we use to perform immunohistochemical analysis for *hMLH1* and *hMSH2* expression.

From: *Methods in Molecular Medicine, vol. 50: Colorectal Cancer: Methods and Protocols*
Edited by: S. M. Powell © Humana Press Inc., Totowa, NJ

2. Materials

1. Probe On Plus™ charged and precleaned glass slides (Fisher Scientific, Pittsburgh, PA).
2. Oven for drying slides at 60°C (VWR Scientific Products, West Chester, PA).
3. Xylene (Sigma, St. Louis, MO).
4. Absolute ethanol, 95% ethanol.
5. 3% Hydrogen peroxide (Humco, Texarkana, TX).
6. HPLC grade methanol (EM Science, Gibbstown, NJ).
7. Hydrogen peroxide/methanol solution (50/50): Equal parts of 3% hydrogen peroxide and HPLC grade methanol. Prepare fresh daily.
8. Vegetable steamer (Black & Decker Handy Steamer Plus, Shelton, CT).
9. Tissue-Tek 24 count slide rack and reagent tank (Allegiance, McGaw Park, IL).
10. EDTA, disodium salt (Sigma, St. Louis, MO).
11. 1 mM EDTA, pH 8.0.
12. Normal goat serum (Jackson ImmunoResearch Laboratories Inc., West Grove, PA).
13. Tween-20 (Sigma).
14. NaCl (Sigma).
15. NaH_2PO_4 (Sigma).
16. K_2HPO_4, (Sigma).
17. PBS/Tween-20 solution: 9.5 mL 1 M NaH_2PO_4, 40.5 mL 1 M K_2HPO_4, 9.0 g NaCl, 5.0 mL Tween-20, 945.0 mL H_2O.
18. 5% and 1% normal goat serum in PBS/Tween-20: 5 or 1 mL of normal goat serum added to 95 or 99 mL PBS/Tween-20 solution.
19. *hMLH1* antibody, clone G168-728 (PharMingen, San Diego, CA): 2 µg/mL in 1% normal goat serum/PBS/Tween-20.
20. *hMSH2* antibody, clone FE11 (Oncogene Sciences, Cambridge, MA): 0.5 µg/mL in 1% normal goat serum/PBS/Tween-20.
21. Nonimmune mouse IgG (2 µg/mL for MLH1; 1 µg/mL for MSH2) (Jackson ImmunoResearch Laboratories Inc., West Grove, PA).
22. Humidified chamber (Tupperware container with damp paper towel at bottom).
23. Biotinylated goat antimouse IgG (Vector, Burlingame, CA). Dilute 1:100 in 1% goat serum/PBS/Tween-20.
24. Elite avidin-biotin complex (Vector).
25. Diaminobenzidine (DAB) substrate solution: One 10 mg tablet of DAB (Sigma), 50 mM Tris-Imidazole buffer, pH 7.65 (Gibco-BRL, Gaithersburg, MD), 0.15 mL 3% hydrogen peroxide. Prepare fresh for each batch of slides!
26. 0.1% Mayer's hematoxylin (Stephen's Scientific, Riverdale, NJ).
27. Mounting media, Cytoseal XYL (Stephens).
28. Light microscope with 10×, 40×, and 63× objectives.

3. Methods

3.1. Slide Preparation

1. Cut sections at 6 microns and mount on Probe On charged slides.
2. Dry paraffin slides in 60°C oven for minimum of 60 min.

3. Deparaffinize in 2 changes of xylene—5 min each.
4. Rehydrate with 10 dips in absolute ethanol, 10 dips in 95% ethanol, and then 1–2 min rinse in tap water.
5. Block endogenous peroxidase activity in 3% hydrogen peroxide/methanol solution for 10 min at room temperature.
6. Rinse in running tap water for 2 min.

3.2. Antigen Retrieval

The following is called the "Steam EDTA Protocol." It is a heat-induced epitope retrieval method.

1. Ten to 15 min prior to the completion of the blocking of the endogenous peroxidase activity, fill the lower chamber of a Black & Decker™ Handy Steamer Plus with 1000 mL of distilled water.
2. Place a reagent reservoir containing 200 mL of 1 mM EDTA, pH 8.0 in the upper chamber of the steamer.
3. Turn the timer on the steamer to the maximum time setting.
4. After the distilled water in the lower chamber of the Black & Decker Handy Steamer has reached a full boil (~10–12 min) place the slides into the 1 mM EDTA in the upper chamber of the steamer.
5. Steam slides for 30 min.
6. Open steamer and allow to stand for 5 min with the steamer turned off.
7. Rinse slides in running cool tap water for 1 min.

3.3. Immunostaining (see Note 1)

1. Block nonspecific protein binding sites by incubating in 5% normal goat serum/PBS/Tween-20 for 10 min at room temperature.
2. Blot off goat serum. Do not rinse!
3. Add 50–500 µL (depending on size of tissue section) of *hMLH1* antibody or *hMSH2* antibody to the test slides.
4. Add 50–500 µL (depending on size of tissue section) of nonimmune mouse IgG 2 µg/mL to the negative control slide(s).
5. Be sure that the sections are completely covered with antibody solution.
6. Incubate for 1 h at room temperature in a humidified chamber.
7. Drain off antibody and rinse twice in tap water—2 min each, then once in PBS/Tween-20 for 2 min.
8. Add biotinylated goat antimouse IgG diluted 1:100 in 1% goat serum/PBS/Tween-20.
9. Incubate for 30 min at room temperature.
10. Drain off antibody and rinse twice in tap water (2 min each), then once in PBS/Tween-20 for 2 min.
11. Add avidin-biotin complex and incubate for 30 min at room temperature.
12. Drain and rinse twice in tap water (2 min each).
13. Place slides in DAB substrate solution and incubate for 5 min at room temperature.

14. Rinse in tap water (2 min).
15. Counterstain in light hematoxylin for 10 s.
16. Rinse in running tap water for 3 min.
17. Dehydrate through graded alcohols to xylene.
18. Apply mounting media and coverslip.

3.4. Slide Interpretation (see Notes 2–5)

1. Assess slides for *hMLH1* and/or *hMSH2* immunostaining with a light microscope equipped with 10 or 20×, 40×, and 63× objectives.
2. A case is considered positive for *hMLH1* or *hMSH2* expression if the nuclei of the tumor cells exhibit a homogenous or finely punctate brown nuclear stain (**Fig. 1A** and **C**). Cytoplasmic staining is generally artifactual and should not be regarded as evidence of *hMLH1* or *hMSH2* expression.
3. A case is considered to show an absence of *hMLH1* or *hMSH2* expression if the nuclei of the normal colonic epithelial cells or lymphocytes (i.e., the internal controls) show evidence of *hMLH1* or *hMSH2* expression but the nuclei of the tumor cells do not (**Fig. 1B** and **D**).

4. Notes

1. Nonspecific background staining can result if the slides are allow to dry between steps or there is inadequate rinsing between steps.
2. Interpretation. Our practice has been to score a case as positive for *hMLH1* or *hMSH2* expression if any focus of the tumor exhibits positive staining. Negative staining in other areas of the tumor is usually an artifact that results either from incomplete tissue fixation or possibly due to inadequate contact of one of the antibodies with that focus of the tissue. Rare cases may show true intratumoral heterogeneity for *hMLH1* or *hMSH2* expression. If this appears to be the case, carefully assess the see that the tumor infiltrating lymphocytes stain positively in the focus of tumor that appears to be staining negatively.
3. Internal controls. The best internal controls for evidence of positive staining are normal colonic epithelium and lymphocytes. Endothelial cells will also stain positively but are not as good as internal controls since they sometimes stain nonspecifically (cytoplasmic) positive. If the internal controls do not stain positively repeat the staining procedure on a new section. Occasional cases will not stain despite repeated attempts. This is most frequently the result of inadequate tissue fixation prior to paraffin-embedding.
4. Staining artifacts. Occasional cases exhibit punctate nuclear staining with <10 large "granules" of staining in an otherwise negatively staining nucleus. These cases are generally showing a true absence of *hMLH1* or *hMSH2* expression. However, if doubt remains as to the interpretation of the stain, repeat the immunostain and/or perform microsatellite analysis to determine the MSI phenotype of the tumor.
5. Quality control. If there is any doubt as to whether a tumor is showing a true loss of *hMLH1* or *hMSH2* expression, assess the tumor for evidence of a "high level"

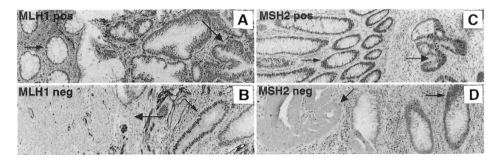

Fig. 1. Examples of colorectal carcinomas exhibiting positive or negative immuno-histochemical staining for *hMLH1* (**A** and **B**) or *hMSH2* (**C** and **D**). Small arrows point to positively staining normal colonic epithelium (positive internal control). Large arrows point to positively (A and C) or negatively (B and D) staining tumor cells.

MSI (MSI-H) phenotype (i.e., MSI at >30% of the loci examined). Tumors with a loss of *hMLH1* or *hMSH2* staining should exhibit an MSI-H phenotype. The fastest way to assess tumors for evidence of an MSI-H phenotype is with the microsatellite marker BAT-26. MSI at this marker is strongly correlated with an MSI-H phenotype and defective DNA MMR *(17)*.

Acknowledgments

The authors would like to thank Dr. Larry Burgart and Linda Murphy, M.T. (ASCP) for help in the preparation of this manuscript.

References

1. Aaltonen, L. A., Peltomaki, P., Leach, F. S., Sistonen, P., Pylkkanen, L., Mecklin, J. P., et al. (1993) Clues to the pathogenesis of familial colorectal cancer. *Science* **260,** 812–816.
2. Thibodeau, S. N., Bren, G., and Schaid, D. (1993) Microsatellite instability in cancer of the proximal colon. *Science* **260,** 816–819.
3. Liu, B., Parsons, R., Papadopoulos, N., Nicolaides, N. C., Lynch, H. T., Watson, P., et al. (1996) Analysis of mismatch repair genes in hereditary non-polyposis colorectal cancer patients. *Nature Med.* **2,** 169–174.
4. Moslein, G., Tester, D. J., Lindor, N. M., Honchel, R., Cunningham, J. M., French, A. J., et al. (1996) Microsatellite instability and mutation analysis of hMSH2 and hMLH1 in patients with sporadic, familial and hereditary colorectal cancer. *Hum. Molec. Genet.* **5,** 1245–1252.
5. Kane, M. F., Loda, M., Gaida, G. M., Lipman, J., Mishra, R., Goldman, H., et al. (1997) Methylation of the hMLH1 promoter correlates with lack of expression of hMLH1 in sporadic colon tumors and mismatch repair-defective human tumor cell lines. *Cancer Res.* **57,** 808–811.

6. Herman, J. G., Umar, A., Polyak, K., Graff, J. R., Ahuja, N., Issa, J. P., et al. (1998) Incidence and functional consequences of hMLH1 promoter hypermethylation in colorectal carcinoma. *Proc. Natl. Acad. Sci.USA* 6870–6875.

7. Cunningham, J. M., Christensen, E. R., Tester, D. J., Kim, C.-Y., Roche, P. C., Burgart, L. J., and Thibodeau, S. N. (1998) Hypermethylation of the hMLH1 promoter in colon cancer with microsatellite instability. *Cancer Res.* **58,** 3455–3460.

8. Thibodeau, S. N., French, A. J., Roche, P. C., Cunningham, J. M., Tester, D. J., Lindor, N. M., et al. (1996) Altered expression of hMSH2 and hMLH1 in tumors with microsatellite instability and genetic alterations in mismatch repair genes. *Cancer Res.* **56,** 4836–4840.

9. Thibodeau, S. N., French, A. J., Cunningham, J. M., Tester, D., Burgart, L. J., Roche, P. C., et al. (1998) Microsatellite instability in colorectal cancer: different mutator phenotypes and the principlal involvment of hMLH1. *Cancer Res.* **58,** 1713–1718.

10. Löthe, R. A., Peltomäki, P., Meling, G. I., Aaltonen, L. A., Nyström-Lahti, M., Pylkkänen, L., et al. (1993) Genomic instability in colorectal cancer: relationship to clinicopathological variables and family history. *Cancer Res.* **53,** 5849–5852.

11. Bubb, V. J., Curtis, L. J., Cunningham, C., Dunlop, M. G., Carothers, A. D., Morris, R. G., et al. (1996) Microsatellite instability and the role of hMSH2 in sporadic colorectal cancer. *Oncogene* **12,** 2641–2649.

12. Cawkwell, L., Li, D., Lewis, F. A., Martin, I., Dixon, M. F., and Quirke, P. (1995) Microsatellite instability in colorectal cancer: improved assessment using fluorescent polymerase chain reaction. *Gastroenterology* **109,** 465–471.

13. Lukish, J. R., Muro, K., DeNobile, J., Katz, R., Williams, J., Cruess, D. F., et al. (1998) Prognostic significance of DNA replication errors in young patients with colorectal cancer. *Ann. Surg.* **227,** 51–56.

14. Aebi, S., Kurdi-Haidar, B., Gordon, R., Cenni, B., Zheng, H., Fink, D., et al. (1996) Loss of DNA mismatch repair in acquired resistance to cisplatin. *Cancer Res.* **56,** 3087–3090.

15. Fink, D., Nebel, S., Aebi, S., Zheng, H., Cenni, B., Nehmé, A., et al. (1996) The role of DNA mismatch repair in platinum drug resistance. *Cancer Res.* **56,** 4881–4886.

16. Fink, D., Zheng, H., Nebel, S., Norris, P. S., Aebi, S., Lin, T.-P., et al. (1997) *In vitro* and *in vivo* resistance to cisplatin in cells that have lost DNA mismatch repair. *Cancer Res.* **57,** 1841–1845.

17. Hoang, J. M., Cottu, P. H., Thuille, B., Salmon, R. J., Thomas, G., and Hamelin, R. (1997) BAT–26, an indicator of the replication error phenotype in colorectal cancers and cell lines. *Cancer Res.* **57,** 300–303.

10

Mutation Detection in Colorectal Cancers

Direct Sequencing of DNA Mismatch Repair Genes

Julie M. Cunningham, David J. Tester, and Stephen N. Thibodeau

1. Introduction

The detection of unknown mutations has proved complex and time consuming, and this is certainly the case for HNPCC. Germline mutations have been detected in five of the six human DNA mismatch repair genes (in *hMLH1*, *hMSH2*, *hMSH6*, *hPMS1*, *hPMS2*, but not *hMSH3)* in HNPCC patients *(1–7)* with *hMLH1* and *hMSH2* being the most frequently affected *(8–11)*. Point mutations resulting in missense, nonsense and frameshift alterations are found in HNPCC, as well as mutations leading to splicing alterations *(9)*. The detection of mutations in these genes has relied upon direct sequencing of genomic DNA. Scanning or prescreening methods have been investigated *(12–15)*, but at this stage direct sequencing is the gold standard by which these methods are generally judged. One caveat however, is that this method does not detect deletions that span exons or entire genes, the frequency of which may be up to 6.5% of HNPCC cases *(16)*. To be rigorous, it would be prudent to include direct sequencing along with Southern analysis. This chapter will focus on the direct sequencing of *hMLH1* and *hMSH2*, although the overall strategy may also be used for the analysis of the other mismatch repair genes.

2. Materials
2.1. DNA Isolation

1. Puregene DNA isolation kit from Gentra (Minneapolis, MN), using the normal white blood cell count of 3.5 to 10.5×10^6 cells/mL whole blood.
2. 0.5% Toluidine blue in 100% ethanol.

From: *Methods in Molecular Medicine, vol. 50: Colorectal Cancer: Methods and Protocols*
Edited by: S. M. Powell © Humana Press Inc., Totowa, NJ

3. Lysis buffer: 250 µL 2X lysis buffer (ABI, Foster City, CA), 230 µL CDTA buffer (10 mM CDTA, 100 mM NaCl, 50 mM Tris-HCl, pH 7.5) and 20 µL protease K 20 mg/mL (ABI).
4. Phenol-chloroform solution: 25:24:1 (v/v/v) phenol/chloroform/isoamyl alcohol.
5. 3 M Sodium acetate, pH 5.2.
6. TE: 10 mM Tris, 1 mM EDTA, pH 8.0.
7. 70%, 100% Ethanol.
8. Isopropanol.

2.2. Preparation of Sequencing Template

1. 10X PCR buffer with magnesium (Perkin Elmer, Foster City, CA): 100 mM Tris-HCl (pH 8.3), 15 mM MgCl$_2$, 500 mM KCl.
2. 10 mM stocks dATP, dCTP, dGTP, and dTTP (Perkin Elmer, Foster City, CA). Prepare a 5X buffer by adding 100 µL of each dNTP to 500 mL 10X PCR buffer and 100 µL sterile H$_2$O.
3. 25 mM MgCl$_2$ (Perkin Elmer).
4. Oligonucleotide primers (20 pmol/µL) (*see* **Table 1**).
5. Sterile water.
6. Ampli*Taq* gold DNA polymerase, 5 U/µL (Perkin Elmer).
7. Exonuclease I (10 U/mL) and shrimp alkaline phosphatase (2 U/mL).
8. NuSieve agarose (F.M.C., Rockland, ME) and agarose (Boehringer Mannhein, Indianapolis, IN).
9. 50X TAE buffer: 2.0 M Tris-acetate, 50 mM EDTA (National Diagnostics, Atlanta, GA).
10. Ethidium bromide, 10 mg/mL.
11. 6X Loading buffer: 0.125 g bromophenol blue and 7.5 g Ficoll type 400 to 50 mL with sterile purified H$_2$O. This will remain stable at room temperature for 1 yr.

2.3. Sequencing Reaction

1. Thermosequenase kit (Amersham-Pharmacia, Piscataway, NJ)
2. Loading buffer: 95% formamide, 20 mM EDTA, 0.05% bromophenol blue, 0.05% xylene cyanol FF.

2.4. Gel Electrophoresis

1. Gel solution: Add 48 mL purified H$_2$O to each of 2×30 g bottles of Acrylamide/ *Bis* powder (19:1, Bio-Rad, Hercules, CA) and stir for 1 h to dissolve. Add 100 mL of 10X TBE buffer (*see* **step 2**) and 420 g of urea. Stir to dissolve, adjust volume to 1 L, filter and store protected from light at 4°C. Degas before use. The solution will remain stable for 6 mo if properly stored (*see* **Notes 1** and **2**).
2. 1X TBE buffer: 0.089 M Tris-borate, 2 mM EDTA, pH 8.3, made from 10X buffer stock (National Diagnostics).
3. Ammonium persulfate (10 mg/mL), TEMED (Bio-Rad, Richmond, CA).
4. Autoradiography film (Biomax, Kodak-Eastman, Rochester, NY), exposure cassettes.

2.5. Equipment

1. Thermocycler.
2. Microcentrifuge.
3. Sequencing gel apparatus.
4. Agarose gel apparatus.
5. Gel dryer.
6. Film developer and processor.

3. Methods

3.1. Isolation of Genomic DNA from Peripheral Blood Leukocytes

DNA isolation is performed using the Puregene kit.

1. Add 300 µL whole blood to a tube containing 900 µL of red blood cell lysis solution. Invert to mix, wait 5 min, then invert again and wait another 5 min.
2. Centrifuge at maximum speed in a microfuge; remove the supernatant leaving the visible white cell pellet and 10–20 µL of residual liquid. Cap the tube and vigorously vortex to resuspend the cells.
3. Add 300 µL cell lysis solution to the tube and pipet up and down to lyse the cells. Incubate at least 15 min at room temperature; samples are stable in cell lysis solution for at least 18 mo at room temperature.
4. Add 100 µL protein precipitation solution to the cell lysate. Vortex vigorously to mix uniformly.
5. Centrifuge at maximum speed for 3 min in microfuge. Transfer the supernatant (contains the DNA) into a clean flat-bottomed tube containing 300 µL isopropanol. Mix the tube by inverting until white threads of DNA form a visible clump.
6. Centrifuge at room temperature at maximum speed for 5 min, the DNA will be visible as a small white pellet. Pour off as much isopropanol as possible, then add 500 µL 70% ethanol. Invert the tube several times to wash the DNA pellet.
7. Centrifuge at maximum speed for 3 min. Carefully pour off the ethanol, be careful not to lose the pellet.
8. Drain the tube on absorbent paper, and allow to air dry for 15 min. Add sufficient volume of TE, usually 50 µL is sufficient. Allow to sit overnight to dissolve DNA. Adjust to 0.25 mg/mL.

3.2. Isolation of Tumor DNA from Frozen Sections

1. Slides with 10 µm thick frozen sections are immediately fixed in cold 100% ethanol for 15–30 s.
2. The section is then stained in 0.5% Toluidine blue for 8–10 s. Wash the slide twice in 100% ethanol, about 3 s per wash. Air dry slide at room temperature.
3. Using an H&E stained reference slide, mark areas to be microdissected. Microdissect tissue using a scalpel and place in tube containing 500 µL lysis buffer.
4. Digest overnight at 55°C in a shaking incubator. Store at 4°C until extraction.
5. Add an equal volume of phenol:chloroform solution to the digest in a 1.5 mL microtube. Vortex for 10 s, spin at high speed for 15 s.

Table 1
Primer Sequences and PCR Conditions for Preparation of *hMLH1* and *hMSH2* Sequencing Templates

Gene/exon	Oligo	Oligo sequence	[MgCl$_2$] mM	*Taq*Gold (U)	Primer (pmole)	PCR product size (bp)
				PCR amplification conditions[a]		
A. *hMLH1*						
1	sense	AGGCACTGAGGTGATTGGC	2.0	1.25	20	226
	αsense	TCGTAGCCCTTAAGTGAGC				
2	sense	AATATGTACATTAGAGTAGTTG	2.0	1.25	20	214
	αsense	CAGAGAAAGGTCCTGACTC				
3	sense	AGAGATTTGGAAAATGAGTAAC	2.0	1.25	20	207
	αsense	ACAATGTCATCACAGGAGG				
4	sense	AACCTTTCCCTTTGGTGAGG	2.0	1.25	20	236
	αsense	GATTACTCTGAGACCTAGGC				
5	sense	GATTTTCTCTTTTCCCCTGGG	2.0	1.25	20	190
	αsense	CAAACAAAGCTTCAACAATTTAC				
6	sense	GGGTTTTATTTTCAAGTACTTCTATG	3.5	1.25	20	236
	αsense	GTCCAGCAACTGTTCAATGTATGAGC				
7	sense	CTAGTGTGTGTTTTGGC	2.0	1.25	20	185
	αsense	CATAACCTTATCTCCACC				
8	sense	CTCAGCCATGAGACAATAAATCC	3.5	1.25	20	217
	αsense	GGTTCCCAAATAATGTGATGG				
9	sense	CAAAAGCTTCAGAATCTC	2.0	1.25	20	193
	αsense	CTGTGGGTGTTTCCTGTGAGTGG				
10	sense	CATGACTTTGTGTGAATGTACACC	3.0	0.625	20	238
	αsense	GAGGAGAGCCTGATAGAACATCTG				
11	sense	GGGCTTTTCTCCCCTCCC	2.0	1.25	20	288
	αsense	AAAATCTGGGCTCTCACG				

12	sense	AATTATACCTCATACTAGC	3.5	0.3	20	557
	αsense	GTTTTATTACAGAATAAAGGGAGG				
13	sense	TGCAACCCACAAAATTTGGC	2.0	1.25	20	292
	αsense	CTTTCTCCATTTCCAAAACC				
14	sense	TGGTGTCTCTAGTTCTGG	2.0	1.25	20	254
	αsense	CATTGTTGTGTAGTAGCTCTGC				
15	sense	CCCATTTGTCCCAACTGG	3.0	0.625	20	181
	αsense	CGGTCAGTTGAAATGTCAG				
16	sense	CATTTGGATGCTCCGTTAAAGC	2.0	1.25	20	275
	αsense	CACCCGGCTGGAAATTTTATTTG				
17	sense	GGAAAGGCACTGGAGAAATGGG	2.0	1.25	20	227
	αsense	CCCTCCAGCACACATGCATGTACCG				
18	sense	TAAGTAGTCTGTGATCTCCG	2.0	1.25	20	246
	αsense	ATGTATGAGGTCCTGTCC				
19	sense	GACACCAGTGTATGTTGG	2.0	1.25	20	270
	αsense	GAGAAAGAAGAACACATCCC				

B. *hMSH2*

1	sense	GGCGGGAAACAGCTTAGT	2.0	1.25	20	338
	αsense	AAGGAGCCGCGCCACAA				
2	sense	CAGTCTCGGGTATGTCTTTA	2.0	0.3	20	364
	αsense	CCCATTCTACTATCACAATCT				
3	sense	TTTAAAGTATGTTCAAGAGTTTG	2.0	1.25	20	380
	αsense	TTTCCTAGGCCTGGAATCT				
4	sense	ATTCCTTTTCTCATAGTAGTTT	2.0	1.25	20	308
	αsense	TTGAGATAAATATGACAGAAATAT				
5[b]	sense	CCAGTGGTATAGAAATCTTCG	2.0	1.25	20	240
	αsense	CCAATCAACATTTTAACCC				
6	sense	GAGCTTGCCATTCTTTCTAT	3.0	1.25	20	242
	αsense	GGTATAATCATGTGGGTAAC				

(continued)

Table 1 (continued)

Gene/ exon	Oligo	Oligo sequence	PCR amplification conditions[a]			
			[MgCl$_2$] mM	TaqGold (U)	Primer (pmole)	PCR product size (bp)
7	sense	CTAAAATATTTTACATTAATTCAAG	2.5	0.625	20	345
	αsense	ATGTGTCCTAAGAGTGAGTC				
8[b]	sense	GATTTGTATTCTGTAAAATGAGATC	3.5	1.25	20	222
	αsense	GGCCTTTGCTTTTAAAAATAAC				
9[b]	sense	GTCTTTACCCATTATTTATAGG	2.0	1.25	20	217
	αsense	GTATAGACAAAAGAATTATTCC				
10	sense	GTGAGTATGTTGTCATATAATAA	1.5	1.25	20	322
	αsense	GCATTTAGGGAATTAATAAAGG				
11	sense	CATTATTTGGATGTTTCATAGG	2.0	1.25	20	271
	αsense	CATGATTTTCTTCTGTTACCA				
12	sense	TTATTCAGTATTCCTGTGTACA	2.0	1.25	20	324
	αsense	CAAAACGTTACCCCCACAA				
13	sense	CTTGCTTCTGATATAATTTGTT	2.0	1.25	20	327
	αsense	CATGAGAATCTGCAAATATACT				
14	sense	GGCATACCTTCCCAATGTAT	2.0	1.25	20	399
	αsense	AGTAAGTTTCCCATTACCAAG				
15	sense	TCTTCTCATGCTGTCCCT	2.0	0.3	20	263
	αsense	ATAATAGAGAAGCTAAGTTAAAC				
16	sense	ATTTTAATTACTAATGGGACATT	2.0	1.25	20	317
	αsense	CATGGGCACTGACAGTTAA				

[a]Routine PCR volume of 25 μL.
[b]Sequences for these primers were kindly provided by Dr. Kolodner (17).

92

6. The phases (organic and aqueous) should be well separated. If not, spin again for 1–2 min. Carefully remove the aqueous phase containing the DNA and place in a new tube. If a white precipitate is present, re-extract the sample.
7. Add 1/10 vol 3 *M* sodium acetate pH 5.2, vortex to mix. Add 2–2.5 vol of ice-cold 100% ethanol. Vortex to mix and place on crushed dry ice for ≥5 min to precipitate the DNA (or place at –70°C for ≥15 min or at –20°C for ≥30 min).
8. Spin for 5 min in a fixed-angle centrifuge, and remove the supernatant.
9. Add 1 mL 70% ethanol, invert tube several times and spin again.
10. Dry the pellet, then dissolve in an appropriate volume of H_2O (if using right away) or TE (if storing).

3.3. Preparation of Sequencing Template

1. PCR amplify 50 ng DNA for each exon of *hMLH1* and *hMSH2* (*see* **Table 1** for primer sequences and magnesium, primer and Ampli*Taq* Gold concentrations). Keep on ice until placed in thermocycler. All templates are preheated at 95°C for 12 min, then PCR amplified for 35 cycles of (95°C, 30 s; 55°C, 30 s, 72°C for 1 min), with a final extension at 72°C for 10 min.
2. To verify the presence of a PCR product, run 10 µL of the PCR product out on a 3% agarose gel. To 100 mL 1X TAE (made from 20X stock) add 2 g of NuSieve agarose and 1 g of agarose. Microwave at high temperature for 1 min, swirl and heat again for an additional min. After cooling to ~50°C, add 2.5 µL ethidium bromide, swirl to mix and then pour into an 11×14 mm² gel mold, place well combs and allow to set for at least 1 h. Add 2 µL 6X loading buffer to 10 µL PCR product, load into wells and run gel in 1X TAE. Visualize PCR products under UV illumination. Use samples with a positive result for sequencing.
3. To remove remaining oligonucleotides, place 5 µL PCR products in a set of microtubes and add 1 µL exonuclease I (10 U/mL) and 1 µL shrimp alkaline phosphatase (2 U/mL). Incubate at 37°C for 15 min, then heat to 80°C for a further 15 min. Place at 4°C until ready to sequence.

3.4. Sequencing Reaction

Sequencing is performed using the Thermosequenase kit; *see* **Fig. 1** for the overall strategy.

1. Prepare *termination mixes* on ice by adding 2 µL of termination mix (dGTP) and 0.5 µL of $(\alpha\text{-}^{32}P)$ddNTP, one each of G, A, T, and C, for each sample to be sequenced (i.e., 4 tubes per sequence). You should prepare sufficient quantities of each $(\alpha\text{-}^{32}P)$ddNTP for all the samples to be sequenced, then aliquot 2.5 mL to each tubes.
2. Prepare a *sequencing master mix* for each of the sequencing primers by placing 13 µL sterile H_2O, 2 µL reaction buffer, 1 µL sequencing primer (20 µ*M*) and finally 2 µL Thermosequenase DNA polymerase. Vortex gently, then spin briefly in a microfuge. Keep on ice.

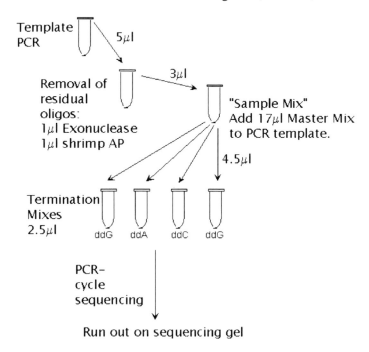

Fig. 1. Sequencing flow chart: from PCR to sequencing gel.

3. Prepare the sequencing reactions: for each exon to be sequenced label 4 PCR tubes with the sample number followed by "G," "A," "T," and "C." Include a set for the positive control.
4. Add 2.5 μL of the appropriate d/ddNTP *termination mix* to each tube, and keep in a PCR rack on ice.
5. Place 3 μL (or 2 μL) of the pretreated PCR template in a labeled microfuge tube for each patient and control. Add 17 μL (or 18 μL) of the *sequencing master mix* to each of the tubes to create a *sample mix*. Vortex gently to mix, then briefly spin.
6. Add 4.5 μL of each *sample mix* to each "G," "A," "T," and "C" labeled tube for each patient and control. Pipet up and down to mix. Keep in PCR rack on ice.
7. Place in thermal cycler and PCR amplify for 30 cycles of (95°C, 30 s; 58°C, 30 s; 72°C for 1 min).
8. Add 4 μL loading buffer to each tube and mix by pipeting up and down. Heat at 72°C and quickly cool in an ice/water slurry. Load within 1 h of heating the samples. Alternatively, store at –20°C until needed (heat before proceeding).
9. Run 3.5 μL of the reaction products out on denaturing 6% polacrylamide/7 *M* urea sequencing gels, using 1X TBE buffer (*see* **Table 2** for run times for individual exons; using 0.4 mm thick, 31 × 38.5 cm² gels). It may be helpful to load each of the individual "G"s, "A"s, "T"s, and "C"s together, to enable easy identification of sequence variations (*see* **Fig. 2** and **Notes 3** and **4**).

Table 2
Sequencing Primers and Subsequent Analysis for *hMLH1* and *hMSH2*

Gene/exon	Sequencing primer	Gel run times[a]
A. *hMLH1*		
1, αsense	TAGCCCTTAAGTGAGCCCGGCTC	1:30/2:45
2, αsense	CCTGACTCTTCCATGAAGCGCACA	1:40
3, sense	AGAGATTTGGAAAATGAGTAACATGATTA	1:40
4, sense	GAGGTGACAGTGGGTGACCCAGC	1:45
5, sense	CCCCTTGGGATTAGTATCTATCTCTC	1:45
6, sense	TTTCAAGTACTTCTATGAATTTACAAGAAA	1:35
7, αsense	AACCTTATCTCCACCAGCAAACTATTA	2:00
8, αsense	CCCAAATAATGTGATGGATGATAAACC	1:40
9, αsense	TTCCTGTGAGTGGATTTCCCATGTG	1:20
10, αsense	GAGAGCCTGATAGAACATCTGTTCC	1:40
11, sense	TTTCTCCCCCTCCCACTATCTAAGG	1:30/3:00
12, αsense	GAATAAAGGAGGTAGGCTGTACTTTTC	1:30/4:00
13, αsense	CTTGGCAGTTGAGGCCCTATGCAT	1:30/3:00
14, sense	GTGCCTGGTGCTTTGGTCAATGAAG	2:10
15, sense	TGTCCCAACTGGTTGTATCTCAAGC	1:40
16, αsense	CCCGGCTGGAAATTTTATTTGGAGAA	1:45/3:00
17, sense	GGCACTGGAGAAATGGGATTTGTTTA	2:00
18, sense	CTGTGATCTCCGTTTAGAATGAGAATG	1:55
19, sense	TTGGGATGCAAACAGGGAGGCTTAT	1:25/3:00
B. *hMSH2*		
1, αsense	CCTCCCCAGCACGCGCCGTCC	1:20/3:00
2, αsense[b]	CTTCACATTTTTATTTTTCTACTCTTAAAA	1:20
3, αsense	GCCTGGAATCTCCTCTATCACTAGA	1:20/3:00
4, αsense	GAAATATCCTTCTAAAAAGTCACTATAGT	2:00
5, sense[b]	CCAGTGGTATAGAAATCTTCGATT	1:30
6, αsense	CATGTGGGTAACTGCAGGTTACATAA	1:30
7, αsense	TTATGAGGACAGCACATTGCCAAGTA	1:40/3:00
8, αsense[b]	GGCCTTTGCTTTTTAAAAATAACTACTGC	2:00
9, αsense[b]	ATAGACAAAAGAATTATTCCAACCTCCA	1:20
10, sense	GTAGTAGGTATTTATGGAATACTTTTTCT	1:30
11, αsense	CCAAAAGCCAGGTGACATTCAGAAC	1:30
12, αsense	CCCCCACAAAGCCCAAAAACCAGGT	1:20/3:00
13, αsense	CAAATATACTTTTCCTTCTCACAGGAC	1:40/3:00
14, sense	GTATGTTACCACATTTTATGTGATGGG	1:30/3:00
15, sense[b]	CTTCTCATGCTGTCCCCTCACGCT	1:20/3:00
16, sense	TACTAATGGGACATTCACATGTGTTTC	1:20/3:00

[a]Hours: minutes, at 70 W/gel.
[b]Sequences for these primers were kindly provided by Dr. Kolodner *(17)*.

hMLH1 exon 7

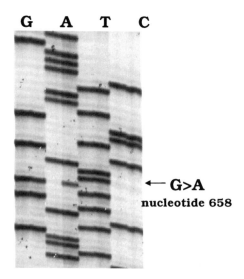

Fig. 2. An example of a sequencing gel. The results of two separate samples are shown, with the second sample demonstrating a G>A substitution (antisense) at codon 658 in exon 7 of *hMLH1*.

4. Notes

The sequencing conditions were designed to allow cycle sequencing at a single temperature for all the exons. There may be times that optimization is required and the following notes may be of help.

1. If when sequencing, you have spurious bands in the gel, it may be helpful to use 35 μM 7-deaza-GTP (Boehringer Mannhein, Indianapolis, IN) in place of dGTP in preparation of the template.
2. For GC-rich sequences, incorporating 30–40% formamide into the gel will help with problems of band compression. Run gels at 80 W/gel.
3. All alterations should be verified with a second PCR amplification and sequencing reaction. To be most stringent, sequencing of both strands is desirable. An alternate sequencing approach with M13-tagged primers used as universal sequencing primers for template production (M13 sense, 5'-TCC CAG TCA CGA CGT-3'; M13 antisense, 5'-AAC AGC TAT GAC CAT G-3), allows sequencing of both strands. This approach may also be particularly useful if there are problems with removal of original primers (i.e., leading to reverse priming in the sequencing reaction).
4. The International Collaborative Group on Hereditary Non-Polyposis Colorectal Cancer maintains a website containing a mutation database for polymor-

phisms and mutations in *hMLH1, hMSH2, hMSH6, hPMS1*, and *hPMS2*: http:/www.nfdht.nl.

References

1. Peltomaki, P. and de la Chapelle, A. (1997) Mutations predisposing to hereditary nonpolyposis colorectal cancer. *Adv. Cancer Res.* **71,** 93–119.
2. Moslein, G., Tester, D. J., Lindor, N. M., Honchel, R., Cunningham, J. M., French, A. J., et al. (1996) Microsatellite instability and mutation analysis of hMSH2 and hMLH1 in patients with sporadic, familial and hereditary colorectal cancer. *Hum. Mol. Genet.* **5,** 1245–1252.
3. Papadopoulos, N., Nicolaides, N. C. , Wei, Y. F., Ruben, S. M., Carter, K. C., Rosen, C. A., et al. (1994) Mutation of a mutL homolog in hereditary colon cancer (see comments). *Science* **263,** 1625–1629.
4. Nicolaides, N. C., Papadopoulos, N., Liu, B., Wei, Y. F., Carter, K. C., Ruben, S. M., et al. (1994) Mutations of two PMS homologues in hereditary nonpolyposis colon cancer. *Nature* **371,** 75–80.
5. Liu, B., Parsons, R., Papadopoulos, N., Nicolaides, N. C., Lynch, H. T., Watson, P., et al. (1996) Analysis of mismatch repair genes in hereditary non-polyposis colorectal cancer patients (see comments). *Nature Med.* **2,** 169–174.
6. Akiyama, Y., Sato, H., Yamada, T., Nagasaki, H., Tsuchiya, A., Abe, R., and Yuasa, Y. (1997) Germ-line mutation of the hMSH6/GTBP gene in an atypical hereditary nonpolyposis colorectal cancer kindred. *Cancer Research,* **57,** 3920–3923.
7. Shin, K. H., Ku, J. L., and Park, J. G. (1999) Germline mutations in a polycytosine repeat of the hMSH6 gene in Korean hereditary nonpolyposis colorectal cancer. *J. Hum. Genet.* **44,** 18–21.
8. Nystrom-Lahti, M., Wu, Y., Moisio, A. L., Hofstra, R. M., Osinga, J., Mecklin, J. P., et al. (1996) DNA mismatch repair gene mutations in 55 kindreds with verified or putative hereditary non-polyposis colorectal cancer. *Hum. Mol. Genet.* **5,** 763–769.
9. Peltomaki, P. and Vasen, H. F. (1997) Mutations predisposing to hereditary nonpolyposis colorectal cancer: database and results of a collaborative study. The International Collaborative Group on Hereditary Nonpolyposis Colorectal Cancer. *Gastroenterology* **113,** 1146–1158.
10. Buerstedde, J. M., Alday, P., Torhorst, J., Weber, W., Muller, H., and Scott, R. (1995) Detection of new mutations in six out of 10 Swiss HNPCC families by genomic sequencing of the hMSH2 and hMLH1 genes. *J. Med. Genet.* **32,** 909–912.
11. Tannergard, P., Lipford, J. R., Kolodner, R., Frodin, J. E., Nordenskjold, M., and Lindblom, A. (1995) Mutation screening in the hMLH1 gene in Swedish hereditary nonpolyposis colon cancer families. *Cancer Res.* **55,** 6092–6096.
12. Farrington, S. M., Lin-Goerke, J., Ling, J., Wang, Y., Burczak, J. D., Robbins, D. J., and Dunlop, M. G. (1998) Systematic analysis of hMSH2 and hMLH1 in young colon cancer patients and controls. *Am. J. Hum. Genet.,* **63,** 749–759.

13. Wu, Y., Nystrom-Lahti, M., Osinga, J., Looman, M. W., Peltomaki, P., Aaltonen, L. A., et al. (1997) MSH2 and MLH1 mutations in sporadic replication error-positive colorectal carcinoma as assessed by two-dimensional DNA electrophoresis. *Genes Chromosomes Cancer* **18,** 269–278.

14. Suspiro, A., Fidalgo, P., Cravo, M., Albuquerque, C., Ramalho, E., Leitao, C. N., and Costa, M. F. (1998) The Muir-Torre syndrome: a rare variant of hereditary nonpolyposis colorectal cancer associated with hMSH2 mutation. *Am. J. Gastroenterol.* **93,** 1572–1574.

15. Borresen, A. L., Lothe, R. A., Meling, G. I., Lystad, S., Morrison, P., Lipford, J., et al. (1995) Somatic mutations in the hMSH2 gene in microsatellite unstable colorectal carcinomas. *Hum. Mol. Genet.* **4,** 2065–2072.

16. Wijnen, J., Vanderklift, H., Vasen, H., Khan, P. M., Menko, F., Tops, C., et al. (1998) MSH2 genomic deletions are a frequent cause of HNPCC. *Nature Genet.* **20,** 326–328.

17. Kolodner, R. D., Hall, N. R., Lipford, J., Kane, M. F., Rao, M. R., Morrison, P., et al. (1994) Structure of the human MSH2 locus and analysis of two Muir-Torre kindreds for msh2 mutations. *Genomics* **24,** 516–526.

11

Mutation Detection in TGF-β Receptors

William M. Grady, Lois L. Myeroff, Hongmei He, and Sanford Markowitz

1. Introduction

1.1. BAT-RII Mutations

The transforming growth factor β (TGF-β) receptors are an important class of tumor suppressor gene. TGF-β markedly inhibits the growth of many epithelial cell types; whereas in contrast, cancers of many different tissue types are commonly TGF-β resistant (10). Many cancer cell lines are resistant to the growth suppressive effects of TGF-β and display evidence of disruption of TGF-β signal transduction (1,4,10). To date, this resistance appears to often result from mutations in the TGF-β receptors or the *smad* family of TGF-β signaling proteins (5,11,12,14,16). In particular, mutation of the type II receptor (RII) is a frequent event responsible for disrupting TGF-β signaling, and it is especially common in microsatellite unstable (MSI) colon cancers (11). The mutations found in MSI colon cancers are frameshift mutations that occur in a microsatellite-like 10 bp polyadenine tract, named BAT-RII, and are present in greater than 90% of MSI colon tumors (14). The name BAT refers to the polyadenine repeat—"Big A Tract;" all the mutations in BAT-RII detected to date are insertions or deletions of one or two adenines. Thus, they shift the reading frame resulting in the expression of a truncated protein that lacks its transmembrane and intracellular kinase domains. BAT-RII mutations also occur commonly in MSI gastric and occasionally in MSI endometrial tumors (12). The BAT-RII PCR assay described below will only detect mutations in this hotspot 10 bp adenine repeat in the RII coding region, bases 709–713 (Genbank accession number M85079). Insertion and/or deletion mutations are detected as a shift in size of the 73-bp band by 1 or 2 bp on a sequencing-type polyacrylamide gel. Of note, the TGF-β RII gene carries another microsatellite-

From: *Methods in Molecular Medicine, vol. 50: Colorectal Cancer: Methods and Protocols*
Edited by: S. M. Powell © Humana Press Inc., Totowa, NJ

like repeat consisting of $(GT)_3$ from basepairs 1931–1936, but this region is only rarely mutated *(14,18)*. Consequently, routine assessment of this region for mutations is not recommended. An optimized protocol for detection of BAT-RII mutations is presented below. This protocol is a modification of the originally published method *(12,14)*, and these changes are described in the methods section.

1.2. TGF-β RII Mutations

In addition to the frameshift mutations observed in MSI cancers, missense mutations in the type II receptor, primarily in the kinase domain, have been detected in MSI and microsatellite stable (MSS) colon carcinomas, head and neck cancers, ovarian cancers, and cutaneous T-cell lymphomas *(3,4,7–9,17)*. Direct sequencing of RT-PCR products is the most sensitive method to detect such mutations *(4)*, and the details of a sequencing protocol for RII is described below. Other laboratories use PCR/SSCP or chemical mismatch cleavage to screen for RII mutations, followed by sequencing of regions displaying abnormalities *(2,3)*; however, these methods are less sensitive for detecting RII mutations.

The RII cDNA is difficult to amplify full length with traditional two-step RT-PCR. Protocol development in our lab has demonstrated that the Titan one-step RT-PCR kit (Roche) is the easiest method to amplify full-length RII coding sequence. This easy-to-use kit utilizes a mixture of reverse transcriptase, Pwo polymerase and Taq polymerase for high fidelity and processivity. However, if the RII amount is low or if the Titan kit is unavailable, it may be preferable to amplify the coding region in two overlapping pieces with AMV reverse transcriptase and PCR (*see* **Subheading 2.2.2.**). The primers specified in the methods section are named according to their position number given in the deposited RII sequence (Genbank accession number M85079). The numbers correspond to the 5' base at which that primer starts, and "s" and "as" refer to "sense" and "antisense," respectively.

1.3. TGF-β RI Mutations

While mutations in the type I receptor (RI) appear to be rare *(2,15)*, the formal possibility of mutations in RI as the causative mechanism for TGF-β resistance can only be excluded by sequencing RI. Of interest, the TGF-β RI sequence does not carry a mutational hotspot like BAT -RII in TGF-β RII, so a strategy like the BAT-RII assay cannot be employed. A RT-PCR protocol and sequencing protocol for assaying RI are described in the methods section. Because of the very GC-rich 5'-end of the RI gene, it is a difficult cDNA to amplify. Many different methods have been assessed, and the protocol listed below is the most consistent. Amplification of the cDNA in 2 pieces, a 1600 bp "full length" piece for sequencing the coding region from about base 240 to the stop codon at base 1586, and a 582 bp 5' end piece to sequence the start site and GC-rich 5' end results in clean sequence. The primers are named according to the positions given in the deposited RI sequence (Genbank accession number L11695). The numbers correspond to the base at which that primer starts, and "s" and "as" refer to sense and antisense, respectively.

2. Materials

2.1. BAT-RII Assay for Mutation Detection in the TGF-β RII Hotspot

2.1.1. Primer Labeling

1. TA10-F1 primer (5'-CTTTATTCTGGAAGATGCTGC-3'); diluted to 300 ng/µL in H_2O.
2. Polynucleotide kinase (PNK) (10 U/µL) and 10X PNK buffer, supplied with enzyme (Roche).
3. γ-^{32}P-ATP (10 µCi/µL) or γ-^{33}P-ATP (10 µCi/µL) (*see* **Note 1**).
4. G-50 (Sephadex) in TE (*see* **Note 2**).
5. 1 mL syringe.
6. Glass wool.

2.1.2. PCR Amplification

1. DNase- and RNase-free H_2O for PCR.
2. 1.25 mM dNTPs for PCR (Perkin Elmer).
3. Pwo enzyme (5 U/µL) and 10X buffer, supplied with enzyme (Roche).
4. TA10-R1 primer. (5'-GAAGAAAGTCTCACCAGG-3'); diluted to 300 ng/µL in H_2O.

2.1.3. Gel Electrophoresis

1. LongRanger gel solution (FMC BioProducts).
2. Urea.
3. APS, 10% in H_2O.
4. TEMED (Sigma).
5. TBE 1X.

2.2. RII RT-PCR and Sequencing

2.2.1. Titan RT-PCR Method (One-Step Method)

1. Titan RT-PCR kit (Roche).
2. RNase- and DNase-free H_2O.
3. 1.25 mM dNTPs for PCR (Perkin-Elmer).
4. Primers RII-297s, RII-2077as (diluted to 300 ng/µL).
5. Qiaquick gel extraction kit (Qiagen).
6. Qiaquick PCR purification kit (Qiagen).
7. Amplification primers, diluted to 4 µM in water (*see* **Notes 7** and **8**):

RII-297s (5'-CGCTGGGGGCTCGGTCTATG-3')
RII-2077as (5'-GCAGCCTCTTTGGACATGC-3')
RII-1160as (5'-CCACTGTCTCAAACTGCTCT-3')
RII-1028s (5'-TGCCAACAACATCAACCACA-3')
RII-2073as (5'-CCTCTTTGGACATGCCCAGCC-3')

8. Sequencing primers, diluted to 4 µM in water (*see* **Note 8**):

RII-297s (5'-CGCTGGGGGCTCGGTCTAT-3')
RII-425s (5'-GTCGGTTAATAACGACATGATAG-3')
RII-719s (5'-GCCTGGTGAGACTTTCTT-3')
RII-926s (5'-GAGTTCAACCTGGGAAACC-3')
RII-1028s (5'-TGCCAACAACATCAACCACAA-3')
RII-1323s (5'-AAGGGCAACCTACAGGAGTACC-3')
RII-1562s (5'-TGTGGATGACCTGGCTAA-3')
RII-463as (5'-CCGTTGTTGTCAGTGACTATC-3')
RII-708as (5'-CTTTCATAATGCACTTTGGA-3')
RII-1160as (5'- CCACTGTCTCAAACTGCTCT-3')
RII-2073as (5'- CCTCTTTGGACATGCCCAGCC-3')

2.2.2. Alternative RT-PCR Two-Step Method (Alternate Method for Doing RT-PCR and Sequencing to be Used in Place of Titan RT-PCR One-Step Method)

1. Random hexamers, 2 mg/mL.
2. AMV Reverse Transcriptase and 5X buffer (Roche, 25 U/µL).
3. Taq polymerase and 10X buffer (Roche).
4. Primers RII-297s, RII-1160as, RII-1028s, RII-2073as (diluted to 300 ng/µL).
5. Qiaquick gel extraction kit (Qiagen).
6. Qiaquick PCR purification kit (Qiagen).
7. Amplification primers, diluted to 4 µM in water (*see* **Notes 7** and **8**):

RII-297s (5'-CGCTGGGGGCTCGGTCTATG-3')
RII-2077as (5'-GCAGCCTCTTTGGACATGC-3')
RII-1160as (5'-CCACTGTCTCAAACTGCTCT-3')
RII-1028s (5'-TGCCAACAACATCAACCACA-3')
RII-2073as (5'-CCTCTTTGGACATGCCCAGCC-3')

8. Sequencing primers, diluted to 4 µM in water (*see* **Note 8**):

RII-297s (5'-CGCTGGGGGCTCGGTCTAT-3')
RII-425s (5'-GTCGGTTAATAACGACATGATAG-3')
RII-719s (5'-GCCTGGTGAGACTTTCTT-3')
RII-926s (5'-GAGTTCAACCTGGGAAACC-3')
RII-1028s (5'-TGCCAACAACATCAACCACAA-3')
RII-1323s (5'-AAGGGCAACCTACAGGAGTACC-3')
RII-1562s (5'-TGTGGATGACCTGGCTAA-3')
RII-463as (5'-CCGTTGTTGTCAGTGACTATC-3')
RII-708as (5'-CTTTCATAATGCACTTTGGA-3')

RII-1160as (5'- CCACTGTCTCAAACTGCTCT-3')
RII-2073as (5'- CCTCTTTGGACATGCCCAGCC-3')

2.3. RI RT-PCR and Sequencing

1. RNase- and DNase-free water for PCR.
2. 1.25 mM dNTPs for PCR (Perkin-Elmer).
3. Advantage-GC genomic polymerase mix—5X GC genomic PCR reaction buffer and 5.0 M GC-Melt buffer, 25 mM Mg(OAc)$_2$, supplied with enzyme (Clontech) for "full-length" PCR.
4. Advantage-GC cDNA polymerase mix—5X GC cDNA PCR reaction buffer and 5.0 M GC-Melt, supplied with enzyme (Clontech).
5. Primers as listed below, diluted to 5 μM (*see* **Note 8**):

PCR product	Size (bp)	Forward primer	Reverse primer
RI "full length"	1600	RI-75s	RI-1675as
		(5'-CCATGGAGGCGGCGGTCGCTGCTCCGCG-3')	
			(5'-CTCAGTGAGGTAGAACAACTGACCTCCC-3')
RI 5'-end	582	RI-5s	RI-586as
		(5'-AGGCGAGGTTTGCTGGGG-3')	
			(5'-AAAAGGGCGATCTAATGAAGGG-3')

6. Sequencing primers (*see* **Note 8**):

    RI-13s (5'-TTTGCTGGGGGTGAGGCAGCG-3') for sequencing 5' end
    RI-278as (5'-TGTGTATAACTTTGTCTGTGGTCTC-3') for sequencing 5' end
    RI-228s (5'-ATGGGCTCTGCTTTGTCTC-3') for sequencing "full length"
    RI-459s (5'-CTGTCATTGCTGGACCAG-3') for sequencing "full length"
    RI-764s (5'-GCTGTTAAGATATTCTCCT-3') for sequencing "full length"
    RI-828as (5'-GTTTGATAAATCTCTGCCTC-3') for sequencing "full length"
    RI-1669as (5'-GAGGTAGAACAACTGACCT-3') for sequencing "full length"

3. Methods

3.1. BAT-RII Assay

3.1.1. End-Label Primer

The labeling reaction consists of: 7 μL TA10-F1 primer (from 300 ng/mL stock), 7.5 μL 10X PNK buffer, 54 μL water, 6 μL γ-P^{32}-ATP (10 μCi/μL) or γ-P^{33}-ATP (10 μCi/μL), and 0.5 μL polynucleotide kinase (PNK) enzyme, for a total volume of 75 μL.

1. Mix primer, water, buffer and PNK together in a microfuge tube in an area designated for PCR work only, then quickly move to a shielded radioactive area and add the radioactive isotope to the tube. Pipet the reaction mix several times and then immediately incubate at 37°C for 30 min (*see* **Note 1**).
2. After the 37°C incubation, heat at 70°C for 5 min to inactivate the enzyme.

3. Remove unincorporated isotope with a size separation purification column. Removal of the unincorporated nucleotides decreases the amount of radioactivity in the bottom buffer after electrophoresis to low levels (<7 µCi). This step is optional, but significantly simplifies the handling of radioactive waste generated during the labeling.

   To prepare an inexpensive column, remove the plunger from a 1 mL syringe. Insert a small plug of glass wool into the bottom of the syringe, and pack it down with the plunger. Pipet 1 mL of prehydrated G-50 into the glass wool plugged syringe. Place the syringe in a 15 mL disposable plastic tube, and centrifuge for 1 min at 1000 rpm in a tabletop centrifuge. Add more G-50 and repeat centrifugation until the bed volume in the syringe reaches 1 mL. Remove all liquid from the 15 mL tube and place the syringe column back in the tube.

   Add 25 µL water to the radioactive inactivated reaction mix, load the 100 µL volume onto the column, and centrifuge for 1 min at 1000 rpm in a tabletop centrifuge. Next apply 150 µL water, to the column, repeat the centrifugation, and collect all of the effluent.

5. If column purification is not used, add 175 µL water to the inactivated reaction mix to achieve an 8 ng/µL labeled primer solution. The labeled primer can be stored at $-20°C$ for about 1 mo for P^{32}, 2–3 mo for P^{33}.

3.1.2. BAT-RII PCR Reaction

1. In 0.5 mL or 0.2 mL PCR tubes, aliquot approx 50–100 ng of genomic DNA for each sample to be tested (*see* **Note 3**), and add water to achieve a total volume of 7.95 µL in each tube (n = total number of samples).
2. Mix a reaction cocktail for (n + 2) reactions. Multiply the volumes below by (n + 2) to determine the total volume of each item in the cocktail.

   > 0.75 µL TA10-R1 primer, unlabeled
   > 2.4 µL 1.25 mM dNTPs
   > 1.5 µL 10X Pwo buffer

3. Add (n + 2) × 0.15 µL Pwo polymerase to the reaction cocktail, mix briefly and centrifuge in a microfuge quickly. Next, add (n + 2) × 2.25 µL of the end-labeled TA10-F1 to the reaction cocktail. Aliquot 7.05 mL of the cocktail into each sample tube, and then add 15 mL mineral oil to cover the final reaction mix (*see* **Note 4**).
4. Run a "touchdown" PCR program: 95°C 5'; then 3 cycles of (95°C 1', 62°C 30", 72°C 30"), then decrease the annealing temperature 2°C/cycle until an annealing temperature of 56°C is reached. Continue cycling for a total of 30 cycles, followed by a 70°C 10' final extension and 4°C hold. This "touchdown" program is more stringent than a typical, one temperature annealing program and decreases artifact bands (*see* **Note 5**).

3.1.3. Gel Electrophoresis

1. While the thermocycler is running the PCR reaction, prepare a 6% LongRanger/7 M urea sequencing gel with sharks tooth comb. Allow the gel to cure for 45 min. Prerun the gel at 75 W for about 20 min.

2. When the thermocycler has finished, remove the tubes, add 15 μL of a reaction stop solution (95% formamide, 0.05% bromophenol blue, 0.05% xylene cyanol) to each 15 μL PCR reaction mix under oil, incubate at 85°C for 5 min, and immediately place on ice.

3. Immediately prior to loading the samples in the polyacrylamide gel, flush the wells in the polyacrylamide gel with buffer from the top chamber in the electrophoresis chamber. Load 4–6 μL of each sample reaction mix into their designated wells, and run the gel at 75 W constant power (52°C) until the bromophenol blue is about 2 cm from the bottom of the gel. Load the gel asymmetrically to simplify orientation later.

4. Dry the gel at 70°C for 30 min and expose to film or a phosphoimager screen.

3.2. TGF-β-RII RT-PCR and Sequencing

3.2.1. One-Step RT-PCR with Titan Kit with Primers RII-297s and RII-2077as

1. For each reaction, aliquot 1 μL each of primers RII-297s and RII-2077as into PCR tubes, and add 1 μg total RNA. The RNA must be in a volume ≤ 1 μL.

2. For *n* samples (including a water control) multiply the volumes shown below by (*n* + 1) and make the following reaction cocktail (*see* **Note 6**):

> 8 μL dNTPs (1.25 m*M*)
> 2.5 μL DTT
> 10 μL 5X Titan buffer
> 25.5 μL water
> 1 μL Titan enzyme mix

3. Aliquot 47 μL of the reaction cocktail into each RNA sample tube, pipet several times to mix, and transfer to a 50°C preheated PCR block. Run the following program: 50°C × 30', 95°C × 2'; then cycle (95°C × 45", 58°C × 1', 68°C × 2') for 36 cycles, 68°C × 5' final extension, and then a 4°C hold.

4. Run 5 μL of each sample on a 0.8% agarose gel to verify amplification of the 1780 bp expected band. If more than one band or a smear is visible, use the Qiaquick gel extraction kit exactly according to manufacturer's instructions to purify the product. If only one band is visible, use the Qiaquick PCR purification kit to remove primers and nucleotides. Use the Qiaquick PCR purification kit according to manufacturer's directions for preparation of samples for direct sequencing, and elute the DNA with water (not TE). After Qiaquick purification, estimate the concentration of DNA either by agarose gel electrophoresis next to known standards or by spotting 1 μL on an ethidium bromide agarose plate next to standards of known concentration (*see* **Note 7**).

3.2.2. Alternate Method: Two-Step Reverse Transcription and PCR Amplification

3.2.2.1. REVERSE TRANSCRIPTION OF cDNA

1. For each reaction desired, prepare the following reaction cocktail:

8.5 µL total volume of 5 mg total RNA and water
0.5 µL random hexamers (2 mg/mL)
10 µL 1.25 m*M* dNTPs
5 µL 5X AMV RT buffer
1 µL AMV RT (Roche, 25 U/µL)

2. Incubate at 42°C for 1.5 h. Store cDNAs at –20°C for up to several months.

3.2.2.2. RII PCR AMPLIFICATION

PCR product	Size (bp)	Forward primer	Reverse primer
RII-297s/RII-1160as	861	RII-297s	RII-1160as
RII-1028s/RII-2073as	1025	RII-1028s	RII-2073as

1. Aliquot 5 µL of cDNA from the previous step into the PCR tubes.
2. For *n* reactions, prepare a reaction cocktail of (*n* + 1) times the following volumes:

1 µL forward primer (RII-297s or RII-1028s)
1 µL reverse primer (RII-1160as or RII-2073as)
5 µL 1.25 m*M* dNTPs
5 µL 10X PCR buffer
32.8 µL water
0.2 µL Taq (5 U/µL)

3. Aliquot 45 µL of the reaction cocktail into each PCR tube, pipet several times to mix.
4. Run the following PCR program: 95°C × 5' initial denaturation, (95°C × 45", 61°C × 1', 72°C × 2') for 35 cycles, 70°C × 10' final extension, 4°C hold.
5. Run 5 µL of each sample on a 0.8% agarose gel to verify amplification of the expected bands. Prepare the PCR products for direct sequencing as described above in the one-step Titan RT-PCR protocol.

3.2.3. Direct Sequencing (see **Notes 9** and **10**)

RT-PCR products can be sequenced directly, without cloning. The PCR products can be cloned and then sequenced as well (*see* **Note 11**). Automated sequencing can be performed with the ABI system 377, following the manufacturer's directions exactly. The concentration of RT-PCR product is estimated using the method described above, and then a premixed reaction is prepared that contains 10–20 ng of RT-PCR product for each 200 bp of template length, 2 µL of 4 µ*M* primer, and water to achieve a final volume of 24 µL. Different facilities may have different requirements for premixed reactions, and these requirements should be followed. If automated sequencing is not available, another option is manual cycle sequencing with one of the commercial kits, such as the Perkin Elmer Amplicycle kit.

3.3. TGF-β-RI RT-PCR and Sequencing

3.3.1. Reverse Transcription of cDNA

1. For each reaction, mix:

> 8.5 µL total volume for 5 mg total RNA and water
> 0.5 µL random hexamers (2 mg/mL)
> 10 µL 1.25 mM dNTPs
> 5 µL 5X AMV RT buffer
> 1 µL AMV RT (Roche, 25 U/µL)
> 25 µL total volume

2. Incubate 42°C for 1.5 h. Store cDNAs at –20°C for up to several months.

3.3.2. PCR for Full-Length RI (PCR Product is 1600 bp), or the 5' End of RI (PCR Product is 582 bp)

1. Aliquot 5 µL cDNA from the previous step into a PCR tube.
2. For *n* reactions, multiply the volumes below by (*n* + 1) to make a cocktail:

For full length PCR:

> 1 µL forward primer RI-75s (5 µM)
> 1 µL reverse primer RI-1675as (5 µM)
> 5 µL 1.25 mM dNTPs
> 10 µL 5X GC genomic PCR reaction buffer
> 10 µL GC-melt (5.0 M)
> 2.2 µL 25 mM Mg(OAc)$_2$
> 1 µL Advantage-GC genomic polymerase mix
> 14.8 µL water

For 5' end PCR:

> 1 µL forward primer RI-5s (5 µM)
> 1 µL reverse primer RI-586as (5 µM)
> 5 µL 1.25 mM dNTPs
> 10 µL 5X GC cDNA PCR reaction buffer
> 10 µL GC-melt (5.0 M)
> 1 µL Advantage-GC cDNA polymerase mix
> 17 µL water

Aliquot 45 µL of the cocktail into each sample tube, mix briefly and close the tubes.
3. Run the PCR thermocycler programs as follows:

    a. For full length: 5' 95°C;(95°C 30", 64°C 1', 70°C 3') for 38 cycles, 70°C 5' final extension, 4°C hold.
    b. For 5' end PCR: 5' 95°C; (95°C 30", 60°C 1', 70°C 3') for 38 cycles, 70°C 5' final extension, 4°C hold.
4. Run 5–10 µL of each reaction on a 0.8% agarose gel to check amplification. If more than one band or a smear is visible, use the Qiaquick gel extraction kit exactly according to manufacturer's instructions. Use Qiaquick PCR purification kit if only one band is visible to remove primers and nucleotides. Use the

manufacturer's directions for preparation for direct sequencing, and elute the DNA with water (not TE). After Qiaquick purification, estimate the concentration of DNA either by electrophoresis next to standards or by spotting 1 μL on an ethidium bromide agarose plate next to standards of known concentration.

3.3.3. Direct Sequencing (see **Notes 12** and **13**)

RT-PCR products can be sequenced directly, without cloning. The products can be cloned and then sequenced as well (*see* **Note 11**). Automated sequencing can be performed with the ABI system 377, following the manufacturer's directions exactly. The concentration of RT-PCR product is estimated using the method described above, and then a premixed reaction is prepared which contains 10–20 ng of RT-PCR product for each 200 bp of template length, 2 μL of 4 μ*M* primer, and water to achieve a final volume of 24 μL. Different facilities may have different requirements for premixed reactions, and these requirements should be followed. If automated sequencing is not available, another option is manual cycle sequencing with one of the commercial kits, such as the Perkin Elmer Amplicycle kit.

4. Notes

1. Either ^{32}P or ^{33}P can be used for primer labeling. ^{32}P has greater signal strength, which improves the detection of dilute samples, but ^{33}P gives sharp bands that can make interpretation easier, especially for the wt/–1 heterozygous samples.
2. The G-50 sephadex should be incubated in excess TE buffer at least overnight before being used.
3. The amount of genomic DNA used can vary from 25–300 ng, but the most consistent results are achieved with about 50 ng. If the DNA has been extracted from paraffin-embedded fixed tissue, it may be necessary to use more than 50 ng.
4. Use of the proofreading thermostable polymerase Pwo results in a minimal error rate as the polymerase replicates the repetitive A_{10} tract. Thus, Pwo reduces the appearance of an artifact shadow band at the –1 (72 bp) position. However, Pwo polymerase has intrinsic exonuclease activity, which will digest the primers in the absence of genomic DNA, so the reaction mix should be prepared in the following order and used immediately after it is prepared:
   a. If stored at –20°C, thaw the labeled TA10-F1 primer in the PCR radioactive working area.
   b. Aliquot the sample DNA and water into tubes on the PCR bench and set aside.
   c. Prepare the cocktail with cold TA10-R1 primer, 10X buffer and dNTPs, set aside.
   d. Transfer sample tubes to the radioactive PCR working area and open the tube lids.
   e. Preheat the PCR block to 95°C.
   f. Add the Pwo enzyme to the reaction cocktail, mix, centrifuge, and go immediately to the radioactive area. Add labeled TA10-F1 primer to the cocktail,

pipet several times to mix, and start transferring the reaction cocktail into the sample tubes. Perform these steps as quickly as you can safely, with no delays.

    g. Layer on the oil, close the tubes, transfer the tubes to the preheated PCR block, and immediately initiate the thermocycler program. An oil overlay is used even with a heated lid PCR block to minimize the effects of evaporation on the reaction given the small reaction volumes.

5. Use genomic DNA from cell lines with known BAT-RII mutations as standards. RL-952 (wt/–1 heterozygote) and HCT-116 (–1 homozygous) are tumor cell lines available from ATCC that are convenient standards.

6. Because the Titan enzyme mix contains Pwo polymerase, use the reaction mix immediately after adding the enzyme to minimize the exonuclease effect on the primers.

7. If 297/2077 full-length RII does not amplify, the expression levels in the sample may be low and it may be necessary to amplify the cDNA in 2 overlapping pieces, RII-297/RII-1160as and RII-1028s/RII-2073as using the alternate method described above.

8. The PCR amplification primers do not need to be purified, but sequencing primers to be used for direct automated sequencing perform optimally if they are HPLC or reverse phase purified.

9. Sequencing through the A_{10} tract can be difficult. This protocol sequences away from it on either side with RII-708as and RII-719s, and sequences toward it as well with RII-425s and RII-1160as.

10. At base 429, the junction between exons 1 and 2, there may be an in-frame insertion of 75 bp in the cDNA *(6,13)*. This alternatively spliced RII receptor has function indistinguishable from the predominant RII species, and is present at lower levels. However, its presence in the RT-PCR product often causes the sequence after that point to be an unreadable mixture of two sequences. For this reason, the RII-425s sequencing primer has been included to sequence only the predominant RII cDNA.

11. For cloning the RT-PCR product, the TOPO-TA kit (Invitrogen) works well. Cloning with this kit is optimally performed using PCR products as soon as possible after the PCR reaction is finished because the one base overhangs generated by the Taq polymerase, which the cloning enzyme in this kit uses, degrade with time. In addition, if the RT-PCR product used for cloning is generated using the Titan kit, it is necessary to add 3' A-overhangs to the product before using the TOPO-TA kit since PWO does not leave 3' A overhangs like Taq does. This simple method is included in the manufacturer's protocols for the kit.

12. One RT-PCR reaction usually gives enough product to perform 3 sequencing reactions, so multiple RT-PCR reactions from the same template should be amplified to generate enough product for full length sequencing.

13. The 5'-end partial PCR can be used to amplify and sequence the GC-rich 5' end and the region of GCG alanine repeats. The number of alanines is polymorphic, *(15)* and heterozygous individuals create a sequencing problem. To solve this problem, sequencing from both ends of the 5'-end PCR product is performed.

References

1. Alexandrow, M. and Moses, H. (1995) Transforming growth factor β and cell cycle regulation. *Cancer Res.* **55,** 1452–1457.
2. Chen, T., Carter, D., Garrigue-Antar, L., and Reiss, M. (1998) Transforming growth factor β type I receptor kinase mutant associated with metastatic breast cancer. *Cancer Res.* **58,** 4805–4810.
3. Garrigue-Antar, L., Munoz-Antonia, T., Antonia, S., Gesmonde, J., Vellucci, V., and Reiss, M. (1995) Missense mutations of the transforming growth factor β type II receptor in human head and neck squamous carcinoma cells. *Cancer Res.* **55,** 3982–3987.
4. Grady, W., Myeroff, L., Swinler, S., Rajput, A., Thiagalingam, S., Lutterbaugh, J., et al. (1999) Mutational inactivation of transforming growth factor β receptor type II in microsatellite stable colon cancers. *Cancer Res.* **59,** 320–324.
5. Hahn, S., Schutte, M., Shamsul Hoque, A., Moskaluk, C., da Costa, L., Rozenblum, E., et al. (1996) *DPC4*, a candidate tumor supressor gene at human chromosome 18q21.1. *Science* **271,** 350–353.
6. Hirai, R. and Fujita, T. (1996) A human transforming growth factor-β type II receptor that contains an insertion in the extracellular domain. *Exp. Cell Res.* **223,** 135–141.
7. Knaus, P., Lindemann, D., DeCoteau, J., Perman, R., Yankelev, H., Hille, M., et al. (1996) A dominant inhibitory mutant of the type II transforming growth factor β receptor in the malignant progression of a cutaneous T-cell lymphoma. *Mol. Cell. Biol.* **16,** 3480–3489.
8. Lu, S.-L., Zhang, W.-C., Akiyama, Y., Nomizu, T., and Yuasa, Y. (1996) Genomic structure of the transforming growth factor β type II receptor gene and its mutations in hereditary nonpolyposis colorectal cancers. *Cancer Res.* **56,** 4595–4598.
9. Lynch, M., Nakashima, R., Song, H., DeGroff, V., Wang, D., Enomoto, T. and Weghorst, C. (1998) Mutational analysis of the transforming growth factor β receptor type II gene in human ovarian carcinoma. *Cancer Res.* **58,** 4227–4232.
10. Markowitz, S. and Roberts, A. (1996) Tumor supressor activity of the TGF-β pathway in human cancers. *Cytokine Growth Factor Rev.* **7,** 93–102.
11. Markowitz, S., Wang, J., Myeroff, L., Parsons, R., Sun, L., Lutterbaugh, J., et al. (1995) Inactivation of the type II TGF-β receptor in colon cancer cells with microsatellite instability. *Science* **268,** 1336–1338.
12. Myeroff, L., Parsons, R., Kim, S.-J., Hedrick, L., Cho, K., Orth, K., et al. (1995) A transforming growth factor β receptor type II gene mutation common in colon and gastric but rare in endometrial cancers with microsatellite instability. *Cancer Res.* **55,** 5545–5547.
13. Nikawa, J. (1994) A cDNA encoding the human transforming growth factor β receptor suppresses the growth defect of a yeast mutant. *Gene* **149,** 367–372.
14. Parsons, R., Myeroff, L., Liu, B., Willson, J., Markowitz, S., Kinzler, K., and Vogelstein, B. (1995) Microsatellite instability and mutations of the transforming growth factor β type II receptor gene in colorectal cancer. *Cancer Res.* **55,** 5548–5550.

15. Pasche, B., Luo, Y., Rao, P., Nimer, S., Dmitrovsky, E., Caron, P., et al. (1998) Type I transforming growth factor β receptor maps to 9q22 and exhibits a polymorphism and a rare variant within a polyadenine tract. *Cancer Res.* **58,** 2727–2732.

16. Schutte, M., Hruban, R., Hedrick, L., Cho, K., Nadasdy, G., Weinstein, C., et al. (1996) DPC4 gene in various tumor types. *Cancer Res.* **56,** 2527–2530.

17. Takenoshita, S., Tani, M., Nagashima, M., Hagiwara, K., Bennet, W., Yokota, J., and Harris, C. (1997) Mutation analysis of coding sequences of the entire transforming growth factor beta type II receptor gene in sporadic human colon cancer using genomic DNA and intron primers. *Oncogene* **14,** 1255–1258.

18. Togo, G., Toda, N., Kanai, F., Kato, N., Shiratori, Y., Kishi, K., et al. (1996) A transforming growth factor β type II receptor gene mutation common in sporadic cecum cancer with microsatellite instability. *Cancer Res.* **56,** 5620–5623.

12

Direct Analysis for Familial Adenomatous Polyposis Mutations

Steven M. Powell

1. Introduction

Over the past decade, the genes that underlie the development of many human diseases have been identified and the diseases causing mutations within these genes have been unveiled. Many genetic alterations responsible for a variety of human disorders have been characterized. These alterations range from simple Mendelian inherited syndromes to more complex traits such as cancers that involve multiple genetic and environmental factors. Identification and characterization of disease-causing mutations has practical as well as biological implications. As our understanding of these alterations advances, the potential for developing molecular genetic markers with clinical applications increases. This improved understanding also opens new avenues for advances in diagnostic testing, prognostication, and design of preventative strategies or therapeutic interventions. Indeed, direct genetic testing for an inherited colorectal cancer predisposition syndromes, Familial Adenomatous Polyposis (FAP) is currently available to the medical community with appropriate genetic counseling *(1)*.

This chapter describes the application of the in vitro synthesis (IVS) protein assay, which is a sensitive and rapid method for detecting truncating gene mutations *(1,2)*. The importance of mutational analyses that can be applied routinely in clinical practice is highlighted by the IVS protein assay's current use to FAP presymptomatically. This assay may also potentially aid in the diagnosis and management of many other diseases that involve truncating genetic mutations (*see* **Table 1**).

We may soon be entering into an era where mutational analysis and detection become the limiting steps in our diagnosis and care of patients. For instance, we may know the gene(s) involved in a disease, but not have the

From: *Methods in Molecular Medicine, vol. 50: Colorectal Cancer: Methods and Protocols*
Edited by: S. M. Powell © Humana Press Inc., Totowa, NJ

Table 1
Applications of the IVS Protein Assay

Current	
Familial adenomatous polyposis syndromes	APC
Emerging	
Hereditary nonpolyposis colon	DNA repair genes (MMR)[a]
Neurofibromatosis type 1	NF1
Hereditary breast/ovarian cancer	BCRA1
Duchenne muscular	Dystrophin
Potential	
Neurofibromatosis type 2	NF2
Von Hippel-Lindau	VHL
Retinoblastoma	Rb
Becker muscular dystrophy	Dystrophin
β-Thalassemia	β-Globin
Hemophilia B	Factor IX
Cystic fibrosis	CFTR
Osteogenesis Imperfecta	COLIA1/COLIA2
Werner's syndrome	WRN

[a]MMR = mismatch repair genes that include: *hMSH2, hM:LH1, hPMS1, hPMS2.*

ability to conveniently test those individuals who may have or are at risk for having the disease for causative alterations in the responsible gene(s). Currently, identifying the appropriate clinical setting for genetic testing is of paramount importance. The group of patients and relatives for whom genetic testing will be beneficial is presently being defined as we better understand genotype to phenotype relationships and the penetrance of pathologic traits.

Many conventional techniques of mutational analysis, such as direct nucleotide sequencing, ribonuclease protection assays, or other chemical cleavage of nucleotide mismatch methods (i.e., hydroxylamine and osmium tetroxide) that can identify genetic mutations sensitively are labor intensive and usually reserved for the research setting (reviewed in **ref. 3**). Other methods of detecting gene mutations, such as single-strand conformation polymorphism (SSCP) analysis *(4)*, denaturing gradient gel electrophoresis (DGGE) analysis *(5)*, or heteroduplex analysis, may require only a few steps but are limited in their sensitivity of mutation detection. The narrow range of a gene's size that can be analyzed by these methods at any one time also restricts their use for mutation identification, specifically limited are those assays that involve altered heteroduplex migration on gel electrophoresis analysis. Moreover, some methods such as allele-specific amplification (ASA), allele-specific hybridization (ASH), ligation amplification reactions (LAR) *(6)*, or restriction site amplifications are relatively simple to perform, but they are designed to detect only a specific nucleotide change. This specificity limits their usefulness for screening genes that tend to have multiple types of mutations occurring at different locations in the gene.

Additionally, genes can be altered in the noncoding region with important functional effects. For example, changes that occur in the promoter or enhancer regions of a gene or alterations that change methylation patterns might result in abnormal gene expression. Moreover, gross allelic or chromosomal deletions, amplifications, or rearrangements are known to occur at gene loci that result in the loss, disruption, or increased expression of its product. High-resolution cytogenetic analyses such as those involving fluorescent *in situ* hybridization (FISH) and Southern blot-based restriction fragment length polymorphism (RFLP) analysis can facilitate the detection of these alterations *(7)*; however, only a few genes presently allow routine identification of such alterations. Thus, none of these conventional methods of mutation detection are readily applicable for routine screening of large genes with a wide distribution and spectrum of mutations. Therefore, one can see how efficient mutational analysis has become a pressing issue.

The *APC* gene was isolated in 1991 *(8,9)* and so named *Adenomatous Polyposis Coli* when it was found to be altered in the germline of FAP patients and cosegregated with this disease *(10,11)*. FAP is a clinically well-described highly penetrant autosomal dominant trait that has been reported for over a century (reviewed in **ref. 12**). Affected individuals develop hundreds to thousands of colorectal adenomatous polyps, some of which inevitably progress to colorectal carcinomas unless they are removed surgically.

FAP patients harbored multiple types of nucleotide changes widely distributed throughout *APC*'s relatively large coding region with some trend toward concentrating in its mid-portion (the 5' end of the last large exon 15). Conventional genetic screening methods were applied in early research-based studies of the coding region of the *APC* gene. They could detect mutations in the range of 30–60% of patients with FAP depending on the technique used *(13–15)*. The variegated nucleotide changes and wide distribution of *APC* gene mutations presented a formidable obstacle in the development of a rapid mutational assay for this gene by conventional approaches.

It was observed that the overwhelming majority of these *APC* gene mutations would result in a truncated gene product when expressed because of small insertions or deletions producing frameshifts and subsequent premature stop codons, nonsense point mutations, or splice site alterations (reviewed in **ref. 16**). Thus, it was surmised that the examination of an individual's *APC* protein would identify the majority of *APC* mutations. A novel assay was developed to examine *APC*'s gene based on IVS of its protein from a PCR-amplified product *(2,3)*. In this assay, an individual's gene or mRNA transcript, amplified by polymerase chain reaction (PCR) or reverse transcription and polymerase chain reaction (RT-PCR) serves as a nucleotide surrogate template of the *APC* gene for rapid in vitro transcription and translation. The protein synthesized in vitro is then analyzed electrophoretically for its size. This method of mutational detection was shown to sensitively identify the germline truncating *APC* mutations in 82% of 62 unique FAP kindreds.

The IVS protein assay originated in an effort to efficiently identify truncating *APC* mutations. This test was first validated in the analysis of sporadic colorectal tumors containing known truncating *APC* gene mutations. The accuracy of identifying *APC* mutations in this manner was illustrated by the clearly visible mutant protein bands in these samples. The sensitivity of this assay was demonstrated in the detection of *APC* mutations in tiny dysplastic colonic polyps and aberrant crypt lesions *(17)*.

The strength of the IVS protein test lies in its ability to rapidly identify truncating gene mutations irrespective of their origin or nature at the nucleotide level. Truncation of a gene's product is a drastic alteration that is expected generally to have critical effects on the protein's normal function in a cell. Therefore, the ability to identify only these truncating kinds of alterations, while avoiding numerous inconsequential polymorphisms or rare variant changes, is a significant advantage offered by the IVS protein assay in mutational screening.

A variety of mutations at the genetic level such as nonsense point mutations, frameshifts, or alterations producing splice abnormalities that result in a truncated gene product, can be detected sensitively all at once by this method. Additionally, the IVS protein assay can be used to analyze relatively long gene segments. This is especially advantageous for large genes having a widespread distribution of mutations. The ability to generate cDNA from mRNA transcripts by RT-PCR reactions for use as a template in this assay facilitates rapid screening of multiple exons and long regions of coding sequence at one time as well as of the splicing pattern of a particular gene.

Limitations of the IVS protein assay include its inability to identify nontruncating genetic mutations such as missense point mutations. Gross allelic loss, insertion, or rearrangement, which may prohibit the amplification of a genetic locus, also would not be detected by the PCR-based IVS protein assay. Furthermore, alterations in noncoding regions such as those that may occur in the promoter or intron regions and affect gene product expression would not be detected by the IVS protein assay.

Finally, the IVS protein assay would not detect epigenetic alterations, such as methylation changes and imprinting abnormalities, that might affect gene expression. Therefore, additional more broad analyses, such as the allele-specific expression (ASK) assay *(2)*, Southern blot analysis, or Western blot analysis, are needed when these types of mutations are sought. Interestingly, a novel strategy, termed monoallelic mutation analysis (MAMA), which is based on somatic cell hybridization technology, was recently reported to identify germline mutations sensitively and specifically *(18)*.

This assay was readily applied to FAP patients' blood samples in the original quest to identify *APC* mutations efficiently and sensitively for clinical use. This assay lends itself to routine use by utilization of supplies and equipment that are commonly available in most molecular biology laboratories. Moreover, RNA and especially DNA can be extracted by standard means from routinely available clinical samples such as blood and stored stably for analysis at convenient times.

At-risk family members are commonly the greatest beneficiaries of using the IVS protein assay to make a molecular diagnosis of FAP patients (*see* **Fig. 1**). Once a causative *APC* mutation is identified with this assay, one can employ the test presymptomatically to determine with virtually 100% accuracy whether or not a family member has inherited the specific genetic abnormality and the resultant risk of neoplasia associated with this disease. Presymptomatic direct genetic testing greatly aids in the clinical management of FAP kindred members and allows more directed screening for cancer development. Genetic counseling is a prerequisite for this type of testing to convey information appropriately to these patients *(19)*.

Since its emergence in 1993, the IVS protein assay has also been used to identify truncating genetic mutations in other genes, most notably the DNA mismatch repair genes, the Duchennes muscular dystrophy gene, *BRCA1,* and *NF1*. HNPCC is a cancer predisposition syndrome inherited as an autosomal dominant trait with fairly high penetrance which is associated with colorectal and other cancer development (reviewed in **ref. 20**). This disease was recently demonstrated to result from alterations in DNA mismatch repair genes *(21–25)*. The IVS protein assay was used initially to screen the candidate genes in HNPCC patients for deleterious mutations and revealed germline truncating alterations of varied genetic origins in four different genes, namely *hMSH2, hMLH1, hPMS1, and hPMS2,* which reflect the heterogeneity of this disease.

The clinical utility of the IVS protein test in identifying alterations in DNA repair genes is just beginning to be established *(26,27)*. The spectrum of mutations in the DNA repair genes in HNPCC patients suggests that more than half of those identified are truncating in nature and would be amenable to detection by the IVS protein assay. A clinically useful genetic test to identify an HNPCC kindred's causative mutation would have important implications for presymptomatic screening of at-risk family members similar to those described for FAP. An additional subgroup of patients that might benefit from the use of

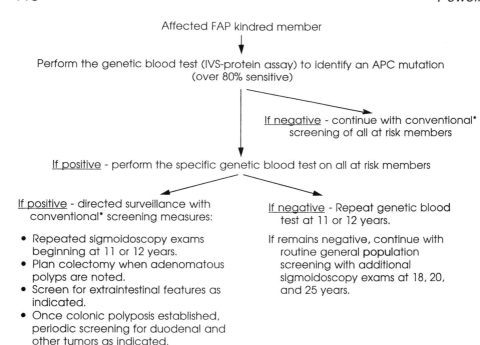

Fig. 1. Algorithm for the management of FAP kindreds. These management guide-lines of FAP kindreds incorporate presymptomatic direct genetic testing for *APC* mutations. The conventional measures of screening for members of FAP kindreds at risk may vary in frequency (e.g., sigmoidoscopic exams usually performed annually until approx 40 yr of age or until significant adenomatous polyposis is noted). Endoscopic surveillance exams once colectomy has been performed is dependent on the surgical procedure performed, severity of polyposis, and amount of remaining colon mucosa left at risk (e.g., sigmoidoscopic exams every 6 mo if the rectum is intact vs annual exams after ileoanal anastomosis procedures). Extraintestina screening examinations advocated by some physicians inclucle fundoscopic exams and radiologic exams of the skull, man-dible, and teeth. Once colonic adenomatous polyposis is established, surveillance for duodenal polyposis is considered every 1–3 yr, although cost to benefit ratios are not well established. Surveillance for other extraintestinal tumors, such as brain, thyroid, and soft tissues (e.g., desmoids), must then be considered, especially in kindreds already manifesting these features (e.g., Gardner's or Turcot's syndrome). Adapted from **ref. *44*** with permission.

the IVS protein assay to identify DNA repair gene mutations are those indi-viduals who display microsatellite instability in their colon tumor and are diag-nosed with colorectal cancer at <35 yr of age. A study found that 5 of 12 such subjects, who were examined for DNA mismatch repair gene abnormalities, harbored germline truncating alterations in *hMSH2* or *hMLH1 (28)*.

Other genes that potentially lend themselves to clinically applicable mutational screening by the IVS protein assay include: the neurofibromatosis 2 gene *(NF2)* *(29,30)*, the von Hippel- Lindau gene *(31)*, Duchenne and Becker muscular dystrophy gene *(32)*, *BCM1* *(33)* collagen genes (e.g., *COL1A1* or *COL1A2*, which cause osteogenesis imperfecta when altered *[34]*), the retinoblastoma gene *(35)*, the beta-thalassemia gene *(36)*, and the hemophilia B gene *(37)*(*see* **Table 1**). All of these genes have a significant proportion (many greater than 50%) of truncating intragenic mutations in the patients examined so far. These mutations appear to be detectable by the IVS protein test. Over 50% of the various cystic fibrosis mutations that have been characterized, other than the common phenylalanine deletion at codon 508, appear to be detectable by the IVS protein assay as well *(38–40)*.

The Neurofibromatosis 1 gene *(NF1),* Duchenne muscular dystrophy gene, and *BCRA1* have been screened for mutations using the methodology of the IVS protein test with successful identification of truncating mutations *(41–43)*. Many of these genes are quite large with widespread genetic changes that could not be screened easily for mutations by conventional approaches, as they are too laborious or cumbersome for routine clinical use.

Of course, before one would decide to perform a genetic test, such as the IVS protein assay, to identify a causative mutation clinically, a benefit would have to be gained in doing so (e.g., enabling more directed screening measures or allowing earlier preventive or therapeutic interventions to be given). Studies are also needed to determine which individuals would be the best to screen and who would gain the most from these direct mutational tests. Sensitivity and cost-to-benefit ratio analyses are needed to help address these issues.

2. Materials
2.1. Blood Processing
1. EDTA anticoagulated (lavender top) blood tubes filled with whole blood (Becton Dickinson [Bedford, MA], Vacutainer Brand).
2. Histopaque-1077 (Sigma, St. Louis, MO).
3. 50-mL and 15-mL polypropylene conical tubes and 1.5-mL tubes (Marsh, Rochester, NY).
4. Hanks balanced saline solution (Gibco-BRL, Gaithersburg, MD).
5. Table-top centrifuge and plastic transfer pipets and 1.5-mL Eppendorf tubes.

2.2. DNA Extraction
1. Chelex-100 (5% stock solution made with sterile water) (Bio-Rad, Hercules, CA).
2. Sterile water (Gibco-BRL, HPLC-purified).
3. Microfuge and Eppendorf tubes.

2.3. RNA Extraction

1. Promega RNagents kit (Promega, Madison, WI).
2. 70% Ethanol solution.
3. Microfuge, Eppendorf tubes, and snap-cap tubes.

2.4. First-Strand cDNA Synthesis

1. Superscript II reverse transcriptase (200 U/μL) (Gibco-BRL).
2. Random hexamers (1 mg/mL stock) (Pharmacia Biotech, Piscataway, NJ).
3. 5X first-strand buffer (Gibco-BRL).
4. dNTPs (100 mM stock) (Pharmacia Biotech).
5. RNasin (40 U/μL) (Promega).
6. Bind-Aid (0.5 U/μL) (USB, Arlington Heights, IL).
7. DTT (0.1 M stock) (Gibco-BRL).
8. Template (total RNA).
9. Heating block (VWR, Bridgeport, NJ).

2.5. PCR Amplifications

1. Ampli*Taq* DNA polymerase (Perkin Elmer, Foster City, CA).
2. Bind-Aid amplification kit (USB).
3. Ampliwax gem beads (Perkin Elmer).
4. Oligonucleotides (10 μM stocks) (*see* **Table 2**).
5. Sterile water.
6. Thermocycler.
7. PCR tubes (Marsh).
8. Template (genomic DNA or cDNA).

2.6. Coupled In Vitro Transcription/Translation

1. TnT-coupled T7 transcription/translation system (Promega).
2. L-[^{35}S]-Methionine Tran^{35}S-label, >1000 Ci/mmol) (ICN, Los Angeles, CA).
3. RNasin (40 U/μL) (Promega).
4. Template (PCR product).
5. Heating block (VWR).

2.7. Gel Electrophoresis and Fluorography

1. Protein sample buffer: 10% glycerol, 5% 2-mercaptoethanol, 2% SDS, 62.5 mM Tris-HCl, pH 6.8, and 0.002% bromophenol blue.
2. Gel electrophoresis rig, accessories, and power supply.
3. SDS-polyacrylamide gel, 10–20% gradient.
4. Stacking gel (5% stock solution, 500 mM Tris-HCl, pH 6.8).
5. Eletrophoresis buffer: 25 mM Tris-HCl, 0.192 M glycine, 0.1% SDS.
6. Ammonium persulfate (10% stock solution) and TEMED (Bio-Rad, Richmond, CA).
7. 10% SDS solution (Gibco-BRL).
8. Fixative solution: 30% methanol, 10% acetic acid.

Table 2
APC Gene PCR Amplification Oligonucleotide Primers

Primer[a]	Sequence (5' to 3')
Segment 1:	
Stage I (Outside-F)	CAA GGG TAG CCA AGG ATG GC
Stage I (Outside-A)	TTG CTA GAC CAA TTC CGC G
Stage II (internal-F)	GGA TCC TAA TAC GAC TCA CTA TAG GGA GAC CAC CAT GGC TGC AGC TTC ATA TGA TC
Stage II (internal-R)	CTG ACC TAT TAT CAT CAT GTC G
Segment 2:	
F	GGA TCC TAA TAC GAC TCA CTA TAG GGA GAC CAC CAT GGA TGC ATG TGG AAC TTT GTG G
R	GAG GAT CCA TTA GAT GAA GGT GTG GAC G
Segment 3:	
F	GGA TCC TAA TAC GAC TCA CTA TAG GGA GAC CAC CAT GGT TTC TCC ATA CAG GTC ACG G
R	GGA GGA TCC TGT AGG AAT GGT ATC TCG
Segment 4:	
F	GGA TCC TAA TAC GAC TCA CTA TAG GGA GAC CAC CAT GGA AAA CCA AGA GAA AGA GGC AG
R	TTC ACT AGG GCT TTT GGA GGC
Segment 5:	
F	GGA TCC TAA TAC GAC TCA CTA TAG GGA GAC CAC CAT GGG TTT ATC TAG ACA AGC TTC G
R	GGA GTG GAT CCC AAA ATA AGA CC

[a]F = forward primers, R = reverse primers of a pair for amplification. All forward primers except stage I outside primer have the T7 transcription and translation nucleotide sequences at its 5' end.

9. ENHANCE (Dupont, NEN, Boston, MA).
10. Gel dryer, autoradiography film (Kodak [Rochester, NY] X-Omat), developer, and processor.
11. ^{14}C-labeled protein molecular weight standards (Gibco-BRL).

3. Methods

3.1. Blood Processing

1. Pipet 30 µL of EDTA anticoagulated whole blood into 1 mL of sterile water for Chelex DNA extraction (*see* **Subheading 3.3.**) (*see* **Note 1**).
2. Pour the rest of the EDTA anticoagulated whole blood (approx 10–20 mL) into a 50-mL conical tube.
3. Carefully pipet 12–15 mL of Histopaque-1077 into the bottom of the same 50-mL conical tube (*see* **Note 2**).
4. Centrifuge the 50-mL conical tube at 400*g* for 30 min at room temperature.

5. Transfer the opaque mononuclear layer (approx 5 mL) with plastic transfer pipet into a 15-mL conical tube and fill tube with Hank's balanced saline solution (HBSS) and invert mix several times (*see* **Note 3**).
6. Centrifuge the 15-mL conical tube at 400g for 5 min at room temperature.
7. Aspirate supernatant off and repeat wash of pellet with HBSS one more time.
8. Resuspend cell pellet in 1–2 mL of guanidinium isothiocyanate solution from Promega RNAgents kit (*see* **Note 4**).

3.2. DNA Extraction

1. Let mix of whole blood and water from **Subheading 3.1., step 1** sit at room temperature for 30 min with occasional mixing.
2. Microfuge at 12,000g for 3 min and pipet off supernatant.
3. Pipet 180 μL of a 5% Chelex solution in and tap mix.
4. Incubate at 56°C for 30 min, then briefly vortex.
5. Seal lids and boil for 8 min.
6. Briefly vortex, then centrifuge at 12,000g for 3 min (*see* **Note 5**).

3.3. RNA Extraction

1. Process 0.5 mL of guanidinium solution from **Subheading 3.1., step 8** above with Promega's RNagents reagents according to manufactures directions (acid quanidinium isothiocyanate-phenol-chloroforrn extraction method).
2. Wash precipitated RNA pellet with 70% ethanol.
3. Resuspend RNA precipitate in 100 μL of sterile water.

3.4. Amplification of APC Gene Segment 1 (RT-PCR)

3.4.1. First-Strand cDNA Synthesis

1. Total RNA of 5–10 μL from **Subheading 3.3., step 3** (approx 5 μg) is mixed with 1 μg of random hexamer, 1 μL of Bind-Aid, and 300 μL of superscript II reverse transcriptase and appropriate buffer containing dNTPs, DTT, and RNasin according to manufacturer's instructions in a 20 μL reaction (*see* **Note 6**).
2. Incubate reaction for 1 h at 37°C.
3. Heat inactivate at 65°C for 10 min, then cool on ice.
4. Use immediately in PCR reaction or store at –20°C.

3.4.2. Two-Stage Nested PCR Amplification

1. cDNA of 4 μL is mixed with 35 ng of each outside segment one primer, 2.5 U of Ampli*Taq*, and appropriate buffer containing dNTPs in a 20 μL PCR reaction according to Bind-Aid amplification kit manufacturer's instructions.
2. Thermocycle for 10 cycles of: 95°C for 30 s, 55°C for 2 min, 70°C for 2 min, then 70°C for 5 min.
3. For the second stage: 30 μL of an additional mix containing 350 ng of internal primers for segment one, 3.75 U of Ampli*Taq*, and appropriate Bind-Aid amplification kit buffer components including dNTPs are added to the 20 μL of first stage reaction.

4. Thermocycle the 50 μL PCR reaction for 30 cycles of: 95°C for 30 s, 62.5°C for 2 min, 70°C for 2 min, then 70°C for 5 min.
5. PCR products can be used immediately in the TnT reaction or stored at –20°C.

3.5. Amplification of APC Segments 2–5 (PCR)

1. Five to ten microliters of chelex treated blood from **Subheading 3.2., step 5** (approx 100 ng of genomic DNA) is mixed with 350 ng of each appropriate primer pair, 5 U of Ampli*Taq*, and appropriate Bind-Aid amplification kit buffer components including dNTPs in 50 μL PCR reactions according to manufacturer's instructions with the addition of Ampliwax gem beads according to manufacturer's instructions for a form of "hot" start amplification (*see* **Note 7**).
2. Thermocycle for 35 cycles of 95°C for 30 s, anneal temp (*see* **Note 8**) for 90 s, 70°C for 90 s, then 70°C for 5 min.
3. PCR products can be used immediately or stored at –20°C.

3.6. Coupled Transcription/Translation Reaction

1. Thaw components of Promega's coupled TnT (T7 polymerase) kit and keep on ice throughout.
2. Mix 3 μL of PCR product from **Subheading 3.4.2., step 5** or **Subheading 3.5., step 3** with 40 μCi of ^{35}S-methionine translabel, 10 U of RNasin, and appropriate components of the TNT kit in a 25 μL reaction according to manufacturer's instructions.
3. Incubate reaction at 30°C for 1 h (*see* **Note 9**).
4. Add 25 μL of protein sample buffer to the reaction tube, then boil for 5 min and give quick spin to bring condensate down off lid (*see* **Note 10**).

3.7. Gel Electrophoresis and Fluorography

1. Rinse precasted 10–20% gradient gel (ISI) and place in casting mount.
2. After adding APS and TEMED, pour in top stacking gel layering over gradient gel.
3. Add comb and let polymerize for approx 45 min.
4. Remove comb and set up gel in electrophoresis apparatus in appropriate buffer.
5. Load samples (5 μL from **Subheading 3.6., step 5**) and electrophores at constant current (approx 30 mAmps) till dye at bottom of gel (approx 2.5 h).
6. Take down apparatus and place gel in fixative solution with gentle shaking for 30 min.
7. Place gel in ENHANCE solution for 60 min.
8. Place gel in water for 30 min.
9. Place gel on Whatman paper, cover with plastic wrap, and dry on gel dryer till dry (*see* **Note 11**).
10. Place dried gel on Whatman paper in film cassette and expose overnight at room temperature or at –80°C, then develop film.

4. Notes

1. Duplicate samples are usually made at this step since blood samples are not always easily obtained.

2. A moppet can be used to slowly add the Histopaque to the bottom of the tube below the blood that rises above the histopaque, being less dense.
3. If a clear layer of mononuclear cells is not formed after the first spin, repeating centrifugation can sometimes help form a better layer to pipet out. Blood that has been in tubes longer than 2 d can be hard to layer out the cells.
4. An aliquot can be extracted immediately for nucleic acids (RNA or DNA) or this solution can be stored frozen for later use. Syringe aspiration with a 23-gage needle can be used to help decrease viscous solutions.
5. This supernatant contains genomic DNA and can be used immediately in a PCR amplification reaction or stored frozen for later use with repeat vortexing and centrifugation.
6. A mock reverse transcription reaction including everything except the enzyme is performed in parallel and further used as template in PCR amplification to serve as a control to identify any contamination problems.
7. Reaction (40 µL) was first mixed including everything except Ampli*Taq* and Bind-Aid. An Ampliwax gem bead was then added to the tube with a sterile needle and heated at 70°C for several minutes to melt the wax to form a barrier; 10 µL of top mix containing Ampli*Taq* and Bind-Aid was then pipeted onto the solid wax barrier for subsequent thermocyling.
8. Annealing temperatures used for PCR amplification of the various segments of APC included: segment 2, 65°C; segment 3, 60°C; segment 4, 62.5°C; and segment 5, 60°C.
9. Incubating this reaction longer can lead to increased protein degradation products. Protease inhibitors added little to prevent protein degradation.
10. This sample can be loaded for gel electrophoresis immediately or stored at –80°C for subsequent loading and analysis after thawing and reboiling. One tenth of the reaction usually gives adequate signals on fluorography.
11. Gel cracking can be a problem with high-percentage acrylamide gels (i.e., 20%). Therefore, steady heat and vacuum applied to the gel is critical in drying, often requiring several hours.

Acknowledgments

This work was supported in part by a Foundation AGA Research Scholarship award and NIH grant 1R29CA67900-01. I would like to thank Melissa Schmitt for help in preparing this chapter.

References

1. Powell, S. M., Petersen, G. M., and Krush, A. J. (1993) Molecular diagnosis of familial adenomatous polyposis. *N. Engl. J. Med.* **329,** 1982–1987.
2. van der Luijt, R., Khan, P. M., Vasen, H., van Lecuwen, C., Tops, C., Roest, P., den Dunen, J., and Fodde, R. (1994) Rapid detection of translationterminating mutations at the adenomatous polyposis cold *(APC)* gene by direct protein truncation test. *Genomics* **20,** 1–4.
3. Cotton, R. G. H. (1993) Current methods of mutation detection. *Mutat. Res.* **285,** 125–144.

4. Orita, M., Iwahana, H., Kanazawa, H., Hayashi, K., and Sekiya, T. (1989) Detection of polymorphisms of human DNA by gel electrophoresis as single strand conformation polymorphisms. *Proc. Natl. Acad. Sci. USA* **86,** 2766–2770.

5. Myers, R. M., Maniatis, T., and Lerman, L. S. (1987) Detection and localization of single base changes by denaturing gradient gei electrophoresis. *Meth. Enzymol.* **155,** 501–527.

6. Landegran, U., Kaiser, R., Sanders, J., and Hood, L. (1988) A ligase mediated gene detection technique. *Science* **241,** 1077–1080.

7. Schad, C. R., Jalal, S. M., and Thibodeau, S. N. (1995) Genetic testing for Prader-Willi and Angelman syndromes. *Mayo Clin. Proc.* **70,** 1195,1196.

8. Kinzler, K. W., Nilber, M. C., Su, L. K., Vogelstein, B., Bryan, T. M., Levy, D. B., Smith, K. J., Preisinger, A. C., Hedge, P., McKechnie, D., Finniear, R., Markham, A., Groffen, J., Boguski, M. S., Altschul, S. F., Horii, A., Ando, H., Miyoshi, Y., Miki, Y., Nishisho, I., and Nakamura, Y. (1991) Identification of FAP locus genes from chromosome *5q21. Science* **253,** 661–665.

9 Groden, J., Thilveris, A., Samowitz, W., Carlson, M., Gelbert, L., Albertsen, H., Joslyn, G., Stevens, J., Spirio, L., Robertson, M., Sargeant, L., Krapcho, K., Wolff, E., Burt, R., Hughes, J. P., Warrington, J., McPherson, J., Wasmuth, J., LePaslier, D., Abderrahim, H., Cohen, D., Leppert, M., and White, R. (1991) Identification and characterization of the familial adenomatous polyposis cold gene. *Cell* **66,** 589–600.

10. Nishisho, I., Nakamura, Y., Miyoshi, Y., Miki, Y., Ando, H., Horii, A., Koyama, K., Utsunomiya, J., Baba, S., Hedge, P., Markham, A., Krush, A. J., Petersen, G., Hamilton, S. R., Nilbert, M. C., Levy, D. B, Bryan, T. M., Preisinger, A. C., Smith, K. J., Su, L. K., Kinzler, K. W., and Vogelstein, B. (1991) Mutations of chromosome *5q21* genes in FAP and colorectal cancer patients. *Science* **253,** 665–669.

11. Joslyn, G., Carlson, M., Thiliveris, A., Albertsen, H., Gelbert, L., Samowitz, W., Groden, J., Stevens, J., Spirio, L., Robertson, M., Sargeant, L., Krapcho, K., Wolff, E., Burt, R., Hughes, J. P., Warrington, J., McPherson, J., Wasmuth, J., LePaslier, D., Abderrahim, H., Cohen, D., Leppert, M., and White, R. (1991) Identification of deletion mutations and three new genes at the familial polyposis locus. *Cell* **66,** 601–613.

12. Bussey, H. J. R. (1990) Historical clevelopments in familial adenomatous polyposis, in *Familial Adenomatous Polyposis* (Herrera, L., ed.), Liss, New York, pp. 1–7.

13. Miyoshi, Y. Ando, H., Nagase, H., Nishisho, I., Horii, A., Miki, Y., Mori, T., Utsunomiya, J., Baba, S., Petersen, G., Hamilton, S. R., Kinzler, K. W., Vogelstein, B., and Nakamura, Y. (1992) Germ-line mutations of the *APC* gene in 53 familial adenomatous polyposis patients. *Proc. Natl. Acad. Sci. USA* **89,** 4452–4456.

14. Groden, J., Gelbert, L., Thliveris, A., Nelson, L., Robertson, M., Joslyn, G., Samowitz, W., Spirio, L., Carlson, M., Burt, R., Leppert, M., and White, R. (1993) Mutational analysis of patients with adenomatous polyposis: identical inactivating mutations in unrelated individuals. *Am. J. Hum. Genet.* **52,** 263–272.

15. Nagase, H., Miyoshi, Y., Horii, A., Aoki, T., Petersen, G. M., Vogelstein, B., Maher, E., Ogawa, M., Maruyama, M., Utsunomiya, J., Baba, S., and Nakamura, Y. (1992) Screening for germ-line mutations in familial adenomatous polyposis patients: 61 new patients and a summary of 150 unrelated patients. *Hum. Mutat.* **1,** 467–473.

16. Nagase, H. and Nakamura, Y. (1993) Mutations of the *APC* (adenomatous polyposis coli) gene. *Hum. Mutat.* **2,** 425–434.
17. Jen, J., Powell, S. M., Papadopoulos, N., Smith, K. J., Hamilton, S. R., Vogelstein, B., and Kinzler, K. W. (1994) Molecular determinants of cysplasia in colorecal lesions. *Cancer Res.* **54,** 5523–5526.
18. Papadopoulos, N., Leach, F. S., Kinzler, K. W., and Vogelstein, B. (1995) Monoalleli mutation (MAMA) for identifying germline mutations. *Nature Genet.* **11,** 99–102.
19. Petersen, G. M. (1995) Genetic counseling and predictive genetic testing in familial adenomatous polyposis. *Sem. Colon Rectal Surg.* **6/1,** 55–60.
20. Lynch, H. T., Smyrk, T. C., Watson, P., Lanspa, S. J., Lynch, J. F., Lynch, P. M., Cavalieri, R. J., and Boland, C. R. (1993) Genetics, natural history, tumor spectrum, and pathology of hereditary nonpolyposis colorectal cancer. *Gastroenterology* **104,** 1535–1549.
21. Leach, F. S., Nicolaides, N. C., Papadopoulos, N., Liu, B., Jen, J., Parsons, R., Peltomaki, P., Sistonen, P., Aaltonen, L. A., Nystrom-Lahti, M., Guan, X. Y., Zhang, J., Meltzer, P. S., Yu, J. W., Kao, F. T., Chen, D.J., Cerosaletti, K. M., Rournier, R. E. K., Todd, S., Lewis, T., Leach, R. J., Naylor, S. L., Weissenbach, J., Mecklin, J. P., Jarvinen, H., Petersen, G. M., Hamilton, S. R., Green, J., Jass, J., Watson, P., Lynch, H. T., Trent, J. M., de la Chapelle, A., Kinzler, K. W., and Vogelstein, B. (1993) Mutations of a *mutS* homolog in hereditary non-polyposis colorectal cancer. *Cell* **75,** 1215–1225.
22. Fishel, R., Lescoe, M. K., Rao, M. R. S., Copeland, N. G., Jenkins, N. A., Garber, J., and Kolodner, R. (1994) The human mutator gene homolog *MSH2* and its association with hereditary nonpolyposis colon cancer. *Cell* **75,** 1027–1038.
23. Papadopoulos, N., Nicolaides, N. C., Wei, Y. F., Ruben, S. M., Carter, K. C., Rosen, C. A., Haseltine, W. A., Fleischmann, R. D., Fraser, C. M., Adams, M. D., Venter, J. C., Hamilton, S. R., Petersen, G. M., Watson, P., Lynch, H. T., Peltomiki, P., Mecklin, J. P., de la Chapelle, A., Kinzler, K. W., and Vogelstein, B. (1994) Mutation of a *mutL* homolog in hereditary colon cancer. *Science* **263,** 1625–1629.
24. Bronner, C. E., Baker, S. M., Morrison, P. T., Warren, G., Smith, L. G., Lescoe, M. K., Kane, M., Earabino, C., Lipford, J., Lindblom., A., Tannergard, P., Bollag, R. J., Godwin, A. R., Ward, D. C., Nordenskjold, M., Fishel, R., Kolodner, R., and Liskay, R. M. (1994) Mutation in the DNA mismatch repair gene homologue *hMLH1* is associated with hereditary non-polyposis colon cancer. *Nature* **368,** 258–261.
25. Nicolaides, N. C., Papadopoulos, N., Liu, B., Wei, Y. F., Carter, K. C., Ruben, S. M., Rosen, C. A., Haseitine, W. A., Fleischmann, R. D., Fraser, C. M., Adams, M. D., Venter, J. C., Dunlop, M. G., Hamilton, S. R., Petersen, G. M., de la Chapelle, A., Vogelstein, B., Kinzler, K. W. (1994) Mutations of two *PMS* homologues in hereditary nonpolyposis colon cancer. *Nature* **371,** 75–80.
26. Liu, B., Parsons, R., Papadopoulos, N., Nicolaides, N., Lynch, H. T., Wastson, P., Jass, J. R., Dunlop, M., Wyllie, A., Peltomaki, P., De La Chapelle, A., Hamilton,

S. R., Vogelstein, B., and Kinzler, K. W. (1996) Analysis of mismatch repair genes in hereditary non-polyposis colorectal cancer patients. *Nature Med.* **2,** 169–174.

27. Luce, M. C., Marra, G., Chauhan, D. P., Laghi, L., Carethers, J. M., Cherian, S. P., Hawn, M., Binnie, C. G., Kam-Morgan, L. N. W., Cayouette, M. C., Koi, M., and Boland, C. R. (1995) *In vitro* transcription/translation assay for the screening of *hM4H1* and *hMSH2* mutations in familial colon cancer. *Gastroenterology* **109,** 1368–1374.

28. Liu, B., Farrington, S. M., Petersen, G. M., Hamilton, S. R., Parsons, R., Papadopoulos, N., Fijiwara, T., Jen, J., Kinzler, K. W., Wyllie, A. H., Vogelstein, B., and Dunlop, M. G. (1995) Genetic instability occurs in the majority of young patients with colorectal cancer. *Nature Med.* **1/4,** 348–352.

29. Trofatter, J. A., MacCollin, M. M., Rutter, J. L., Murrell, J. R., Duyao, M. P., Parry, D. M., Eldridge, R., Kley, N., Menon, A. G., Pulaski, K., Haase, V. H., Ambrose, C. M., Munroe, D., Bove, C., Haines, J. L., Martuza, R. L., MacDonald, M. E., Seizinger, B. R., Short, M. P., Buckler, A. J., and Gusella, J. F. (1993) A novel moesin-, ezrin-, radixin-like gene is a candidate for the neurofibromatosis 2 tumor suppressor. *Cell* **72,** 791–800.

30. Rouleau, G. A., Merel, P., Lutchrnan, M., Sanson, M., Zucman, J., Marineau, C., Hoang-Xuan, K., Demczuk, S., Desmiaze, C., Plougastel, B., Pulst, S. M., Lenoir, G., Bijlsma, E., Fashold, R., Dumanski, J., de Jong, P., Parry, D., Eldrige, R., Aurias, A., Delattre, O., Thomas, G. (1993) Alteration in a new gene encoding a putative membrane-organizing protein causes neuro-fibromatosis type 2. *Nature* **363,** 515–521.

31. Latif, F., Tory, K., Gnarra, J., Yao, M., Duh, F. M., Orcutt, M. L., Stackhouse, T., Kuzmin, I., Modi, W., Geil, L., Schmidt, L., Zhou, F., Li, H., Wei, M. H., Chen, F., Glenn, G., Choyke, P., Walther, M. M., Weng, Y., Duan, D. S. R., Dean, M., Glavac, D., Richards, F. M., Crossey, P. A., Ferguson-Smith, M. A., Le Paslier, D., Chumakov, L., Cohen, O., Chinault, A. C., Maher, E. R., Linehan, W. M., Zbar, B., and Lerman, M. I. (1993) Identification of the von Hippel-Lindau disease tumor suppressor gene. *Science* **260,** 1317–1320.

32. Malhotra, S. B., Hart, K. A., Klamut, H. J., Thomas, N. S. T., Bodrug, S. E., Burghes, A. H. M., Bobrow, M., Harper, P. S., Thompson, M. W., Ray, P. N., and Worton, R. G. (1988) Frame-shift deletions in patients with Duchenne and Becker muscular dystrophy. *Science* **242,** 755–759.

33. Collins, F. S. (1996) *BRCA1*–Lots of mutations, lots of dilemmas. *N. Engl. J. Med.* **334/3,** 186–188.

34. Kuivaniemi, H., Tromp, G., and Prockop, D. J. (1991) Mutations in collagen genes: causes of rare and some common diseases in humans. *FASEB J.* **5,** 2052–2060.

35. Yandell, D. W., Campbell, T. A., Dayton, S. H., Petersen, R., Walton, D., Little, J. B., McConkie-Rosell, A., Buckley, E. G., and Dryja, T. P. (1989) Oncogenic point mutations in the human retinoblastoma gene: their application to genetic counseling. *N. Engl. J. Med.* **321/25,** 1689–1695.

36. Kazazian, H. H. Jr., Dowlin, C. E., Boehm, C. D, Warren, T. C., Economou, E. P., Katz, J., and Antonarakis, S. E. (1990) Gene defects in beta-thalassemia and their prenatal diagnosis. *Ann. NY Acad. Sci.* **612,** 1–14.

37. Giannelli, F., Green, P. M., High, K. A., Lozier, J. N., Lillicrap, D. P., Ludwig, M., Olek, K., Reitsma, P. H., Goossens, M., Yoshioka, A., Sommer, S., and Brownlee, G. G. (1990) Haemophilia B: database of point mutations and short additions and deletions. *Nucleic Acids Res.* **18,** 4053–4058.

38. Tsui, L. C. (1992) Mutations and sequence variations, detected in the cystic fibrosis transmembrane conductance regulator (CFTR) gene: a report from the cystic fibrosis genetic analysis consortium. *Hum. Mutat.* **1,** 197–203.

39. Tsui, L. C. (1992) The spectrum of cystic fibrosis mutations. *Trends Genet.* **8/11,** 392–398.

40. Collins, F. S. (1992) Cystic fibrosis: molecular biology and therapeutic implications. *Science* **256,** 775–779.

41. Heim, R. A., Silverman, L. M., Farber, R. A., Kam-Morgan, L. N. W., and Luce, M. C. (1994) Screening for truncated *NF1* proteins. *Nature Genet.* **8,** 218, 219.

42. Roest, P. A. M., Roberts, R. G., Sugino, S., van Ommen, G. B., and Dunnen, J. T. (1993) Protein truncation test (PTT) for rapid detection of translation-terminating mutations. *Hum. Mol. Genet.* **2,** 1719–1721.

43. Hogervorst, F. B. L., Cornelis, R. S., Bout, M., van Vliet, M., Oosterwijk, J. C. Olmer, R., Bakker, B., Klijn, J. G. M., Vasen, H. F. A., Meijers-Heijboer, H., Menko, F. H., Cornelisse, C. J., den Dunnen, J. T., Devilee, P., and van Ommen, G. J. B. (1995) Rapid detection of *BRCA1* mutations by the protein truncation test. *Nat. Genet.* **10,** 208–212.

44. Powell, S. M. (1995) Clinical applications of molecular genetics in colorectal cancer. *Sem. Colon. Rectal Surg.* **6(1),** 2–18.

13

I1307K Mutation Detection by Allele-Specific PCR in Familial Colorectal Cancer

Perry S. Chan and Steven L. Gersen

1. Introduction

Familial colorectal cancer (FCC) is a hereditary form of colorectal cancer that accounts for 15–50% of all colorectal cancers (1,2). FCC patients generally have one or two family members affected with colon polyps or cancer. A mutation (I1307K) in the *APC* gene has been associated with colorectal cancer in Ashkenazi Jews (3). This specific mutation is detected in approx 6% of the Ashkenazic Jewish population. The frequency increases to about 28% in Ashkenazim with a family history of colorectal cancer. A person carrying this mutation will have a twofold increased risk, over the general Ashkenazic Jewish population, of developing colorectal cancer in his or her lifetime (3). This risk is estimated to be approx 18–30% (3). Screening for this mutation is therefore important preventative care in this high-risk population.

A cost-effective method to screen for this mutation is vital. The following method to detect the I1307K mutation is based on the amplification refractory mutation system (ARMS) (4). The ARMS concept is based on the inability of Taq DNA polymerase to extend if a nucleotide mismatch occurs at the 3' end of the primer, and on the absence of 3'-exonucleolytic proofreading activity. Primers are constructed for the mutated and wild-type alleles and PCR reactions are performed separately. Internal control primers, which amplify the growth hormone gene, are used to confirm the reliability and reproducibility of each assay.

2. Materials
2.1. DNA Isolation

1. Red blood cell lysis buffer (RBC lysis buffer): 0.32 M sucrose, 10 mM Tris-HCl, pH 7.5, 5 mM MgCl$_2$, 1% Triton X-100.

From: *Methods in Molecular Medicine, vol. 50: Colorectal Cancer: Methods and Protocols*
Edited by: S. M. Powell © Humana Press Inc., Totowa, NJ

2. Cell lysis solution: 0.2 *M* Tris-HCl, pH 8.5, 0.1 *M* EDTA and 35 m*M* sodium dodecyl sulfate (SDS).
3. Proteinase K (10 mg/mL).
4. RNase A solution (4 mg/mL; activity: >30 U/µg).
5. 6 *M* NaCl.
6. 70% ethanol.
7. Isopropanol.
8. TE buffer: 10 m*M* Tris-HCl, 0.2 m*M* EDTA, pH 7.5.
9. Glycogen solution (20 mg/mL).

2.2. PCR Amplification

1. Sterile water.
2. 10X PCR buffer: 20 m*M* $MgCl_2$, 500 m*M* KCl, 100 m*M* Tris-HCl, pH 8.3 and 0.01% (w/v) gelatin.
3. 25 m*M* stocks of deoxynucleotide mix, prepared by adding 250 µL of each 100 m*M* dATP, dTTP, dCTP, and dGTP stock (Pharmacia Biotech) to a total volume of 1 mL.
4. *Taq* polymerase (5 U/µL)
5. Oligonucleotide primers are diluted to 10 m*M* with sterile water. Primers, HGH-5 and HGH-3 *(5)*, used to amplify the growth hormone gene are, 5'-TGCCTTCCC-AACCATTCCCTTA-3' (forward) and 5'-CCACTCACGGATTTCTGTTGTG-TTTC-3' (backward) respectively. Primers, APC-1, APC1307W and APC1307M *(3,6,7)*, used to amplify the APC gene are, 5'-GATGAAATAGGATGTA-ATCAGACG-3' (forward), 5'-CAGCTGACCTAGTTCCAATCTTTTCTTTCA-3' (backward) and 5'-CAGCTGACCTAGTTCCAATCTTTTCTTTCT-3' (backward) respectively (*see* **Note 1**).
6. Sterile 0.2 mL PCR reaction tubes.

2.3. Agarose Gel Electrophoresis

1. Agarose.
2. 1X TAE buffer: 0.04 *M* Tris-acetate, 0.001 *M* EDTA, pH 8.0.
3. Sample loading buffer: To a 50 mL graduated cylinder, add 25 mL glycerol, 25 mL TE buffer and 0.25 g bromophenol blue.
4. DNA marker.
5. Polaroid 667 film.

3. Methods
3.1. DNA Extraction (8,9)
3.1.1. From Blood Samples

1. Transfer one tube of blood (5–10 mL) into a 50 mL conical tube.
2. Bring volume up to 25 mL with the RBC lysis solution.
3. Gently invert tubes to mix and allow red blood cells to lyse for 30 min at room temperature.

4. Spin tube at room temperature for 15 min at 2000*g*.
5. Carefully pour off the RBC lysis buffer and vortex the pellet to resuspend the cells.
6. Add 5 mL cell lysis buffer and 100 µL of proteinase K. Incubate at 55°C for at least 1 h until no clumps remain.
7. When cell lysis is complete, add 20 µL of RNase A solution. Invert several times to mix and incubate at 55°C for 15 min.
8. Add 1 mL of NaCl solution and shake vigorously for 30 s.
9. Spin tube at room temperature for 20 min at 2000*g*.
10. Transfer the DNA solution into a clean tube and add an equal amount of isopropanol. Leave the solution at –20°C for at least 1 h.
11. Use an inoculating loop to transfer the DNA pellet to a 2 mL microcentrifuge tube.
12. Wash the DNA pellet two times with 1 mL 70% ethanol.
13. Carefully drain off excess ethanol and air-dry the pellet.
14. Add 0.5 mL TE buffer. Leave the DNA to dissolve at 55°C for at least 2 h or overnight.

3.1.2. From Buccal Swabs

1. To a 1.5 mL microcentrifuge tube, add 300 µL cell lysis solution and 1.5 µL proteinase K solution.
2. Dip the buccal brush containing cells up and down 10 times in the microcentrifuge tube.
3. Incubate the sample at 55°C for at least 1 h or overnight.
4. Add 1.5 µL RNase A solution to the cell lysate.
5. Mix the sample by inverting the tube 25 times and incubate at 37°C for 15 min.
6. Cool the sample to room temperature before adding 60 µL 6 *M* NaCl solution.
7. Vortex vigorously for 20 s and place the tube in an ice bath for 5 min.
8. Centrifuge for 5 min at 10,000*g* at room temperature.
9. Transfer the DNA solution into a clean 1.5 mL microcentrifuge tube containing 300 µL isopropanol and 0.5 µL glycogen solution.
10. Mix by inverting the tube gently 50 times and incubate at room temperature for at least 5 min.
11. Centrifuge for 5 min at 10,000*g* at room temperature.
12. Decant the supernatant and add 1 mL of 70% ethanol.
13. Invert the tube several times to wash the pellet and centrifuge at 10,000*g* for 1 min.
14. Drain off the ethanol and air dry for 15 min.
15. Add 20 mL of TE buffer. Leave the DNA to dissolve at 55°C for at least 2 h or overnight.

3.2. PCR Amplification

1. Prepare master mixes of PCR reagents for detection of the wild type and mutant alleles according to the following (*see* **Note 2**):

Wild-Type Master Mix

10X PCR buffer	2.0 µL
25 mM dNTP	0.16 µL
25 mM MgCl$_2$	1.6 µL
10 µM HGH-5	1 µL
10 µM HGH-3	1 µL
10 µM APC-1	1 µL
10 µM APC1307W	1 µL
Taq (5 U/µL)	0.1 µL
H$_2$O	10.14 µL
	18 µL

Mutant Master Mix

10X PCR buffer	2.0 µL
25 mM dNTP	0.16 µL
25 mM MgCl2	1.6 µL
10 µM HGH-5	1 µL
10 µM HGH-3	1 µL
10 µM APC-1	1 µL
10 µM APC1307W	1 µL
Taq (5 U/µL)	0.1 µL
H$_2$O	10.14 µL
	18 µL

2. Pipet 18 µL of the master mix into a 0.2 mL PCR tube.
3. Add 2 µL of sample DNA (5 ng/µL) to the appropriately labeled PCR tube. For buccal swab samples, 1 µL of the DNA solution is used directly without prior determination of DNA concentration.
4. Amplify the sample according to the following cycling program (*see* **Note 2**):
   Initial denaturation: 94°C, 3 min. Followed by 35 cycles of: 94°C, 30 s; 61°C, 30 s; 72°C, 30 s. Hold: 72°C, 5 min.
5. Store PCR products at 4°C until electrophoresis.
6. Before electrophoresis, add 2 mL of gel loading buffer to each sample.

3.3. Agarose Gel Electrophoresis of PCR Products

1. Prepare a 2.5% agarose gel by measuring 2.5 g agarose and 100 mL of 1X TAE buffer.
2. Melt to dissolve the agarose. To the cooling agarose, add 5 µL of 10 mg/mL ethidium bromide and mix well.
3. After the agarose is solidified, load 11 µL of the PCR products onto the gel.
4. Electrophoresis until the bromophenol blue dye has migrated two-third of the length of the gel.
5. Photograph the gel using a Polaroid camera by sliding the gel off the gel tray onto a medium wave UV transilluminator.

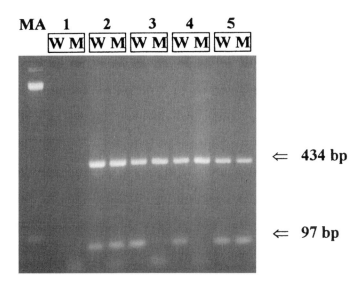

Fig. 1. I1307K mutation detection by allele specific PCR. Samples from four different patients (lanes 2 to 5) were subjected to PCR detection using either the wild type (W) or mutant (M) master mixes. Lanes 2 and 3 are blood samples and lanes 4 and 5 are buccal swabs. Lane 1 is a reagent blank control, with TE buffer substituted for DNA. A 123 bp DNA marker (MA) was used, and 2.5% agarose gel electrophoresis was performed to separate the PCR products. Growth hormone gene amplification shows a 434 bp band whereas *APC* gene amplification shows a 97 bp band. Primer-dimer running in front of the 97 bp band can be seen in some lanes. Patients 2 and 5 are heterozygous for the I130K mutation, whereas patients 3 and 4 do not carry the mutation.

3.4. Interpretation of Results

1. The reagent blank should not show any bands unless there is cross contamination. The growth hormone gene internal control should show a distinct band of 434 bp for all samples analyzed (*see* **Fig. 1**). The APC PCR product should show a distinct band of 97 bp. For a normal individual, the 97 bp PCR product will only be detected when the wild type PCR mix is used. Similarly, an individual who is heterozygous for the I1307K mutation will have the 97 bp band detected when either the wild type or mutant PCR mix is used.

2. The internal control is used to confirm the presence of amplifiable DNA in the sample and to monitor the efficiency of the amplification. In an individual who is a heterozygote for the mutation, the internal control bands in both wild type and mutant PCR mixes should be of equal intensities, and the same is true for the APC bands. If the internal control bands are of equal intensities but the APC bands in the wild type and mutant PCR mixes show a significant difference in intensity, one has to be cautious about the possibility of nonspecific amplification. DNA samples may need to be purified further before being subjected to

amplification. Occasionally, for various reasons, the internal control bands for the two different mixes may not show the same intensity, and it is important to consider such differences when interpreting the results for the APC amplification.

3. Occasionally, primer-dimers may appear in the gel. These primer-dimers migrate in front of the 97 bp APC band and should not be confused with the APC band. A higher percentage of agarose gel may be used to achieve a better separation.

4. Notes

1. The ARMS concept utilizes the inability of *Taq* polymerase to extend mismatched primers from the 3'-OH terminus. A mismatch is made more refractory to amplification by substituting a C for a T adjacent to the 3' nucleotide in both the wild type and mutant-specific primers. Using large primers 30-mer (30 nucleotide in length), further enhances specificity of primer annealing so that a higher annealing temperature can be used.

2. The final magnesium concentration and the annealing temperature in the cycling program are crucial to the success of this technique. The magnesium concentration and the annealing temperature have been optimized for DNA isolated using the above protocols. Different DNA isolation protocols may result in different degree of nonspecific amplification and may give false positive results. Optimization of magnesium concentration and annealing temperature may be required if different DNA isolation method is used.

Acknowledgment

I would like to thank Dr. Alex Chiu for critical reading of this chapter.

References

1. Cannon-Albright, L. A., Skolnick, M. H., Bishop, D. T., Lee, R. G., and Burt, R. W. (1988) Common inheritance of susceptibility to colonic adenomatous polyps and associated colorectal cancers. *N. Engl. J. Med.* **319,** 533–537.

2. Houlston, R. S., Collins, A., Slack, J., and Morton, N. E. (1992) Dominant genes for colorectal cancer are not rare. *Ann. Hum. Genet.* **56,** 99–103.

3. Laken, S. J., Peterson, G. M., Gruber, S. B., Oddoux, C., Ostrer, H., Giardiello, F. M., et al. (1997) Familial colorectal cancer in Ashenazim due to a hypermutable tract in APC. *Nature Genet.* **17,** 79–83.

4. Newton, C. R., Graham, A., Heptinstall, L. E., Powell, S. J., Summers, C., Kalsheker, N., et al. (1989) Analysis of any point mutation in DNA. The amplification refractory mutation system (ARMS). *Nucleic Acids Res.* **17,** 2503–2516.

5. Chen, E. Y., Liao, Y. C., Smith, D. H., Barrera-Saldana, H. A., Gelinas, R. E., and Seeburg, P. H. (1989) The human growth hormone locus: nucleotide sequence, biology, and evolution. *Genomics* **4,** 479–497.

6. Kinzler, K. W., Nilbert, M. C., Su, L. K., Vogelstein, B., Bryan, T. M., Levy, D. B., et al. (1991) Identification of FAP locus genes from chromosome 5q21. *Science* **253,** 661–665.

7. Nishisho, I., Nakamura, Y., Miyoshi, Y., Miki, Y., Ando, H., Horii, A., et al. (1991) Mutations of chromosome 5q21 genes in FAP and colorectal cancer patients. *Science* **253,** 665–669.
8. Buffone, G. J. (1985) Isolation of DNA from biological specimens without extraction with phenol. *Clin. Chem.* **31,** 164–165.
9. Miller, S. A., Dykes, D. D., and Polesky, H. F. (1988) A simple salting out procedure for extracting DNA from human nucleated cells. *Nucleic Acids Res.* **16,** 1215.

14

Microsatellite Analysis
of the Insulin-Like Growth Factor II Receptor
in Colorectal Carcinomas

Rhonda F. Souza and Stephen J. Meltzer

1. Introduction

The insulin-like growth factor II (IGFII) growth control pathway is comprised of three major components: IGFII ligand, insulin-like growth factor I receptor (IGFIR), and insulin-like growth factor II receptor (*IGFIIR*). IGFIR and *IGFIIR* work together to maintain constant circulating levels of IGFII. IGFII is a potent mitogen, produced by epithelial cells, which stimulates cell growth and prevents apoptosis by binding to IGFIR *(1,2)*. IGFIR is a member of the receptor tyrosine kinase family *(3)* Upon binding IGFII, IGFIR autophosphorylates tyrosine residues, thereby initiating signaling (**Fig. 1**) *(3)*. Both mitogenic and anti-apoptotic signaling pathways are initiated by the binding of IGFII to IGFIR *(3)*. Both of these pathways require the presence of insulin receptor substrate-1 (IRS-1), which is also phosphorylated by activated IGFIR. In the mitogenic pathway, phosphorylated IRS-1 attracts a linker molecule known as Grb2; Grb2 then activates a series of mitogenic proteins through the Ras/Raf pathway. The second pathway activated by IGFIR prevents apoptosis *(4)*. *IGFIIR* counterbalances the mitogenic and anti-apoptotic effects of IGFII, but unlike IGFIR, *IGFIIR* is not involved in intracellular signaling. Instead, *IGFIIR* binds, internalizes, and allows the degradation of IGFII, with a resulting inhibition of cell division and augmentation of apoptosis *(5)*. Because *IGFIIR* antagonizes the growth-stimulatory and anti-apoptotic effects of IGFII, it is reasonable to postulate that *IGFIIR* plays a tumor-suppressive role. In fact, there is much evidence from primary tumors to support this role in a variety of human cancers *(6)*.

From: *Methods in Molecular Medicine, vol. 50: Colorectal Cancer: Methods and Protocols*
Edited by: S. M. Powell © Humana Press Inc., Totowa, NJ

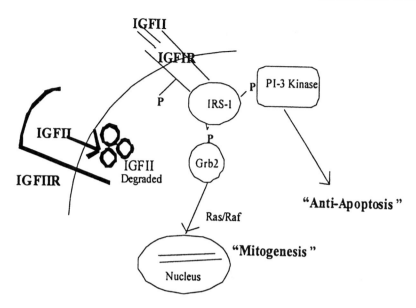

Fig. 1. The Insulin-Like Growth Factor II pathway. IGFII ligand binds IGFIR thereby initiating a signaling cascade which is both mitogenic and anti-apoptotic. IGFIIR counterbalances these mitogenic and anti-apoptotic effects by binding, internalizing, and degrading IGFII thus making IGFII unavailable to activate IGFIR. IGFIR and IGFIIR work together to maintain constant circulating leveles of IGFII.

The gene for *IGFIIR*, mapped to 6q26–27, has been implicated as a tumor suppressor gene in various human cancer types *(7)*. *IGFIIR* exerts its putative antineoplastic effects via two ligands, latent TGF-β1 and IGFII. The binding of secreted TGF-β1 latent complex to *IGFIIR* is essential for cleavage to its active state *(8–10)*. In this active form, TGF-β1 primes a growth-suppressive cascade in epithelial cells; therefore, inactivation of *IGFIIR* (and paralysis of TGF-β1 in its latent, inactive form) should remove normal inhibitory controls on epithelial cell growth. Additionally, *IGFIIR* controls cell division by binding, internalizing and degrading IGFII, a potent cell mitogen which acts on the cell via the insulin-like growth factor I receptor *(11,12)* (**Fig. 1**). Therefore, by increasing levels of active TGF-β1 and by decreasing levels of IGFII, *IGFIIR* apparently tips the balance of forces toward growth suppression.

Clinical evidence supports the role of *IGFIIR* as a tumor suppressor gene. Breast cancer, ovarian cancer, malignant melanoma, and hepatoma frequently display chromosomal deletions and loss of heterozygosity (LOH) at 6q26–27, the *IGFIIR* locus *(13–17)*. Moreover, in *in situ* breast cancers as well as a hepatocellular cancer which both manifested LOH at 6q26–27, missense mutations and an intronic donor splice site mutation of the remaining *IGFIIR* allele were detected, respectively *(15,16)*. Moreover, colorectal carcinoma cells expressed elevated levels of *IGFIIR* mRNA during differentiation; however, despite this increase in receptor levels, IGFII ligand levels remained high, suggesting a dysfunctional IGFIIR *(18)*. Recently, our laboratory and others reported frame-shift mutations in coding region microsatellites within the *IGFIIR* gene in colorectal, gastric, and endometrial carcinomas manifesting microsatellite instability (MSI) *(19,20)*. Furthermore, we showed that expression of exog-enous wild-type *IGFIIR* in colorectal carcinoma cells possessing a mutant endogenous *IGFIIR* allele resulted in growth suppression and increased apoptosis *(21)*.

Finally, loss of function of the *IGFIIR* gene appears to constitute an early event (in vivo). In rats, N-nitrosodiethylamine-induced preneoplastic hepato-cellular lesions did not express *IGFIIR* or TGF-β1 proteins on immunohis-tochemical analysis *(22)*. Moreover, the majority of frankly malignant murine hepatocellular lesions were partially or completely negative for both of these proteins by immunohistochemical staining *(22)*. However, whether preneoplastic lesions lacking *IGFIIR* or TGF-β1 expression preferentially progress to carcinomas has not yet been determined.

Microsatellite instability (MSI) refers to mutations in oligonucleotide repeat sequences; these repeat sequences (microsatellites) are present throughout the human genome *(23–25)*. During DNA replication, the repetitive nature of these microsatellite tracts renders them susceptible to slipped-strand mispairing of bases, which creates small loops in the DNA. These small DNA loops prima-rily cause insertion or deletion mutations. Erroneously paired or unpaired nucleotides are recognized, excised and corrected by DNA mismatch repair (MMR) genes. To date, there have been described six human genes involved in mismatch repair: hMLH1, hMSH2, hMSH3 (DUG), hMSH6 (GTBP), PMS1, and PMS2 *(26–32)*. Tumors demonstrating frequent mutations within micro-satellite tracts are characterized as MSI-positive (MSI+). MSI can occur in both coding and noncoding regions of the genome; however, current opinion regards only MSI within the protein-encoding portions of genes as potentially clinically significant. Therefore, recent interest has focused on identifying genes containing these coding region microsatellite tracts that are targeted by MSI. MSI within these regions creates frameshift mutations, resulting in trun-cated, nonfunctional protein products. The most significant example of this type of mutation occurs within a 10-deoxyadenine tract within TGF-β1RII in gastrointestinal tumors demonstrating MSI *(33–35)*. Interestingly, *IGFIIR* con-tains 17 coding region microsatellite tracts; mutations of these tracts would be predicted to result in a truncated, nonfunctional protein. Examples of *IGFIIR* coding region microsatellites are illustrated below (**Fig. 2**), and the complete *IGFIIR* sequence is available in GenBank (accession # Y00285).

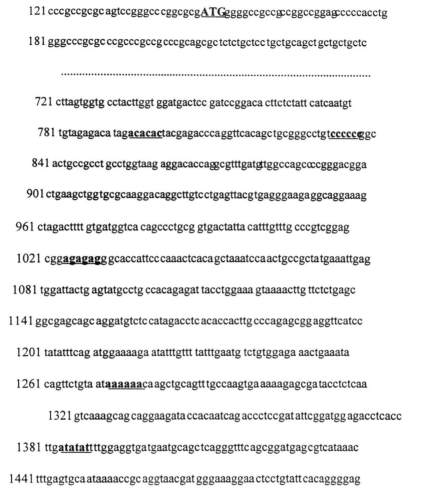

Fig. 2. Examples of *IGFIIR* gene microsatellites. The start codon is "ATG." Microsatellite tracts are bold-underlined, with 5 protein-encoding microsatellites shown - *viz.*, poly-AC, poly-C, poly-AG, poly-A, and poly-AT tracts, respectively.

Among the 17 coding region microsatellite tracts within *IGFIIR*, our laboratory has attempted genomic DNA-based PCR amplification of 10 of these tracts (**Table 1**). Microsatellite tracts were PCR-amplified using primer pairs corresponding to known exonic sequence (**Table 1**). To date, the complete genomic sequence of *IGFIIR*, inclusive of all intron-exon boundaries, has not been submitted into the GenBank registry; however, the genomic sequence of murine *IGFIIR* is available. Using the murine intron-exon boundaries of *IGFIIR* as a guide, we approximated the corresponding intron-exon boundaries of human

Table 1
Primer Sequences Used to Amplify Microsatellites within IGFIIR

Primer sequence		Nucleotides	Repeats	Annealing temperature
B1	5'-TGT GAC GTT TTG CAG-3' 5'-TCC TTG CGC ACC AGC TTC AG-3'	intron 5-920	$(AC)_3$	58°C
B2	5'-TAC GAG ACC CAG GTT CAC AG-3' 5'-TCC TTG CGC ACC AGC TTC AG-3'	800-920	$(C)_6$	No product
R1	Intron interrupts the microsatellite tract	N/A	$(AG)_3$	N/A
R2	5'-TGT CTG TGG AGA AAC TGA AA-3' 5'-GCT GCA TTC ATC ACC TCC AA-3'	1239-1410	$(A)_6$	No product
B3	5'-ATT CGG ATG GAG ACC TCA CC-3' 5'-GTT TAT GAC GCT CAT CCG CT-3'	1361-1471	$(AT)_3$	No product
B4	5'-GGT GCC TAT AAA GTT GAG AC-3' 5'-TTT TTG CCA CCT GGC AGG CT-3'	2089-2197	$(TG)_4$	61°C
B5	5'-GGA TGA TCC AAC TGA ACT AC-3' 5'-TGA TAT TCA GGG AAG CCC AC-3'	2210-2375	$(AC)_4$	61°C
R4	5'-GCA GGT CTC CTG ACT CAG AA-3' 5'-GAA GAA GAT GGC TGT GGA GC-3'	4030-4140	$(G)_8$	58°C
R6	5'-GTA TGC CAT GGA CAA CTC AGG-3' 5'-TGG CAA GCC GAT GCA TAT CGG-3'	2529-2639	$(GT)_3$	54°C
R7	5'-CCT GTG ACC TTT CAG AAC TGG-3' 5'-TAT CCG TCG TTG TCT GAA TGG-3'	intron 19-2935	$(GT)_3$	No product
R5	5'-GAA ACA CAA AAC CTA CGA CC-3' 5'-AGA ACC CAA AAG AGC CAA CC-3'	6141-intron 40	$(CT)_5$	58°C
R8	5'-CAG CTG GTG TAC AAG GAT GGG-3' 5'-AGC GGC GTG TGC CAG GAG AAG-3'	4912-5078	$(CT)_3$	56°C

IGFIIR. Therefore, for microsatellite tracts less than 20 bp from the intron-exon boundary, murine intronic sequence was used to design either the forward or reverse primer (**Table 1**). Not surprisingly, some microsatellite tracts could not be amplified by these murine-derived primer pairs.

We have analyzed 12 of the 17 coding region microsatellite tracts within *IGFIIR* in a group of MSI+ colorectal carcinomas. Our laboratory and others have previously reported frameshift mutations in 2 of these 17 tracts (locus R4 and R5, **Table 1**) in MSI+ colorectal, gastric and endometrial carcinomas *(19,20)*. We examined a total of 51 MSI+ colorectal tumors, of which 5 (9%) demonstrated *IGFIIR* mutation. Grouped by specific tissue type, these included 1/8 HNPCC tumors (12.5%), 3/35 MSI+ sporadic colorectal cancers (9%), and 1/8 MSI+ ulcerative colitis (UC)-associated colorectal cancers (12.5%). All mutations occurred within an 8 poly-deoxyguanine (8G) tract spanning nucleotides 4089 to 4096 of the *IGFIIR* coding sequence (locus R4, **Table 1**, **Fig. 3**). The poly-G tract mutations comprised a one-basepair deletion within this microsatellite region, causing a frameshift and a premature stop codon downstream. None of the MSI+ colorectal carcinomas demonstrated mutation within a poly-CT tract (locus R5, **Table 1**); mutation of this tract was seen only in one MSI+ gastric carcinoma *(19)*. Subsequently, we also detected MSI within a poly-GT tract spanning nucleotides 2529 to 2639 (locus R6, **Table 1**) in 2/27 MSI+ colorectal carcinomas (7%) (unpublished data). This poly-GT mutation comprised a two-basepair deletion within the repetitive tract, causing a truncated, putatively nonfunctional protein. Of the remaining 9 microsatellite tracts investigated, 5 could not be amplified by PCR (**Table 1**). This failure to generate PCR product was probably a result of intervening intronic sequences. The final 4 microsatellite tracts were successfully amplified; however, only wild-type alleles were identified in our colorectal carcinomas (**Table 1**). The remaining 5 coding region microsatellite tracts, which are located in the distal-most 3' region of *IGFIIR*, were not analyzed.

Since submission of this chapter, the complete genomic sequence of human IGFIIR has been sequenced *(36)*. The intron-exon boundries of human IGFIIR and intronic primer sequences designed to amplify all 48 exons of human IGFIIR are now available in print *(36)* and at www.geneimprint.com.

2. Materials

2.1. Tissue Homogenization and DNA Extraction

1. Tissue.
2. Liquid nitrogen.
3. Mortar and pestle (Fisher Scientific, Houston, TX).
4. Proteinase K (Gibco-BRL, Gaithersburg, MD).

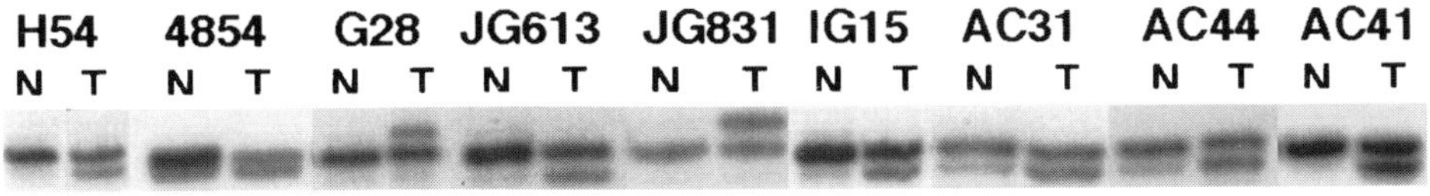

Fig. 3. Mutation of *IGFIIR* . H54 (N and T), normal and tumor DNAs from a patient with ulcerative colitis-associated colorectal cancer; 4854, G28, JG613, JG831, and IG15 (N and T), DNAs from patients with gastric cancer; AC31and AC44 (N and T), DNAs from patients with sporadic colorectal adenocarcinoma; AC41 (N and T), DNAs from a patient with HNPCC. Mutations were demonstrated using primer set R4, except for 4854 N,T (with a mutation demonstrated using primer set R5). An abnormally migrating band, located just above or below the wild-type band, is visible in each of the tumor (T) lanes.

5. TE buffer: Tris-HCl base 10 mM and EDTA 1 mM, adjusted to pH 8.0 (Sigma, St. Louis, MO).
6. 20% SDS (Sigma).
7. Saturated phenol buffer, pH 8.0 (Gibco-BRL).
8. Chloroform (Fisher Scientific).
9. 5 M NaCl (Sigma).
10. Microfuge tubes.

2.2. PCR Amplifications

1. Recombinant Taq polymerase (Gibco-BRL).
2. Oligonucleotides (stock 100–150 ng/µL) (**Table 1**).
3. Deoxynucleotide triphosphates (dATP, dCTP, dTTP, dGTP) (stock 12.5 mM) (Gibco-BRL).
4. Sterile water.
5. Robocylcer (Stratagene, La Jolla, CA).
6. 0.5 mL microfuge tubes.
7. Mineral oil (Sigma).
8. ^{32}P-labeled dCTP (New England Nuclear, Boston, MA).
9. Template (genomic DNA).

2.3. Gel Electrophoresis and Autoradiography

1. Sequencing buffer: to formamide add 0.5 M EDTA, 10% bromophenol blue, and 10% xylene cyanol.
2. Gel electrophoresis apparatus, accessories, and power supply.
3. Sequagel sequencing system: Sequagel concentrate, Sequagel diluent, and Sequagel buffer (National Diagnostics, Atlanta, GA).
4. 10X TBE buffer: Tris base 0.89 M, boric acid 0.89 M, and EDTA 0.02 M (Sigma).
5. Ammonium persulfate (stock 25%) (Sigma) and TEMED (Sigma).
6. Whatman filter paper (Fisher Scientific).

7. Film cassette 14 × 17 inches (Fisher Scientific).
8. Plastic wrap.
9. Autoradiographic film (Kodak X-Omat, Rochester, NY), developer and processor.

3. Methods

3.1. DNA Extraction

3.1.1. Proteinase K Digestion of Tissue

1. Pour 5–10 mL of liquid nitrogen into mortar followed by tissue sample (*see* **Note 1**).
2. Using pestle, homogenize tissue specimen into finely ground powder.
3. Scrape tissue into 2 mL microfuge tube.
4. Pipet 900 μL of TE, pH 8.0 and 50 μL of 20% SDS into the microfuge tube containing the homogenized tissue. Incubate in 37°C water bath for 1 h.
5. Pipet 50 μL of 10mg/mL Proteinase K solution into the microfuge tubes and incubate overnight at 56°C.

3.1.2. Phenol-Chloroform Extraction of DNA

1. Split each 1 mL volume into two 1.5 mL tubes containing 500 μL each (*see* **Note 2**).
2. Pipet one volume of buffer-saturated phenol (pH 8.0) and 10 μL of 5M NaCl into each tube containing overnight-digested sample.
3. Shake 20 times to mix.
4. Centrifuge for 4 min at 3000*g*.
5. Transfer aqueous phase to a fresh tube.
6. Pipet one volume of phenol/chloroform to the aqueous phase of **step 5** and add 10 μL of NaCl.
7. Shake 20 times to mix.
8. Centrifuge for 4 min at 3000*g*.
9. Transfer aqueous phase to a fresh tube.
10. Pipet 1 vol of chloroform to the aqueous phase of **step 9** and add 10 μL of NaCl.
11. Shake 20 times to mix.
12. Centrifuge for 4 min at 3000*g*.
13. Transfer aqueous phase to a fresh tube.

3.1.3. Ethanol Precipitation of DNA

1. Pipet 2.5–3 vol of 100% ethanol to the clear sample of **step 13**.
2. Place sample in –80°C overnight to precipitate the DNA.
3. Centrifuge at 4°C for 30 min at 10,000*g*.
4. Wash the pellet with cold 70% alcohol, centrifuge for 5 min at 10,000*g*, dispose of the supernatant, and allow to air-dry.
5. Dissolve in 50–100 μL of water or TE.
6. Measure OD with spectrophotometer.

3.2. PCR Amplification

1. Approximately 100 ng of genomic DNA is mixed with 0.1 µL of specific *IGFIIR* primer (stock 100–150 ng/µL) (**Table 1**), 0.25 µL of recombinant *Taq* polymerase, 1 µL of buffer, 0.6 µL of 50 m*M* MgCl$_2$, 1.5 µL of 12.5 m*M* dNTPs, and 0.2 µL of P^{32} in a 10 µL reaction (*see* **Note 3**).
2. One drop of mineral oil is added to each reaction tube above, the tubes are then centrifuged for 5–10 s.
3. PCR conditions are 94°C for 1 min, specific annealing temperature depending on the primer used (**Table 1**) for 1 min, and 72°C for 2 min for 35 cycles.
4. PCR products can be electrophoresed immediately or stored at –20°C.

3.3. Gel Electrophoresis and Autoradiography

3.3.1. Preparation of the Sequencing Gel

1. Combine 15 mL of Sequenase buffer, 36 mL of Sequenase concentrate, and 99 mL of Sequenase diluent into 500 mL beaker and mix.
2. Remove 50 mL to be used to pour the base of the gel and add 150 µL of 25% APS and 150 µL of TEMED. Quickly pour into the base of the sequencing apparatus to seal the bottom and allow to polymerize for approximately 30 min.
3. To the remaining 100 mL of gel mix in **step 1**, add 320 µL of 25% APS and 40 µL of TEMED.
4. Using a 50 mL pipet, pour the gel mix between the two glass plates of the sequencing apparatus (*see* **Note 4**).
5. Add comb and allow to polymerize for 1.5–2 h.
6. Following polymerization, fill the apparatus with 1X TBE running buffer and preheat the gel to 55°C.

3.3.2. Electrophoresis and Autoradiography

1. Pipet 10 µL of sequencing buffer and 1 µL of radiolabeled PCR product into a 0.5-mL tube.
2. Boil at 94°C for 2 min.
3. Load 3.5 µL of sample into the preheated gel.
4. Electrophorese at a constant current (approx 100 W) till the blue dye is at the bottom of the gel (approx 2–2.5 h) (*see* **Note 5**).
5. Take down apparatus and place gel on Whatman paper, cover with plastic wrap, and place into film cassette with Kodak X-Omat film.
6. Expose overnight at –80, then develop film.

4. Notes

1. Homoginization of the tissue in liquid nitrogen is to prevent degradation of the RNA and DNA during the extraction process. As the liquid nitrogen evaporates, continue to add more to the mortar until the tissue is ground to a fine powder.
2. Splitting each 1 mL volume into 2 tubes with 500 µL each allows the phenol:chloroform extraction centrifugation steps to be carried out easily in a microfuge.

3. As a negative control, add all the reagents for the PCR reaction but eliminate the genomic DNA; there should be no resultant PCR product from this reaction tube. The presence of a PCR product from this reaction tube signals contamination of your reagents by genomic DNA or PCR product. As a positive control, add all the reagent for the PCR reaction with a known primer such as β-action or GADPH that easily amplifies to ensure there has been no technical error during the reaction setup.

4. When pouring the gel, place the gel apparatus at an angle. An easy method that works well is to lay an empty pipet tip box on its side and rest the sequencing apparatus on top of the pipet tip box. Pour the gel slowly between the plates avoiding bubble formation. If bubbles do form, raise up the gel apparatus such that the bubble rises to the top of the unpolymerized gel solution and dissapate. Then return the apparatus to its resting angled position and finishing slowing pouring the remainder of the gel.

5. Electrophoresis time for each PCR product will vary slighly based on differences in size of the various products. The blue dye used in the sequence buffer will migrate at approximately the same rate as a PCR product of 100 bp. Using this approximation as a guide will assist in adjusting electrophoresis times for the various PCR products.

Acknowledgments

This work was supported by CA73782 and the Medical Research Office, Department of Veterans Affairs (Rhonda F. Souza); CA85069, CA78843, CA77957, DK47717, DK53620, and the Medical Research Office, Department of Veterans Affairs (Steven J. Meltzer).

References

1. Kulik, G., Klippel, A., and Weber, M. J. (1997) Antiapoptotic signalling by the insulin-like growth factor I receptor, phosphatidylinositol 3-kinase, and Akt. *Mol. Cell. Biol.* **17,** 1595–1606.
2. Stewart, C. E. and Rotwein, P. (1996) Insulin-like growth factor-II is an autocrine survival factor for differentiating myoblasts. *J. Biol. Chem.* **10,** 11,330–11,338.
3. Blakesley, V. A., Stannard, B. S., Kalebic, T., Helman, L. J., and LeRoith D. (1997) Role of the IGF-I receptor in mutagenesis and tumor promotion. *J. Endo.* **152,** 339–344.
4. Sell, C., Baserga, R., and Rubin, R. (1995) Insulin-like grwoth factor I (IGF-I) and the IGF–1 receptor prevent etoposide-induced apoptosis. *Cancer Res.* **55,** 303–306.
5. Oka, Y., Rozek, L. M., and Czech, M. P. (1985) Direct demonstration of rapid insulin-like growth factor II receptor internalization and recycling in rat adipocytes. *J. Biol. Chem.* **260,** 9435–9442.
6. Ellis, M. J. C., Leav, B. A., Yang, Z., et. al. (1996) Affinity for the insulin-like growth factor-II (IGF-II) receptor inhibits autocrine IGF-II activity in MCF-7 breast cancer cells. *Mol. Endo.* **10,** 286–297.

7. Laureys, G., Barton, D. E., Ullrich, A., et al. (1988) Chromosomal mapping of the gene for the type II insulin-like growth factor receptor/cation-independent mannose 6-phosphate receptor in man and mouse. *Genomics* **3**, 224–229.

8. Purchio, A. F., Cooper, J. A., Brunner, A. M., Lioubin, M. N., et al. (1988) Identification of mannose 6-phosphate in two asparagine-linked sugar chains of recombinant transforming growth factor-beta1 precursor. *J. Biol. Chem.* **263**, 14,211–14,215.

9. Kojima, S., Nara, K., and Rifkin, D. B. (1993) Requirement for transglutaminase in the activation of latent transforming growth factor-beta in bovine endothelial cells. *J. Cell. Biol.* **121**, 439–448.

10. Dennis, P. A. and Rifkin, D. B. (1991) Cellular activation of latent transforming growth factor β requires binding to the cation-independent mannose 6-phosphate/insulin-like growth factor type II receptor. *Proc. Natl. Acad. Sci. USA* **88**, 580–584.

11. Kornfeld, S. (1992) Structure and function of the mannose 6-phosphate/insulin-like growth factor II receptors. *A. Rev. Biochem.* **61**, 307–330.

12. Dahms, N. M., Lobel, P., and Kornfeld, S. (1989) Mannose 6-phosphate recceptors and lysosomal enzyme targeting. *J. Biol. Chem.* **264**, 12,115–12,118.

13. Devilee, P., van Vliet, M., van Sloun, P., et al. (1991) Allelotype of human breast caracinoma: a second major site for loss of heterozygosity is on chromosome 6q. *Oncogene* **6**, 1705–1711.

14. Millikin, D., Meese, E., Vogelstein, B., Witkowski, C., and Trent, J. (1991) Loss of heterozygosity for loci on the long arm of chromosome 6 in human malignant melanoma. *Cancer Res.* **51**, 5449–5453.

15. De Souza, A. T., Hankins, G. R., et al. (1995) Frequent loss of heterozygosity on 6q at the mannose 6-phosphate/insulin-like growth factor II receptor locus in human hepatocellular tumors. *Oncogene* **10**, 1725–1729.

16. Hankins, G. R., De Souza, A. T., Bentley, R. C., et al. (1996) M6P/IGF2 receptor: a candidate breast tumor suppressor gene. *Oncogene* **12**, 2003–2009.

17. De Souza, A. T., Hankins, G.R., Washington, M. K., et al. (1995) M6P/IGF2R gene is mutated in human hepatocellular carcinomas with loss of heterozygosity. *Nature Genet.* **11**, 447–449.

18. Hoeflich, A., Yang, Y., Rascher, W., et al. (1996) Coordinate expression of insulin-like growth factor II (IGF-II) and IGF-II/mannose–6-phosphate receptor mRNA and stable expression of IGF-I receptor mRNA during differentiation of human colon carcinoma cells (Caco-2). *Europ. J. Endo.* **135**, 49–59.

19. Souza, R. F., Appel, R.,Yin, J., et al. (1996) Microsatellite instability in the insulin-like growth factor II receptor gene in gastrointestinal tumors. *Nature Genet.* **14**, 255–257.

20. Ouyang, H., Shiwaku, H., Hagiwara, H., et al. (1997) The insulin-like growth receptor gene is mutated in genetically unstable cancers of the endometrium, stomach and colorectum. *Cancer Res.* **57**, 1851–1854.

21. Souza, R. F., Wang, S., Thakar, M., et al. (1999) Expression of the wild-type insulin-like growth factor II receptor gene suppresses growth and causes death in colorectal carcinoma cells. *Oncogene* **18**, 4063–4068.

22. Jirtle, R. L., Hankins, G. R., Reisenbichler, H., and Boyer, I. J. (1994) Regulation of mannose 6-phosphate/insulin-like growth factor-II receptors and transforming growth factor βeta during liver tumor promotion with phenobarbital. *Carcinogenesis* **15**, 1473–1478.

23. Thibodeau, S. N., Bren, G., and Schaid, D. (1993) Microsatellite instability in cancer of the proximal colon. *Science* **260**, 816-819.

24. Ionov, Y., Peinado, M. A., Malkhosyan, S., Shibata, D., and Perucho, M. (1993) Ubiquitous somatic mutations in simple repeated sequences reveal a new mechanism for colonic carcinogenesis. *Nature* **363**, 558–561.

25. Aaltonen, L. A., Paltomaki, P., Meling, G. I., et al. (1993) Clues to the pathogenesis of familial colorectal cancer. *Science* **260**, 812–816.

26. Fishel, R., Lescoe, M. K., Rao, M. R. S., Copeland, N. G., Jenkins, N. A., Garber, J., Kane, M., and Kolodner, R. (1993) The human mutator gene hololog MSH2 and its association with hereditary nonpolyposis colon cancer. *Cell* **75**, 1027–1038.

27. Bronner, C. E., Baker, S. M., Morrison, P. T., Warren, G., Smith, L. G., Lescoe, M. K., Kane, M., et al. (1994) Mutation in the DNA mismatch repair gene homologue hMLH1 is associated with hereditary nonpolyposis colon cancer. *Nature* **368**, 258.

28. Leach, F., Nicolaides, N. C., Papodopoulous, N., Liu, B., Jen, J., Parson, R., Peltomaki, P., Sistonen, P., Aaltonen, L. A., et al. (1993) Mutations of a mutS homolog in hereditary nonpolyposis colorectal cancer. *Cell* **75**, 1215–1225.

29. Papadopoulos, N., Nicolaides, N. C., Wei, Y.-F., Ruben, S. M., et al. (1994) Mutation of a mutL homolog in hereditary colon cancer. *Science* **263**, 1625.

30. Palombo, F., Gallinari, P., Iaccarino, I., Lettiere, T., Hughes, M., D'Arrigo, A., Truong, O., Hsuan, J. J., and Jiricny, J. (1995) GTBP, a 160-kilodalton protein essential for mismatch-binding activity in human cells. *Science* **268**, 1912–1914.

31. Malkhosyan, S., Rampino, N., Yamamoto, H., and Perucho, M. (1996) Frameshift mutator mutations. *Nature* **382**, 499–500.

32. Nicolaides, N. C., Papadopoulos, N., Liu, B., Wei, Y.-F., Carter, K. C., Ruben, S. M., et al. (1994) Mutations of two PMS homologues in hereditary nonpolyposis colon cancer. *Nature* **371**, 75–84.

33. Parsons, R., Myeroff, L. L., Liu, B., et al. (1995) Microsatellite instability and mutations of the transforming growth factor β type II receptor gene in colorectal cancer. *Cancer Res.* **55**, 5548–5550.

34. Myeroff, L. L., Parsons, R., Kim, S. J., et al. (1995) Transforming growth factor B receptor type II gene mutation common in colon and gastric but rare in endometrial cancers with microsatellite instability. *Cancer Res.* **55**, 5545–5547.

35. Souza, R. F., Lei, J., Yin, J., Appel, R., Zou, T.-T., Zhou, X.-L., Wang, S., Rhyu, M.-G., et al. (1997) A transforming growth factor β1 receptor type II mutation in ulcerative colitis-associated neoplasms. *Gastroenterology* **112**, 40–45.

36. Killian, J. K. and Jirtle, R. L. (1999) Genomic structure of the human M6P/IGF2 receptor. *Mammalian Genome* **10**, 74–77.

15

Molecular Detection of *Smad2/Smad4* Alterations in Colorectal Tumors

Sam Thiagalingam

1. Introduction

The signaling pathways mediated by the transforming growth factor-β (TGF-β) family of factors are implicated in a wide array of biological processes including cell differentiation and proliferation, determination of cell fate during embryogenesis, cell adhesion and cell death. The recent discovery of the SMAD family of signal transducer proteins as mediators of TGF-β relaying signals from cell membrane to nucleus has revolutionized the understanding of the molecular basis of these processes *(1,2)*. To date, at least eight homologues of the *Smad* genes have been identified and shown to be downstream of the serine/threonine kinase receptors (**Table 1**). SMADs are molecules of relative mass 42K–60K composed of two regions of homology at the amino and carboxy terminals of the protein. The activation of SMADs by receptors upon TGF-β binding results in the formation of hetero-oligomeric complexes and translocation to the nucleus where transcription of target genes is effected. However, some of the SMADs apparently inhibit rather than mediate, TGF-β signaling. These inhibitory SMADs are also induced by TGF-β stimulation suggesting that there is an intracellular negative–feedback loop.

The SMAD family of proteins is divided into three distinct classes based on their structure and function *(1)*. The first category consists of pathway-restricted or receptor regulated Smads (R-Smads): Smad1, Smad5, and Smad8 are specifically involved in bone morphogenetic protein (BMP) signaling whereas Smad2 and Smad3 are TGF-β/activin pathway restricted. These Smads are directly phosphorylated by a type I receptor upon the latter's activation by ligating to a type II receptor bound to the ligand. The pathway restricted Smads have a characteristic Ser-Ser-X-Ser (SSXS) motif in their C-terminal region.

From: *Methods in Molecular Medicine, vol. 50: Colorectal Cancer: Methods and Protocols*
Edited by: S. M. Powell © Humana Press Inc., Totowa, NJ

Table 1
Human SMAD Genes and Cancers

Gene	Map position	Affected cancers	Reference(s)
SMAD1	4q28–31	None	24
SMAD2	18q21	Colon	24,26,32
SMAD3	15q21–22	None	24,33
SMAD4	18q21	Lung, pancreatic, and colon	22–25,33
SMAD5	5q31	None	24,33
SMAD6	15q21–22	None	24,33
SMAD7	18q21	None	24,33,34
SMAD8/MADH6	13q12–14	None	35

The two-most C-terminal serine residues of these Smads are phosphorylated by type I receptors. Unlike the R-Smads, the common-mediator Smads (Co-Smads) belonging to the second class, are required by all distinct pathways and play a central role by forming heteromeric complexes with the R-Smads, translocate into the nucleus, and each complex activates a specific set of genes through cooperative interactions with DNA and other DNA-binding proteins such as FAST1, FAST2, and Jun/Fos. Smad4 is the only member of this class of Smads known in mammals. However, the recent identification of two Smad4 proteins (XSmadα and XSmadβ) in *Xenopus* opens up the possibility that analogues of Smad4 may exist in mammals *(3)*. Smad4 lacks the C-terminal SSXS motif and is not phosphorylated by type I receptors. The third class includes Smad6 and Smad7 which were identified as anti-Smads due to their ability to act as inhibitors of TGF-β signaling. Smad6 and Smad7 associate stably with type I receptors inhibiting phosphorylation of R-Smads in TGF-β signaling. Furthermore, it has been postulated that Smad6 may compete with Smad4 to associate with Smad1 in BMP signaling *(4)*. A model for the current thinking illustrating the different roles of the Smads in TGF-β signaling is outlined in **Fig. 1**.

Although TGF-β was originally discovered for its positive role in transformation and tumor progression, most of the recent effort has focused on the mechanism of epithelial cell growth inhibition *(2,5,6)*. It has been shown that TGF-β induces expression and activation of the cdk inhibitors p15, p27, and p21 suggesting that growth inhibition may be mediated through these effectors. TGF-β overexpression is often seen in advanced human carcinomas *(7–10)*. It is not clear whether these observations represent the cause or consequence of tumor formation. One possibility is that it induces the vigor of tumor progression aiding in increased severity of the disease by somehow promoting tumor proliferation by direct action on the tumor cell *per se*. On the other hand, it may represent insensitivity of the tumor cell to growth inhibition by TGF-β due to defects in the receptors or down stream signaling pathway components such as the SMADs.

Insensitivity to TGF-β is found to be common in a variety of human cancers, emphasizing the importance of pathways mediated by this polypeptide to the neoplastic process *(11–13)*. The early investigations to understand the molecular basis of this resistance were concentrated at the level of TGF-β receptors. A correlation between resistance to TGF-β growth inhibition due to lack of TGF-β receptor expression was established and reported in a variety of human cancer cell lines *(14–17)*. The first genetic evidence for inactivation of the TGF-β signaling pathway due to mutations causing structural defects in the TGF-β receptor type II (RII) revolutionized the understanding of the molecular basis of this defect *(15,17,18)*. Although RII mutations were initially reported in colon cancer with microsatellite instability (MSI) resulting from frame shifts clustered in a naturally occurring 10 bp microsatellite-like polyadenine tract in the 5' coding half of the gene, subsequent studies demonstrated that additional sites such as residues in the kinase domain could also be inactivated in both MSI and non-MSI colon tumors *(17–19)*. Furthermore, there is also evidence that TGF-β receptor type I (RI) could become inactivated in a subset of other cancers *(13)*. However these alterations alone do not explain the mechanism of inactivation of the TGF-β signaling pathway in an overwhelming number of tumors that are resistant to TGF-β. The recent discovery of the *Smad* genes as downstream effectors of TGF-β signaling pathway and mutations in these genes could be regarded as a major breakthrough in the understanding of the molecular basis of insensitivity to TGF-β mediated effects *(20–26)*.

The isolation of the *Smad4* gene itself was based on identification of target tumor suppressor genes localized to frequent homozygous deletions affecting 18q21.1 in pancreatic carcinomas *(25)*. In addition to pancreatic cancer, *Smad4* mutations were also found in a subset of colon and lung cancers but rarely in others *(20–24;* **Table 2**). We have recently isolated five novel *Smad* genes in addition to the *Smad4* gene isolated by our colleagues as a candidate tumor suppressor gene localized to chromosome 18q21 *(26;* **Table 1**). One of the novel genes isolated by us, *Smad2*, also localized to 18q21 and became a legitimate alternate candidate for tumor suppressor genes localized to this region. We were able to demonstrate that *Smad2* is also inactivated in additional colorectal tumors of the same set with LOH at 18q21 analyzed by us for *Smad4* inactivation *(26;* **Table 3**).

Interestingly, the association of chromosome 18q loss with advanced stages of human cancer and the observation of increased malignant conversion frequency and decreased carcinoma latency in mice expressing the TGF-β receptor RII deletion, illustrate that disabling the TGF-β signaling pathway may be a critical late event in the multistep cancer progression *(22,27–31)*. Further-more, the clustering of related genes in a critical region of chromosome 18q21 loss raises an intriguing possibility that there may be additional genes of this kind localized to this region in addition to potentially unrelated target genes *(22,26)*. This is a testable hypothesis but requires more effort of positional cloning directed to this region as well as genomic sequencing efforts targeting the MLR (Minimally Lost Region) identified in our study. Since, *Smad4* and *Smad2* were identified as genes localized to 18q21 and harbor a significant degree of genetic alterations in colorectal cancers, here we provide detailed protocols for detecting these abnormalities.

1.1. Experimental Procedures
to Detect Molecular Alterations in Smad2/Smad4

Inactivation of SMAD genes is presumed to occur *via* two hits in a classical model for inactivation of tumor suppressor genes *(40,41)*. The analysis con-sisted of the determination of LOH (loss of heterozygosity) for 18q by deter-mining allelic loss in tumors or their derivative cell lines or Xenografts with the adjacent matched normal tissue followed by RT-PCR analysis to determine any defects at the level of transcription. Subsequently, searching for mutations is initially conducted by the "in vitro synthesized protein" (IVSP) assay to scan for truncating mutations *(22,24,42)*. This assay detects nonsense mutations, insertions or deletions creating frameshifts, splice site alterations, and in-frame deletions or insertions of greater than 25 bp. The only type of mutations unde-tectable by this method are missense mutations which could be detected by direct sequencing. Since truncating mutations are more definite proof of gene inactivation, it should serve as an indicator of whether the gene is altered in tumors by mutations.

Fig. 1. *(opposite page)* A model for the Smad connection to the TGF-β signaling pathway. TGF-β binds a type-II receptor kinase, which phosphorylates a type I recep-tor kinase that initiates signaling via the Smad proteins. The activated type I receptor kinase recognizes the receptor regulated Smads (R-Smad), such as Smad2, Smad3 or others, and phosphorylates them at the carboxy-terminal serine residues. The phos-phorylated R-Smad forms a heteromeric complex with the common-mediator Smads (Co-Smad) such as Smad4, and translocate into the nucleus. In the nucleus, the R-Smad/ Co-Smad heterodimer, by themselves or by associating with a heterologous Smad interacting DNA binding protein (SIDBP) such as FAST-1, mediates specific tran-scriptional responses. The inhibitory Smads (I-Smad), such as Smad6, lack the C-terminal motif –SSXS in R-Smads and are able to compete with the latter by stably binding the activated type I receptor kinase effectively blocking the signaling cascade of events.

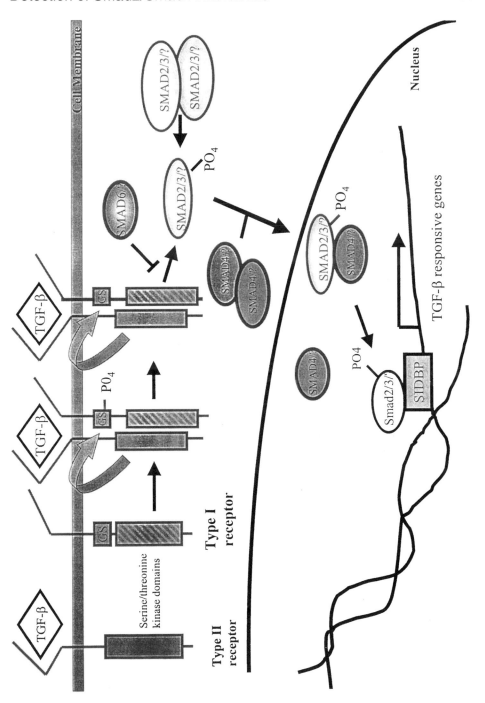

Table 2
Mutations in Smad4

Codon	Mutation	Predicted change	Cancer	Reference(s)
43	TTG to TCG	Leu to Ser	Pancreas	33
100	AGG to ACG	Arg to Thr	Pancreas	23
115	TGT to CGT	Cys to Arg	Colon	36
130	GTC to GAC	Pro to Ser	Colon	22
162	2bp deletion	Frameshift/stop	Pancreas	33
168	GGA to TGA	Gly to stop	Colon	36
195	TACA to TAA	Tyr to stop	Pancreas	33
195	TAC to TAA	Tyr to stop	Colon	36
202–203	4bp deletion	Frameshift/stop	Lung	20
269–270	ACT to ACTT	Frameshift/stop	Colon	36
336–338	2bp deletion(GA)	Frameshift/stop	Colon (HNPCC)	36
339–343	15bp deletion	Frameshift	Colon	36
343	TCA to TGA	Ser to stop	Pancreas	23
343	2bp deletion	Frameshift/stop	Pancreas	23
351	GAT to CAT	Asp to His	Pancreas	23
358	GGA to TGA	Gly to stop	Colon, pancreas	22,25
361	CGC to TGC	Arg to Cys	Colon	22
361	CGC to CAC	Arg to His	Colon	36
363	TGT to AGT	Cys to Ser	Colon	36
369	AAT to GAT	Asn to Asp	Pancreas	37
370	GTC to GAC	Val to Asp	Colon	22
406	GCG to ACG	Ala to Thr	Pancreas	33
412	TAC to TAG	Tyr to Stop	Pancreas	25
415–416	4bp deletion	Frameshift/stop	Colon	36
420	CGT to CAT	Arg to His	Lung	20
441	CGT to CCT	Arg to Pro	Lung	20
442	CAG to TAG	Gln to Stop	Colon	36
445	CGA to TGA	Arg to Stop	Colon	36
447–455	25bp deletion	Frameshift/stop	Colon	36
450–459	28bp deletion	Frameshift/stop	Colon	36
457	GCA to TCA	Ala to Ser	Pancreas	37
483	AGT to AAT	Aberrant splicing	Pancreas	25
493	GAT to CAT	Asp to His	Pancreas	25
497	CGC to CAC	Arg to His	Colon	36
507	AAA to CAA	Lys to Gln	Colon	36
515	AGA to GGA	Arg to Gly	Colon	36
515	AGA to TGA	Arg to Stop	Pancreas	25,37
516	CAG to TAG	Gln to Stop	Colitis	38
516–518	8 bp deletion	Frameshift/stop	Pancreas	25
525	ATT to GTT	Ile to Val	Head and neck	39
526	GAA to TAA	Glu to Stop	Head and neck	39
528/529	4bp deletion	Frameshift/stop	Pancreas	37
540–542	7bp deletion	Frameshift/stop	Colon	36

Table 3
Mutations in *Smad2*

Codon	Mutation	Predicted change	Cancer	Reference(s)
133	CGC to TGC	Arg to Cys	Colon	*32*
345–358	42 bp in deletion	In frame deletion	Colon	*26*
346	TTT to GTT	Phe to Val	Colon	*36*
431–454	9 bp in deletion	In frame deletion	Lung	*21*
440	CTT to CGT	Leu to Arg	Colon	*32*
445	CCT to CAT	Pro to His	Colon	*32*
450	GAC to GAG	Asp to Glu	Colon	*32*
450	GAC to CAC	Asp to His	Lung	*21*

The mutant products identified by RT-PCR and IVSP analysis are tested once again by independent experiments to confirm the observed abnormality *(22)*. Such confirmed alterations are further investigated by direct sequencing of the RT-PCR product. In the case of splice site variants, genomic DNA is sequenced to confirm such an abnormality. If the target gene is a tumor suppressor gene, these methods should be sufficient to detect an alteration indicating an inactivation.

1.2. Genomic DNA and Total RNA from Colorectal Cancer Cell Lines/Xenografts

Surgically-removed colorectal tumors are disaggregated and implanted into nude mice or into in vitro culture conditions as previously described *(22,43)*. The tumor derived lines passaged in vitro (passages <3) and in nude mice following their establishment, are used to prepare RNA and DNA. Total RNA is purified using the guanidine thiocyanate method. The kit from Promega (Madison, WI) works equally well. DNA is purified using standard sodium dodecyl sulfate-proteinase K digestion and phenol-chloroform extraction.

1.3. Allelic Loss Analysis

The microsatellite markers used for LOH analysis in our study are listed *(22)*. The markers encompassing the MLR for 18q21 include D18S535, D18S851, and D18S858. The primers for each of the markers analyzed could be synthesized based on the sequence information available from CHLC (The Cooperative Human Linkage Center) or obtained from Research Genetics (Huntsville, AL). One primer of each pair is end-labeled with ^{32}P-γ-ATP and T4 polynucleotide kinase and PCR amplifications are carried out in 96 well plates in a 10 μL reaction *(22)*. The reaction mixture contains 67 mM Tris-HCl, pH 8.8, 16.6 mM ammonium sulfate, 6.7 mM magnesium chloride, 10 mM

Table 4
RT-PCR Primers for *Smad2* and *Smad4*

Primer ID	Sequence
Smad2 RT-FP	5'-GGA TCC TAA TAC GAC TCA CTA TAG GGA GAC CAC CAT GGG TAA GAA CAT GTC CAT C-3'
Smad2 RT-RP	5'-TTT CCA TGG GAC TTG ATT GG-3'
Smad4 RT-FP	5'-GGA TCC TAA TAC GAC TCA CTA TAG GGA GAC CAC CAT GGA CAA TAT GTC TAT TAC GAA TAC-3'
Smad4 RT-RP	5'-TTT TTT ATA AAC AGG ATT GTA TTT TGT AGT CC-3'

β-mercaptoethanol, 6% dimethyl sulfoxide, 100 μM each of dATP, dGTP, dCTP, and dTTP, 0.02 mM each of the primers, 10 ng of DNA template and 0.5 μL of Platinum Taq (Gibco-BRL). An initial denaturation at 95°C for 2 min is followed by 30 cycles, each carried out at 95°C for 30 s, 55–60°C for 1 min, and 70°C for 1 min.

1.4. RT-PCR

Total RNA from the appropriate samples are used as templates for the synthesis of the first strand cDNA using SuperScriptII (Gibco-BRL) and random hexamers (Amersham-Pharmacia Biotech). Every sample should have a pair of reactions, one with the addition of enzyme (RT+) and the other with water substituted for enzyme (RT–). Since, the forward primers contain signals to enable in vitro transcription and translation, the PCR products generated for *Smad2* and *Smad4* using the indicated primers are also used as templates for IVSP (**Table 4**). The composition of the PCR reaction mixture is as described in the previous section under allelic loss analysis except the annealing temperatures are 58°C and 60°C for *Smad2* and *Smad4*, respectively.

1.5. IVSP

The cell free transcription coupled translation of the RT-PCR templates derived from the different test samples enable a quick scan of the ORF for truncating mutations. The RT-PCR products from the previous section could be either directly used or gel purified and used as templates in a coupled transcription/translation system (Promega Corp., Madison, WI) in the presence of [^{35}S]methionine (Amersham-Pharmacia Biotech) to generate a polypeptide corresponding to the test template. A shorter polypeptide than the expected size during SDS-polyacrylamide gel analysis would indicate a truncation of the protein due to a nonsense codon resulting either from a point mutation or a frameshift.

Table 5
Genomic PCR Primers for *Smad2* and *Smad4*

Primer ID	Sequence
Smad2 GFP	5'-GTC CAT CTT GCC ATT CAC G -3'
Smad2 GRP	5'-TGG TGA TGG CTT TCT CAA GC-3'
Smad4 GFP1	5'-TGT ATG ACA TGG CCA AGT TAG-3'
Smad4 GRP1	5'-CAA TAC TCG GTT TTA GCA GTC-3'
Smad4 GFP2	5'-CCA AAA GTG TGC AGC TTG TTG-3'
Smad4 GRP2	5'-CAG TTT CTG TCT GCT AGG AGC-3'

1.6. DNA Sequencing

DNA sequence analysis provides the ultimate proof for genetic alterations. Sequence analysis is usually coupled with the other methods to confirm the alterations (e.g., changes at splice junctions, nonsense codons, and so on) detected using the other methods (RT-PCR, IVSP, etc.). Furthermore, this is the only reliable method to detect missense mutations. The current method of choice for the author is to use [^{33}P] ddNTPs in cycle sequencing using ThermoSequanase (USB, Cincinnati, OH). The reactions from the same terminator reactions from the different test samples are loaded on the denaturing gel side by side for easy detection of any sequence alterations.

1.7. Genomic PCR

PCR primers that amplify the different exons could be used to detect homozygous deletions within the genes (**Table 5**). We observed homozygous deletions encompassing the *Smad2* and *Smad4* genes by this method. The initial indication for such a deletion may be obtained from allelic loss analysis and RT-PCR.

2. Materials

2.1. Total RNA Isolation

1. Ice cold denaturing solution (to make 100 mL solution, mix 75 g guanidine isothiocyanate [Gibco-BRL, 15535-016], 1 g N-lauroyl sarcosine [Sigma, L-5777], 4 mL 1 *M* sodium citrate, pH 7.0 and 720 µL β-mercapto ethanol).
2. Phenol:chloroform:isoamyl alcohol (25:24:1 [v/v]).
3. 2 *M* sodium acetate, pH 4.0 solution.
4. 20 mg/mL Glycogen (Boehringer Mannheim; 901393).
5. Isopropanol.
6. 75% Ethanol.
7. DEPC (diethyl pyrocarbonate)-treated water.
8. DEPC-treated tubes.
9. Tissue homogenizer (Brinkmann or Dounce).

2.2. Genomic DNA Isolation

1. SDS-proteinase K solution. To make 20 mL solution, mix 100 mg proteinase K (Gibco-BRL, 25530-015) and 200 mg SDS in 500 mM Tris-HCl, 20 mM EDTA, 10 mM sodium chloride solution, pH 8.9.
2. Phenol:chloroform:isoamyl alcohol (25:24:1 [v/v]).
3. 10 M Ammonium acetate solution.
4. 100% Ethanol (200 proof).
5. 70% Ethanol.

2.3. Kinase Labeling of PCR Primers

1. 10X Kinase buffer (Kinase buffers are usually provided by most of the commercial venders who supply polynucleotide kinase (e.g., Gibco-BRL, Promega, New England Biolabs, Epicentre Tech., and others).
2. [γ-^{32}P] ATP (6000 Ci/mmol, 150 µCi/µL; PB15068, Amersham-Pharmacia Biotech).
3. T4 polynucleotide kinase.
4. Oligonucleotide primer (50–100 ng).
5. 0.5 M EDTA.
6. Chroma spin-10 columns (Clontech; K1300).

2.4. PCR Amplification

1. 10X Buffer (670 mM Tris-HCl, pH 8.8, 166 mM ammonium sulfate and 67 mM magnesium chloride, 10 mM β-mercaptoethanol).
2. Dimethyl sulfoxide (Sigma; D2650).
3. 10 mM dNTP solution (Gibco-BRL; 18427-018).
4. Upstream and downstream primers.
5. 10–20 ng DNA solution.
6. Taq polymerase.
7. Mineral oil (Sigma, M3516).

2.5. First-Strand cDNA Synthesis

1. 5X First strand buffer (Gibco-BRL).
2. Random hexamers (1 µg/µL) (Amersham-Pharmacia Biotech).
3. 25 mM dNTPs (Amersham-Pharmacia Biotech.)
4. DTT (0.1 M) (Gibco-BRL).
5. SuperScriptII (200 U/µL) (Gibco-BRL).
6. RNasin (40 U/µL) (Promega).
7. Binding Protein (SSB) (1.5 µg/µL) (USB Corp., Cleveland, Ohio; E70032Z).
8. Total RNA.
9. DEPC-treated water.

2.6. IVSP Assay

1. T$_N$T system (Promega; L1170).
2. [^{35}S]-Pro-mix™ (14 µCi/µL, 1000 Ci/mmol; Amersham-Pharmacia Biotech; SJQ0079) or [^{35}S]methionine (15 µCi/µL, 1000 Ci/mmol; Amersham-Pharmacia Biotech; SJ1515).

3. cDNA template generated using primers with T7 transcription and translation start sites.
4. 2X SDS sample buffer. To make 10 mL, mix 1.25 mL 1 *M* Tris-HCl, pH 6.8, 2 mL 20% SDS, 1 mL 0.2% bromophenol blue, 2 mL glycerol, 0.5 mL β-mercaptoethanol and 3.25 mL dH$_2$O.
5. Gel fixing solution. To make 1 L, mix 300 mL methanol, 80 mL glacial acetic acid in 620 mL dH$_2$O.

2.7. Cycle Sequencing

1. Thermo Sequenase radiolabeled terminator cycle sequencing kit (USB Corp., Cleveland, Ohio; 188403). Thermo Sequanase with thermostable pyrophosphatase, [α-^{33}P]-labaled ddGTP, ddATP, ddTTP, and ddCTP terminators (each 0.3 μ*M*, 1500 Ci/mmol, 450 μCi/mL, 11.25 μCi), 10X reaction buffer, stop solution, dGTP nucleotide master mix and dITP nucleotide master mix.
2. 50–200 ng DNA template (RT+ or genomic PCR product).
3. Oligonucleotide primer of choice (0.5–2.5 pmol).
4. Mineral oil (Sigma, M3516).

3. Methods
3.1. RNA Preparation

1. Place 500 mg of tissue (fresh or frozen) or cell pellet (approx 1 × 10^8 cells) in a DEPC-treated tube.
2. Add 600 μL of denaturing solution and chill on ice.
3. Disrupt the tissue using a homogenizer (high speed for 30–60 s).
4. Add 60 μL 2 *M* sodium acetate, pH 4.0 solution and mix thoroughly until most of the tissue goes into solution.
5. Add 10 μL glycogen.
6. Add 600 μL phenol:chloroform:isoamyl alcohol, mix vigorously and chill on ice for 15 min.
7. Centrifuge at top speed for 30 min.
8. Carefully transfer the top aqueous phase into a new DEPC-treated tube.
9. Add equal volume of isopropanol and incubate at –20°C for 15 min to overnight.
10. Centrifuge at top speed for 30 min at 4°C.
11. Wash the pellet with 75% ice-cold ethanol and centrifuge at top speed for 15 min at 4°C.
12. Dry the pellet in the vacuum desiccator or speed-vac for 10–15 min and resuspend in 100–500 μL DEPC water.

3.2. Genomic DNA Preparation

1. Place 250–500 mg of tissue (fresh, frozen or micro-dissected from sections) or cell pellet (approx 1 × 10^8 cells) in a sterile DNase free tube.
2. Add 500 μL SDS-proteinase K (5 mg/mL) solution, mix vigorously by vortexing and incubate at 56–60°C for 24–48 h with occasional mixing to allow all the tissue get into solution.

3. Add equal volume of phenol:chloroform:isoamyl alcohol (25:24:1 [v/v]), mix vigorously and centrifuge at top speed for 5 min.
4. Carefully transfer the top aqueous phase into a new sterile tube.
5. Repeat **steps 3** and **4**.
6. Add 1/3 volume of 10 *M* ammonium acetate solution.
7. Add equal volume of 100% ethanol.
8. Centrifuge at top speed for 15–30 min.
9. Wash the pellet with 70% ethanol and centrifuge at top speed for 5 min.
10. Repeat **step 9**.
11. Dry the pellet in the vacuum desiccator for 5–10 min and resuspend in 1–2 mL sterile water.

3.3. Setting Up Kinase Reactions

Kinase reaction volumes are determined by the need. A typical reaction volume is 20 µL.

1. Mix 2 µL 10X kinase buffer, 6 µL [γ-^{32}P] ATP, 10 µL Oligonucleotide primer (10 ng/µL), 1 µL water and 1 µL T4 polynucleotide kinase (1–10 µ/µL depending on the supplier).
2. Incubate at 37°C for 30 min.
3. Terminate reaction by the addition of 2 µL 0.5 EDTA or by incubating at 68°C for 10 min.
4. Add 20–40 mL TE and load onto pre-spun chroma spin-10 column or any equivalent column to remove unincorporated radionucleotides. The labeled primer is collected in a tube at the end of the spin.
5. Determine the incorporation of label by Cerenkov counting.
6. For microsatellite marker analysis 10^6 cpm of labeled primer is typically used in a 10 µL reaction.

3.4. Setting Up PCR Reactions

1. PCR reaction volumes are determined by the need. A typical reaction volume is 50 µL. However, volumes as low as 10 µL could be used for microsatellite marker analysis. To make a reaction mixture of 50 µL: Mix 5 µL 10X PCR buffer, 2 µL 10 m*M* dNTPs, 3 µL dimethyl sulfoxide, 100 pmol of each primer (upstream and downstream), 10 ng of DNA template and Taq polymerase (e.g., 0.5 µL of Platinum Taq (Gibco-BRL, 10966-034)/50 µL reaction). An overlay of 1–2 drops (20–50 µL) of nuclease free mineral oil is added to prevent evaporation and condensation.
2. A typical amplification consists of an initial denaturation at 95°C for 2 min followed by 30 cycles, each carried out at 95°C for 30 s, 55–65°C for 1 min, and 70°C for 1 min. The annealing temperatures are specific for the primer pairs as indicated in the specific sections.

3.5. +/– First-Strand cDNA Synthesis

A typical reaction mixture consists of 20 µL each for +/– SuperScript for each template.

1. Make a hexamer mix by mixing 4 μL random hexamers, 2 μL Binding Protein (SSB), 10 μg total RNA and DEPC-treated water to bring up the volume to 25 μL.
2. Heat the hexamer mix to 70°C for 3 min and cool on ice.
3. Make a reaction mix of 13.2 μL by mixing 8 μL 5X first strand buffer, 4 μL 0.1 M DTT, 0.8 μL 25 mM dNTPs and 0.4 μL RNasin.
4. Divide the reaction mix into two equal halves (6.6 μL each) and label + and – reactions respectively.
5. To the + and – reactions, add 2.5 μL each of the hexamer mix from **step 2**.
6. To the + reaction, add 1.5 μL of SuperScriptII and to the – reaction, add 1.5 μL of dH$_2$O.
7. Incubate both the + and – reactions at 37°C for 1 h.
8. Heat the reactions to 65°C for 10 min.
9. Dilute 1:5 with DEPC-water.
10. The + and – first strand cDNA is ready for amplification to test expressed genes (+/– RT-PCR).

3.6. Protein Truncation Assay

1. Thaw on ice the TNT system and [^{35}S]-Pro-mix™ or [^{35}S]methionine stored at –70°C.
2. Mix 16 μL of TNT T7 quick mix, 0.8 μL [^{35}S]methionine, and 3.2 μL of cDNA template (+RT).
3. Incubate the reaction at 30°C for 1–2 h.
4. Terminate the reaction with 10–15 μL 2X SDS sample buffer.
5. Separate the protein products on an appropriate SDS-PAGE gel.
6. Fix the gel in the fixing solution by shaking for 30 min with one change of fixing solution.
7. Dry the gel on a GB002 (Schleicher & Schuell) paper and expose to film.

3.7. Setting Up Sequencing Reactions

1. For each of the four termination reactions corresponding to a specific template, aliquot 2 μL of the master dNTP mix (dGTP or dITP) and 0.5 μL of appropriate [α-^{33}P]-ddNTP to PCR tubes or a 96-well plate.
2. Make the reaction mix by mixing 2 μL 10X reaction buffer, 0.5–2.5 pmol primer and 50–200 ng DNA template, bring up the volume to 18 μL and finally add 2 μL Thermo Sequenase (4 U/mL).
3. To each of the four-terminator reactions for a particular template add 4.5 μL of reaction mixture from **step 2**.
4. Overlay with 10–20 μL mineral oil.
5. 20–30 cycles of PCR cycling is set up for 95°C for 30 s, annealing temperature of the primer-3°C for 30 s and 72°C for 1 min.
6. Add 4 μL of stop solution to each termination reaction.
7. Heat the reactions to 95°C for 2 min, cool to room temperature.
8. Load the sequencing gels in sets of 3–6 of the same terminator reactions (A, C, G, and T) in a row and separate the bands.

9. The gel is fixed, dried and exposed to film using standard procedures.
10. The loading of the same terminator reactions in a row, side by side enables easy detection of sequence abnormalities and hence genetic alterations.

Acknowledgments

I would like to thank Bert Vogelstein, Ken Kinzler, Fred Bunz and Greg Riggins for their discussions; Jerry Brody, Joe Ponte, Arunthi Thiagalingam, Kuang-hung Cheng, Keya Sau, Steve Powell, and Rebecca Foy for their helpful comments; and Kuang-hung Cheng for expert assistance with illustration.

References

1. Heldin, C-H., Miyazono, K., and Dijke, P. T. (1997) TGF-β signalling from cell membrane to nucleus through SMAD proteins. *Nature* **390,** 465–471.
2. Massague, J. (1998) TGF-βeta signal transduction. *Annu. Rev. Biochem.* **67,** 753–791.
3. Masuyama. N., Hanafusa. H., Kusakabe, M., Shibuya, H., and Nishida, E. (1999) Identification of two Smad4 proteins in Xenopus. Their common and distinct properties. *J. Biol. Chem.* **274,** 12,163–12,170.
4. Hata, A., Lagna, G., Massague, J., and Hemmati-Brivanlou, A. (1998) Smad6 inhibits BMP/Smad1 signaling by specifically competing with the Smad4 tumor suppressor. *Genes Dev.* **12,** 186–197.
5. Roberts, A. B. (1998) Molecular and cell biology of TGF-β. *Miner. Electrolyte Metab.* **24(2–3),** 111–119.
6. Sporn, M. B. and Roberts, A. B. 1988. Peptide growth factors are multifunctional. *Nature* **332,** 217–219.
7. Derynck, R., Jarrett, J. A., Chen, E. Y., Eaton, D. H., Bell, J. R., Assoian. R. K., Roberts, A. B., Sporn, M. B., and Goeddel, D. V. (1985) Human transforming growth factor-β complementary DNA sequence and expression in normal and transformed cells. *Nature* **316,** 701–705.
8. Arrick, B. A., Lopez, A. R., Elfman, F., Ebner, R., Damsky, C. H., and Derynck, R. (1992) Altered metabolic and adhesive properties and increased tumorigenesis associated with increased expression of transforming growth factor beta 1. *J. Cell Biol.* **118,** 715–726.
9. Glynne-Jones, E., Harper, M. E., Goddard, L., Eaton, C. L., Matthews, P. N., and Griffiths, K. (1994) Transforming growth factor beta 1 expression in benign and malignant prostatic tumors. *Prostate* **25,** 210–218.
10. Guise, T. A. and Mundy, G. R. (1998) Cancer and bone. *Endocr. Rev.* **19,** 18–54.
11. Sporn, M. B. and Roberts, A. B. (1985) Autocrine growth factors and cancer. *Nature* **313,** 745–747.
12. Roberts, A. B. and Sporn, M. B. (1993) Physiological actions and clinical applications of transforming growth factor-beta (TGF-βeta). *Growth Factors* **8,** 1–9.
13. Kim, I. Y., Ahn, H.-J., Zelner, D. J., Shaw, J. W., Sensibar, J. A., Kim, J-.H., Kato, M., and Lee, C. (1996) Genetic change in transforming growth factor β

(TGF-β) receptor type I gene correlates with insensitivity to TGF-β1 in human prostate cancer cells. *Cancer Res.* **56,** 44–48.

14. Kimchi, A., Wang, X.-F., Weinberg, R., Cheifetzn, S., and Massague, J. (1988) Absence of TGF-β receptors and growth inhibitory responses in retinoblastoma cells. *Science* **240,** 196–199.

15. Park, K., Kim, S.-J., Bang. Y.-J., Park, J.-G., Kim, N. K., Roberts, A. B., and Sporn, M. B. (1994) Genetic changes in the transforming growth factor beta (TGF-β) type II receptor gene in human gastric cancer cells: correlation with sensitivity to growth inhibition by TGF-β. *Proc. Natl. Acad. Sci.* USA **91,** 8772–8776.

16. Sun, L., Wu, G., Willson, J. K. V., Zborowska, E., Yang, J., Rajkarunanayake, I., Wang, J., Centry, L. E., Wang, X.-F., and Brattain, M. G. (1994) Expression of transforming growth factor beta type II receptor leads to reduced malignancy in human breast cancer MCF-7 cells. *J. Biol. Chem.* **269,** 26,449–26,455.

17. Markowitz, S., Wang, J., Myeroff, L., Parsons, R., Sun, L. Z., Lutterbaough, J., Fan, R. S., Zborowska, E., Kinzler, K. W., Vogelstein, B., Brattain, M. G., and Willson, J. K. V. (1995) Inactivation of the type II TGF-β receptor in colon cancer cells with microsatellite instability *Science* **268,** 1336–1338.

18. Parsons, R., Myeroff, L. L., Liu, B., Willson, J. K., Markowitz, S. D., Kinzler, K. W., and Vogelstein, B. (1995) Microsatellite instability and mutations of the transforming growth factor beta type II receptor gene in colorectal cancer. *Cancer Res.* **55,** 5548–5550.

19. Grady, W. M., Myeroff, L. L., Swinler, S. E., Rajaput, A., Thiagalingam, S., Lutterbaugh, J. D., Neumann, A., Brattain, M. G., Chang, J., Kim, S.-J., Kinzler, K. W., Vogelstein, B., Willson, J. K. V., and Markowitz, S. (1999) Mutational inactivation of transforming growth factor beta receptor type II in microsatellite stable colon cancers *Cancer Res.* **59,** 320–324.

20. Nagatake, M., Takagi, Y., Osada, H., Uchida, K., Mitsudomi, T., Saji, S., Shimokawa, K., Takahashi, T., and Takahashi, T. (1996) Aberrant hypermethylation at the bcl-2 locus at 18q21 in human lung cancers. *Cancer Res.* **56,** 2718–2720.

21. Uchida, K., Nagatake, M., Osada, H., Yatabe, Y., Kondo, M., Mitsudomi, T., Matsuda, A., Takahashi, T., and Takahashi, T. (1996) Somatic in vivo alterations of the JV18-1 gene at 18q21 in human lung cancers. *Cancer Res.* **56,** 5583–5585.

22. Thiagalingam, S., Lengauer, C., Leach, F. S., Schutte, M., Hahn, S. A., Overhauser, J., Willson, J. K. V., Markowitz, S., Hamilton, S. R., Kern, S. E., Kinzler, K. W., and Vogelstein, B. (1996) Evaluation of candidate tumour suppressor genes on chromosome 18 in colorectal cancers. *Nature Genet.* **13,** 343–346.

23. Schutte, M., Hruban, R. H., Hedrick, L., Cho, K. R., Nadasdy, G. M., Weinstein, C. L., Bova, G. S., Isaacs, W. B., Cairns, P., Nawroz, H., Sidransky, D., Casero, R. A., Jr., Meltzer, P. S., Hahn, S. A., and Kern, S. E. (1996) DPC4 gene in various tumor types. *Cancer Res.* **56,** 2527–2530.

24. Riggins, J. G., Kinzler, K. W., Vogelstein, B., and Thiagalingam, S. (1997) Frequency of *Smad* gene mutations in human cancers. *Cancer Res.* **57,** 2578–2580.

25. Hahn, S. A, Schutte, M., Hoque, A. T., Moskaluk, C. A., da Costa, L. T., Rozenblum, E., Weinstein, C. L., Fischer, A., Yeo, C. J., Hruban, R. H, and Kern,

S. E. (1996) DPC4, a candidate tumor suppressor gene at human chromosome 18q21.1. *Science* **271**, 350–353.

26. Riggins, J. G., Thiagalingam, S., Rozenblum, E., Weinstein, C. L., Kern, S. E., Hamilton, S. R., Willson, J. K. V., Markowitz, S., Kinzler, K. W., and Vogelstein, B. (1996) *MAD*-related genes in the human. *Nature Genet.* **13**, 347–349.

27. Vogelstein, B., Fearon, E. R., Hamilton, S. R., Kern, S. E., Preisinger, A., Leppert, M., Nakamura, Y., White, R., Smith, A. M. M., and Boss, J. L. (1988) Genetic alterations during colorectal-tumor development. *N. Engl. J. Med.* **319**, 525–532.

28. Yogota, J. and Sugimura, T. (1993) Multiple steps in carcinogenesis involving alterations of multiple tumor suppressor genes. *FESEB J.* **7**, 920–925.

29. Ueda, T., Komiya, A., Emi, M., Suzuki, H., Shiraishi, T., Yatani, R., Masai, M., Yasuda, K., and Ito, H. (1997) Allelic losses on 18q21 are associated with progression and metastasis in human prostate cancer. *Genes Chromosom. Cancer* **20**, 140–147.

30. Amendt, C., Schirmacher, P., Weber, H., and Blessing, M. (1998) Expression of a dominant negative type II TGF-β receptor in mouse skin results in an increase in carcinoma incidence and acceleration of carcinoma development. *Oncogene* **17**, 25–34.

31. Takei, K., Kohno, T., Hamada, K., Takita, J., Noguchi, M., Matsuno, Y., Hirohashi, S., Uezato, H., and Yokota, J. (1998) A novel tumor suppressor locus on chromosome 18q involved in the development of human lung cancer. *Cancer Res.* **58**, 3700–3705.

32. Eppert, K., Scherer, S. W., Ozcelik, H., Pirone, R., Hoodless, P., Kim, H., Tsui, L. C., Bapat, B., Gallinger, S., Andrulis, I. L., Thomsen, G. H., Wrana, J. L., and Attisano, L. (1996) MADR2 maps to 18q21 and encodes a TGF-β-regulated MAD-related protein that is functionally mutated in colorectal carcinoma. *Cell* **86**, 543–552.

33. Jonson, T., Gorunova, L., Dawiskiba, S., Andren-Sandberg, A., Stenman, G., ten Dijke, P., Johansson, B. and M. Hoglund. (1999) Molecular analyses of the 15q and 18q SMAD genes in pancreatic cancer. *Genes Chromosomes Cancer* **24**, 62–71.

34. Nakao, A., Afrakhte, M., Moren, A., Nakayama, T., Christian, J. L., Heuchel, R., Itoh, S., Kawabata, M., Heldin, N. E., Heldin, C. H., and ten Dijke, P. (1997) Identification of Smad7, a TGF-β-inducible antagonist of TGF-β signalling. *Nature* **389**, 631–635.

35. Watanabe, T. K., Suzuki, M., Omori, Y., Hishigaki, H., Horie, M., Kanemoto, N., Fujiwara, T., Nakamura, Y., and Takahashi, E. (1997) Cloning and characterization of a novel member of the human Mad gene family (MADH6). *Genomics* **42**, 446–451.

36. Miyaki, M, Iijima, T., Konishi, M., Sakai, K., Ishii, A., Yasuno, M., Hishima, T., Koike, M., Shitara, N., Iwama, T., Utsunomiya, J., Kuroki, T., and Mori, T. (1999) Higher frequency of Smad4 gene mutation in human colorectal cancer with distant metastasis. *Oncogene* **18**, 3098–3103.

37. Bartsch, D., Hahn, S. A., Danichevski, K. D., Ramaswamy, A., Bastian, D., Galehdari, H., Barth, P., Schmiegel, W., Simon, B., and Rothmund, M. (1999) Mutations of the DPC4/Smad4 gene in neuroendocrine pancreatic tumors. *Oncogene* **18**, 2367–2371.

38. Hoque, A. T., Hahn, S. A., Schutte, M., and Kern, S. E. (1997) DPC4 gene mutation in colitis associated neoplasia. *Gut* **40,** 120–122.

39. Kim, S. K., Fan, Y., Papadimitrakopoulou, V., Clayman, G., Hittelman, W. N., Hong, W. K., Lotan, R., and Mao, L. (1996) *DPC4*, a candidate tumor suppressor gene, is altered infrequently in head and neck squamous cell carcinoma. *Cancer Res.* **56,** 2519–2521.

40. Fearon, E. R. and Vogelstein, B. (1990) A genetic model for colorectal tumorigenesis. *Cell* **61,** 759–767.

41. Knudson, A. G. (1996) Hereditary cancer: two hits revisited. *J. Cancer Res. Clin. Oncol.* **122,** 135–140.

42. Powell, S. M., Peterson, G. M., Krush, A. J., Booker, S., Jen, J., Giardiello, F. M., Hamilton, S. R., Vogelstein, B., and Kinzler, K. W. Molecular diagnosis of familial adenomatous polyposis. *N. Engl. J. Med.* **329,** 1982–1987.

43. Willson, J. K. V., Bittner, G. N., Oberley, T. D., Meisner, L. F., and Weese, J. L. (1987) Cell culture of human colon adenomas and carcinomas. *Cancer Res.* **47,** 2704–2713.

16

Direct Sequencing for Juvenile Polyposis Gene *SMAD4/DPC4* Mutations

Lauri A. Aaltonen and Stina Roth

1. Introduction

Juvenile polyposis (JP) is a rare dominantly inherited tumor predisposition syndrome, the typical lesion being a benign hamartomatous intestinal polyp with dilated crypts. Solitary juvenile polyps are relatively common in childhood, and appear not to be associated with neoplasia *(1,2)*. There is no consensus of how many polyps in one patient would justify the diagnosis for the condition. The number of polyps usually present is low compared to familial adenomatous polyposis where typically hundreds of lesions are found in the fully developed disease. Five histologically confirmed juvenile polyps in one patient have been proposed as a sufficient number to establish juvenile polyposis diagnosis *(3)*. Juvenile polyposis usually presents in childhood, most often with rectal bleeding. In some cases associated congenital defects such as malformations of the heart and the cranium occur *(4,5)*.

Tumor predisposition is not limited to tendency to develop juvenile polyps. Affected individuals have a high, perhaps more than 50% lifetime risk of colorectal cancer, and also other malignancies such as pancreatic cancer may be associated with the syndrome *(6–9)*. While formal proof lacks due to the rarity of the syndrome, it is possible that the patients benefit from colonoscopic tumor screening similar to hereditary nonpolyposis colon cancer patients *(10)*.

The molecular background of juvenile polyposis has not been fully clarified. While one report has proposed that mutations in the *PTEN (MMAC1)* tumor suppressor gene underlie the syndrome *(11),* others have found no evidence to support that notion *(12,13)*. Recent reports have established the involvement of germline mutations of *SMAD4/DPC4* gene, originally identi-

From: *Methods in Molecular Medicine, vol. 50: Colorectal Cancer: Methods and Protocols*
Edited by: S. M. Powell © Humana Press Inc., Totowa, NJ

fied as a pancreatic cancer suppressor *(14),* in juvenile polyposis *(15).* However, it is likely that other, yet unidentified genes play a role in a considerable subset of the families *(16).*

SMAD4/DPC4 is a relatively small gene consisting of 11 exons and encoding a protein of 552 amino acids. The gene product is an important intracellular player in the TGFβ signal transduction pathway. *SMAD4/DPC4* is an obligate partner for SMAD2 and SMAD3 proteins in signalling, and these proteins mediate, e.g., growth inhibitory signals from TGFb type I and II receptor complex to the nucleus; to facilitate transcription of the target genes (reviewed in **ref. *17*).** Impairment of this growth regulatory pathway is a common cause of cancer.

As the gene is small, we recommend direct genomic sequencing as the method of choice in germline mutation analysis. Unexpectedly, one particular mutation in exon 9, a four base deletion causing a stop codon at codon 434, appears to be common in apparently unrelated caucasian JP families *(15).* Thus in the absence of other clues regarding the putative mutation site, analyses should start from exon 9.

The interpretation of positive findings is facilitated by the fact that most germline mutations are truncating *(15,18).* Missense mutations also occur *(15,16),* and it is often impossible to evaluate the significance of such changes through functional analyses. Analysis of control individuals, and sequence alignments to evaluate whether the affected codon has been conserved through evolution, are helpful. If changes occur in conserved amino acids and identical variants are not observed in 50 control individuals, the change is likely to be associated with the disease. Obviously, direct genomic sequencing of the coding area cannot detect mutations such as large deletions and rearrangements, and promotor area mutations. Interpretation of negative results (mutation not found) is hampered by the strong possibility of genetic heterogeneity. Once a mutation has been detected in a family, the testing is robust.

SMAD4/DPC4 mutations have been found in multiple different tumor types. The gene was identified in 1996 in studies focusing on chromosome 18q deletions in pancreatic cancers *(14).* In addition to pancreatic cancer, *SMAD4/DPC4* mutations appear to play an important role in colorectal tumorigenesis, especially in advanced cancers *(19,20).* 18q deletions are very common in colorectal cancer as well, and evidence is accumulating that *SMAD4/DPC4* is one of the major targets of these deletions, if not the most important. *SMAD4/DPC4* mutations are frequent also in tumors of the neuroendocrine pancreas *(21) SMAD4/DPC4* alterations have been described in a small subset of lung *(22),* breast, ovarian *(23),* head and neck squamous cell *(24),* and endometrial cancer *(25).*

2. Materials

2.1. Blood Processing and DNA Extraction

1. EDTA anticoagulated blood tubes filled with whole blood (Vacuette, Greiner Labortechnik, Frickenhausen, Germany).
2. 15-mL polypropylene tubes (Greiner Labortechnik).
3. TKM 1 buffer: 10 mM Tris-HCl, pH 7.6, 10 mM KCl, 10 mM MgCl$_2$, 2 mM EDTA pH 7.6.
4. TKM 2 buffer: 10 mM Tris-HCl, pH 7.6, 10 mM KCl, 10 mM MgCl$_2$, 2 mM EDTA, pH 7.6, 0.4 M NaCl.
5. TKM 1 + Nonidet buffer: 2.5 mL Nonidet in 100 mL TKM1.
6. Nonidet P-40 (Sigma Chemical Company, St. Louis, MO).
7. 20% SDS.
8. 5 M NaCl.
9. Tris-EDTA, pH 8.0 (TE).
10. Centrifuge.
11. 2-mL Eppendorf tubes.
12. Ethanol (99.5%).
13. Pasteur pipets.
14. Microfuge.
15. 1.8 mL cryo tubes (Greiner Labortechnik).

2.2. PCR Amplifications

1. Ampli*Taq* Gold DNA polymerase (Perkin Elmer Applied Biosystems Division PE/ABI, Foster City, CA).
2. 10X PCR reaction buffer (PE/ABI, Foster City, CA).
3. Oligonucleotides (*see* **Table 1**).
4. Sterile water.
5. dNTP-mix (Finnzymes, Espoo, Finland).
6. 15 mM MgCl$_2$ (PE/ABI).
7. Thermocycler.
8. PCR tubes (Robbins Scientific, Sunnyvalley, CA).
9. Template (genomic DNA).
10. QIAquick PCR purification kit (Qiagen).

2.3. Gel Electrophoresis

1. Agarose (NuSieve, Bioproducts, Rockland, ME).
2. Tris-borate (TBE) buffer (0.09 M Tris-borate, 0.002 M EDTA, pH 8.0).
3. Ethidium bromide (EtBr) solution in water (10 mg/mL).
4. Gel-loading buffer (0.05% bromphenol blue, 0.05% xylene cyanole FF, 30% glycerol in water).
5. ϕX174 DNA/*Hae* III marker (Promega, Madison, WI).
6. Gel electrophoresis tank, accessories, and power supply.

Table 1
SMAD4/DPC4 Gene PCR Amplification Oligonucleotide Primers

Primer[a]	Sequence (5' → 3')	Product size, bp
Exon 1F	CGTTAGCTGTTGTTTTTCACTG	469
Exon 1R	AGAGTATGTGAAGAGATGGAG	
Exon 2F	TGTATGACATGGCCAAGTTAG	530
Exon 2R	CAATACTCGGTTTTAGCAGTC	
Exon 3F	CTGAATTGAAATGGTTCATGAAC	308
Exon 3R	GCCCCTAACCTCAAAATCTAC	
Exon 4F	TTTGGTTTTCTATATAGCTCCATCA	321
Exon 4R	CTTACTTGGAGTTTCCCCCA	
Exon 5/6F	CATCTTTATAGTTGTGCATTATC	557
Exon 5/6R	TAATGAAACAAAATCACAGGATG	
Exon 7F	TTTACTGAAAGTTTTAGCATTAGACAA	191
Exon 7R	GCCTGTGTTTGTCGTTTCAA	
Exon 8F	CTGTGTTGTGGAGTGCAAGTG	280
Exon 8R	ATCTGACTATACAATCAATACCTTGCT	
Exon 9F	TATTAAGCATGCTATACAATCTG	332
Exon 9R	CTTCCACCCAGATTTCAATTC	
Exon 10F	AGGCATTGGTTTTTAATGTATG	293
Exon 10R	CTGCTCAAAGAAACTAATCAAC	
Exon 11F	CCAAAAGTGTGCAGCTTGTTG	508
Exon 11R	CAGTTTCTGTCTGCTAGGAG	

[a]F=forward primers, R=reverse primers of a pair for amplification (reference http://24.3.32.113/geneticsweb/DPL4pmr.htm, except for exons 4, 7, and 8 which were designed using the Primer3 server; http://www-genome.wi.mit.edu/cgi-bin/primer/primer3.cgi).

2.4. PCR Product Purification

1. QIAquick PCR purification kit (Qiagen, Valencia, CA).
2. Ethanol (99.5%).
3. Eppendorf tubes (1.5 mL).
4. Microfuge.

2.5. Automated Sequencing

1. ABI prism dye terminator cycle sequencing ready reaction kit (Perkin-Elmer Corp., Foster City, CA).
2. ABI big dye terminator kit (Perkin-Elmer Corp.).
3. Long Ranger gel solution (FMC Bioproducts, Rockland, ME).
4. Urea.
5. Ammonium persulfate.
6. N,N,N',N'-Tetramethylethylene diamine (TEMED).

7. Primers (2 µ*M*).
8. Sterile water.
9. 0.5 mL PCR tubes (Robbins).
10. Template (PCR product).
11. Tris-borate (TBE) buffer: 0.09 *M* Tris-borate, 0.002 *M* EDTA, pH 8.3.
12. Gel electrophoresis equipment (Perkin-Elmer Corp.) and power supply.
13. Applied Biosystems model 373A or 377 automated sequencer (Perkin-Elmer Corp.).

3. Methods
3.1. Blood Processing and DNA Extraction (see Note 1)

1. Take 5 mL of whole blood to the 15 mL polypropylene tube and add 5 mL of TKM-1+Nonidet buffer. Mix blood and buffer carefully and let them stay few minutes in room temperature.
2. Centrifuge tubes at 1000*g* for 10 min at room temperature.
3. Pour the supernatant carefully away and wash the nuclei pellet with 10 mL of TKM-1 buffer. Centrifuge at 1000*g* for 10 min. Repeat this step if needed.
4. Pour the supernatant away and add 800 µL TKM-2 buffer. Transfer the nuclei pellet and buffer to 2-mL Eppendorf tube by Pasteur-pipet. Break the nuclei pellet by pipeting.
5. Add 50 µL 20% SDS and vortex carefully.
6. Incubate tubes at +55°C over night.
7. After incubation add 360 mL 5 *M* NaCl and mix well.
8. Centrifuge at 14,800*g* for 10 min at +4°C (in microfuge).
9. Pipet supernatant into 10 mL polypropylene tubes and add 5 mL of ice cold absolute ethanol. Turn tubes up and down until DNA is precipitating.
10. Transfer DNA into 15 mL tube containing 10 mL of 70% ethanol. Wash DNA in a slow rotating wheel mixer over night.
11. Wind the DNA around the thin glass stick and let it dry until ethanol has evaporated. Dissolve the DNA in Tris-EDTA (pH 8.0) in cryo tubes (100–1500 mL).
12. Dissolve DNA by mixing it in rotating wheel mixer at +4°C (1–3 d).

3.2. Amplification of SMAD4/DPC4 Exons 1-11 (PCR)

1. The reactions are carried out in 50 µL reaction volume containing 100 ng of genomic DNA (*see* **Note 2**), 1X PCR reaction buffer, 200 µ*M* of each dNTP, each primer at 0.8 µ*M*, 1 U of Ampli*Taq* Gold polymerase. The MgCl$_2$ concentration was 1.5 m*M* in all reactions.
2. Use the following cycling conditions: exons 1, 2, and 11: 10 min at 95°C, 40 cycles of 45 s at 95°C, 45 s at 57°C, 1 min at 72°C; for exons 3, 5, and 6: 10 min at 95°C, 40 cycles of 45 s at 95°C, 45 s at 58°C, 1 min at 72°C; for exons 7, 8, 9, and 10: 10 min at 95°C, 40 cycles of 45 s at 95°C, 45 s at 56°C, 1 min at 72°C, for exon 4: 10 min at 95°C, 40 cycles of 45 s at 95°C, 1 min 15 s at 55°C, 1 min 15 s at 72°C. Use final extension of 10 min at 72°C for all exons.

3.3. Agarose Gel Electrophoresis

1. Seal the edges of the plastic tray with tapes and put the comb 2.0–3.0 mm above the tray.
2. Prepare 3% agarose solution in 1X TBE buffer.
3. Cool the solution to 60°C, add EtBr solution to a final concentration of 0.5 μg/mL and mix thoroughly, pour the solution into the plastic tray.
4. Leave the gel for 45 min to solidify. After remove the comb and tapes.
5. Insert the tray with the gel in the electrophoresis tank filled with 1X TBE buffer.
6. Mix 5 μL of the PCR product with 1 μL of gel-loading buffer. Load the mixture into the well. Use 0.5 mg of φX DNA/HaeIII marker.
7. Perform electrophoresis for 1.5 h at 100 V.
8. Check the specificity of the PCR product (*see* **Note 3**).

3.4. PCR Product Purification

If the PCR product is specific, purify the rest of the reaction product using QIAquick PCR purification kit according to the protocol provided by the manufacturer.

3.5. Sequencing

1. Mix 40 ng of the PCR product with 3.2 pmol of the sequencing primer in a volume of 12 μL. The PCR products are sequenced with the primers used in the PCRs (Note: for exons 5 and 6 use only forward primer) (*see* **Note 4**).
2. Sequencing reactions are performed using ABI prism dye terminator cycle sequencing ready reaction kit (373A automated sequencer) or ABI big dye terminator kit (377 automated sequencer) according to the manufacturer's instructions. Cycling conditions are indicated in the protocol provided by the manufacturer. Precipitate the sequencing reaction product with ethanol/sodium acetate according to the procedure in the manual.
3. Sequencing reactions are electrophoresed either on 6% Long Ranger gels, containing 8 *M* urea, or 5% Long Ranger gels, containing 6 *M* urea, and analyzed on an Applied Biosystems model 373A or 377 automated DNA sequencers, respectively (*see* **Notes 5** and **6**).

4. Notes

1. The above is especially true when searching for somatic mutations in tumor tissue, where contaminating normal cell DNA further reduces the proportion of the mutant allele in the template. Before tumor DNA extraction, the tumor percentage of the sample should be evaluated and recorded.
2. When performing the *SMAD4/DPC4* exon PCRs always include a control mix lacking template, to detect contaminations by genomic or previously amplified DNA.
3. If after **Subheading 3.3.**, **step 8** you see the expected band, but also some unspecific amplification, you may consider optimizing the reaction. If this is not of help, the correct band can be cut from the gel and DNA purified with QIAquick

Gel Extraction Kit (Qiagen). Note the possibility that a small genomic deletion may show as an extra band on the agarose gel.

4. Sequencing the samples to both forward and reverse directions increases mutation detection rate and is helpful in clarifying sequencing artifacts.

5. *SMAD4/DPC4* germline mutations are typically heterozygous; software designed for mutation detection does not always pick these up. Evaluation by eye is also obligatory.

6. Further measures to clarify ambiguous results (typically a poorly reproducible double peak indicating a possible heterozygous one base change) include restriction enzyme digestion and allelic specific oligonucleotide analyses. These are rarely needed.

References

1. Nugent, K. P., Talbot, I. C., Hodgson, S. V., and Phillips, R. K. (1993) Solitary juvenile polyps: not a marker for subsequent malignancy. *Gastroenterology* **105,** 698–700.
2. Wu, T. T., Rezai, B., Rashid, A., Luce, M. C., Cayouette, M. C., Kim, C., et al. (1997) Genetic alterations and epithelial dysplasia in juvenile polyposis syndrome and sporadic juvenile polyps. *Am. J. Pathol.* **150,** 939–947.
3. Jass, J. R., Williams, C. B., Bussey, H. J., and Morson, B.C. (1988) Juvenile polyposis—a precancerous condition. *Histopathology* **13,** 619–630.
4. Phillips, R. K. S., Spigelman, A. D., and Thomson, J. P. S. (eds.) (1994) *Familial Adenomatous Polyposis and Other Polyposis Syndromes.* Edward Arnold, London, pp. 204,205.
5. Desai, D. C., Murday, V., Phillips, R. K., Neale, K. F., Milla, P., and Hodgson, S. V. (1998) A survey of phenotypic features in juvenile polyposis. *J. Med. Genet.* **35,** 476–481.
6. Coburn, M. C., Pricolo, V. E., DeLuca, F. G., and Bland, K. I. (1995) Malignant potential in intestinal juvenile polyposis syndromes. *Ann. Surg. Oncol.* **2,** 386–391.
7. Sharma, A. K., Sharma, S. S., and Mathur, P. (1995) Familial juvenile polyposis with adenomatous-carcinomatous change. *J. Gastroenterol. Hepatol.* **10,** 131–134.
8. Howe, J. R., Mitros, F. A., and Summers, R. W. (1998) The risk of gastrointestinal carcinoma in familial juvenile polyposis. *Ann. Surg. Oncol.* **5,** 751–756.
9. Agnifili, A., Verzaro, R., Gola, P., Marino, M., Mancini, E., Carducci, G., et al. (1999) Juvenile polyposis: case report and assessment of the neoplastic risk in 271 patients reported in the literature. *Dig. Surg.* **16,** 161–166.
10. Järvinen, H. J., Mecklin, J.-P., and Sistonen, P. (1995) Screening reduces colorectal cancer rate in families with hereditary nonpolyposis colorectal cancer. *Gastroenterology* **108,** 1405–1411.
11. Olschwang, S., Serova-Sinilnikova, O. M., Lenoir, G., and Thomas, G. (1998) PTEN germline mutations in juvenile polyposis coli. *Nature Genet.* **18,** 12–14.
12. Marsh, D. J., Roth, S., Lunetta, K. L., Hemminki, A., Dahia, P. L., Sistonen, P., et al. (1997) Exclusion of PTEN and 10q22-24 as the susceptibility locus for juvenile polyposis syndrome. *Cancer Res.* **57,** 5017–5021.

13. Kurose, K., Araki, T., Matsunaka, T., Takada, Y., and Emi, M. Variant manifestation of Cowden disease in Japan: hamatomatous polyposis of the digestive tract with mutation of the PTEN gene. *Am. J. Hum. Genet.* **64,** 308–310.

14. Hahn, S. A., Schutte, M., Hoque, A. T., Moskaluk, C. A., da Costa, L. T., Rozenblum, E., et al. (1996) DPC4, a candidate tumor suppressor gene at human chromosome 18q21.1. *Science* **271,** 350–353.

15. Howe, J. R., Roth, S., Ringold, J. C., Summers, R. W., Järvinen, H. J., Sistonen, P., et al. Mutations in the Smad4/DPC4 gene in juvenile polyposis. *Science* **280,** 1086–1088.

16. Houlston, R., Bevan, S., Williams, A., Young, J., Dunlop, M., Rozen, P., et al. (1998) Mutations in DPC4 (SMAD4) cause juvenile polyposis syndrome, but only account for a minority of cases. *Hum. Mol. Genet.* **7,** 1907–1912.

17. Heldin, C. H., Miyazono, K., and ten Dijke, P. (1997) TGF-βeta signalling from cell membrane to nucleus through SMAD proteins. *Nature* **390,** 465–471.

18. Roth, S., Sistonen, P., Hemminki ,A,. Salovaara, R., Loukola, A., Johansson, M., et al. *Smad* genes in juvenile polyposis. *Gene. Chrom. Cancer* **26,** 54–61.

19. Takagi, Y., Kohmura, H., Futamura, M., Kida, H., Tanemura, H., Shimokawa, K., and Saji, S. (1996) Somatic alterations of the DPC4 gene in human colorectal cancers in vivo. *Gastroenterology* **111,** 1369–1372.

20. Miyaki, M., Iijima, T., Konishi, M., Sakai, K., Ishii, A., Yasuno, M., et al. (1999) Higher frequency of Smad4 gene mutation in human colorectal cancer with distant metastasis. *Oncogene* **18,** 3098–3103.

21. Bartsch, D., Hahn, S. A., Danichevski, K. D., Ramaswamy, A., Bastian, D., Galehdari, H., et al. (1999) Mutations of the DPC4/Smad4 gene in neuroendocrine pancreatic tumors. *Oncogene* **18,** 2367–2371.

22. Nagatake, M., Takagi, Y., Osada, H., Uchida, K., Mitsudomi, T., Saji, S., et al. (1996) Somatic in vivo alterations of the DPC4 gene at 18q21 in human lung cancers. *Cancer Res.* **56,** 2718–2720.

23. Schutte, M., Hruban, R. H., Hedrick, L., Cho, K. R., Nadasdy, G. M., Weinstein, C. L., et al. (1996) DPC4 gene in various tumor types. *Cancer Res.* **56,** 2527–2530.

24. Kim, S. K., Fan, Y., Papadimitrakopoulou, V., Clayman, G., Hittelman, W. N., Hong, W. K., et al. (1996) DPC4, a candidate tumor suppressor gene, is altered infrequently in head and neck squamous cell carcinoma. *Cancer Res.* **56,** 2519–2521.

25. Zhou, Y., Kato, H., Shan, D., Minami, R., Kitazawa, S., Matsuda, T., et al. (1999) Involvement of mutations in the DPC4 promoter in endometrial carcinoma development. *Mol. Carcinog.* **25,** 64–72.

17

Direct Sequencing for Peutz-Jeghers Gene *LKB1* (*STK11*) Mutations

Lauri A. Aaltonen and Egle Avizienyte

1. Introduction

While Peutz-Jeghers syndrome (PJS) has been acknowledged as a clinical entity for decades (*1,2*), the molecular background for the disease has been unraveled only very recently. PJS has two cardinal features: First, many but not all patients display mucocutaneous melanin pigmentation that is most prominently seen around the mouth, but can also be present for example in the buccal mucosa, lips, palms, feet, and in the anal region. Second, the patients have a predisposition to hamartomatous intestinal polyps. These lesions can occur anywhere in the gastrointestinal tract, but are most commonly seen in the small intestine (*3*). Tumor predisposition is not limited to intestinal hamartomas. The patients have a relatively unfocused increased risk of cancer, which has been reported to be 10- to 18-fold of that of the general population. Especially the relative risk for breast and gynecologic cancers is high (*4,5*). Other sites possibly involved include at least small and large intestine, and pancreas (*3*). Benign testicular tumors also occur commonly in the syndrome (*6*). Some of the malignant tumors may arise from the benign hamartomatous lesions, which appear to have some malignant potential at least in the context of PJS (*7–10*).

Because of the predisposition to tumors, PJS diagnosis is of clinical relevance. Intussusception due to benign intestinal hamartomas occurs frequently at young age, and at older age risk of malignant transformation increases (*11*). While endoscopic cancer screening along the lines shown in hereditary nonpolyposis colorectal cancer (*12*) may be feasible in preventing Peutz Jeghers intestinal cancers occurring in regions that can be reached, the wide spectrum of involved organ systems is a major clinical challenge. Prominent

From: *Methods in Molecular Medicine, vol. 50: Colorectal Cancer: Methods and Protocols*
Edited by: S. M. Powell © Humana Press Inc., Totowa, NJ

mucocutaneous pigmentation is a useful sign of the syndrome, but it must be emphasized that pigment spots around the mouth are common in the general population, and these lesions are not always present in PJS individuals (the pigmentation tends to be most prominent in adolescence, and is often absent at very young or older age). Histopathological features of the polyps give useful clues: PJS polyps display a pathognomonic tree-like smooth muscle cell core *(3)*. For unambiguous uninvasive diagnosis, molecular methods must be used.

The gene for PJS was recently identified as *LKB1 (STK11) (13)*. First clues to the location and function of the gene came from studies showing allelic loss in 19p in PJS polyps *(14)*, suggesting that this locus harbors a PJS predisposition gene and that the wild type allele is somatically inactivated as proposed in Knudson's two-hit hypothesis *(15)*. Subsequent linkage and physical mapping efforts demonstrated that indeed chromosome 19p harbors the PJS gene *(16–19)*, and that the disease is caused by inactivating mutations of the LKB1 serine/threonine kinase *(13,20)*. This was the first example of inactivating mutations in a kinase in hereditary cancer.

Before blood samples are drawn from at risk individuals for the purpose of genetic PJS testing the individuals should undergo genetic counseling, and give an informed consent. We recommend direct genomic sequencing of *LKB1* as the method of choice in PJS diagnostics. The gene is relatively small, and no close human homologues are known *(13)*; the 9 coding exons contain a 1302 base pair open reading frame corresponding to 433 amino acids. Thus genomic sequencing of the gene in nine fragments is not an extensive task. The interpretation of the results is facilitated by frequent occurrence of truncating mutations *(13,21–24)* which are likely to be disease-causing. In the case of missense mutations interpretation is facilitated by sequence comparisons *(25)* to evaluate whether the variant is in a conserved position. In research environment mutations affecting the kinase domain can be evaluated functionally, through an autophosphorylation assay *(23,24)*. This way common polymorphisms can often be excluded as a cause of the disease. While the present notion is that most if not all PJS cases arise from the background of an *LKB1* mutation, mutation detection rate by genomic sequencing is roughly two thirds *(21,22,24)*. A proportion of the remaining one third may be due to other predisposing genes *(17,18,23)*, but another obvious explanation is occurrence of mutations that cannot be detected by sequencing. Large deletions and other rearrangements are usually impossible to detect in direct genomic sequencing, and the promotor area is not evaluated.

LKB1 somatic mutations appear to be rare in most tumor types, but have been described, e.g., in colorectal, endometrial, testicular and pancreatic malignancies, as well as malignant melanomas *(26–32)*. Direct genomic sequencing of *LKB1* is one option for analysis of somatic mutations especially if samples of particular interest are to be scrutinized.

2. Materials
2.1. Blood Processing and DNA Extraction

1. EDTA anticoagulated blood tubes filled with whole blood (Vacuette, Greiner Labortechnik, Frickenhausen, Germany).
2. 15-mL polypropylene tubes (Greiner Labortechnik).
3. TKM 1 buffer: 10 mM Tris-HCl, pH 7.6, 10 mM KCl, 10 mM MgCl$_2$, 2 mM EDTA pH 7.6.
4. TKM 2 buffer: 10 mM Tris-HCl, pH 7.6, 10 mM KCl, 10 mM MgCl$_2$, 2 mM EDTA, pH 7.6, 0.4 M NaCl.
5. TKM 1 + Nonidet buffer (2.5 mL Nonidet in 100 mL TKM1).
6. Nonidet P-40 (Sigma Chemical, St. Louis, MO).
7. 20% SDS.
8. 5 M NaCl.
9. 10 mM Tris-HCl and 1 mM EDTA, pH 8.0.
10. Centrifuge.
11. 2-mL Eppendorf tubes.
12. Ethanol (99.5%).
13. Pasteur pipets.
14. Micro centrifuge.
15. 1.8 mL cryo tubes (Greiner Labortechnik).

2.2. PCR Amplifications

1. Ampli*Taq* Gold DNA polymerase (Perkin Elmer Applied Biosystems Division PE/ABI, Foster City, CA).
2. 10X PCR reaction buffer (PE/ABI).
3. Oligonucleotides (*see* **Table 1**).
4. Sterile water.
5. dNTP-mix (Finnzymes, Espoo, Finland).
6. MgCl$_2$ (15 mM, PE/ABI).
7. Thermocycler.
8. PCR tubes (Robbins Scientific, Sunnyvalley, CA).
9. Template (genomic DNA).
10. QIAquick PCR purification Kit (Qiagen).
11. DMSO (Dimethyl sulfoxide, Sigma).

2.3. Gel Electrophoresis

1. Agarose (NuSieve, Bioproducts, Rockland, ME).
2. Tris-borate (TBE) buffer: 0.09 M Tris-borate, 0.002 M EDTA, pH 8.0.
3. Ethidium bromide (EtBr) solution in water (10 mg/mL).
4. Gel-loading buffer: 0.05% bromphenol blue, 0.05% xylene cyanole FF, 30% glycerol in water.
5. ϕX174 DNA/Hae III marker (Promega, Madison, WI).
6. Gel electrophoresis tank, accessories, and power supply.

Table 1
***LKB1* Gene PCR Amplification Oligonucleotide Primers**

Primer[a]	Sequence (5' → 3')	Product size, bp
Exon 1F	GGAAGTCGGAACACAAGGAA	450
Exon 1R	GGGAGGAGAGAAGGAAGGAA	
Exon 2F	GAGGTACGCCACTTCCACAG	288
Exon 2R	CTTCAAGGAGACGGGAAGAG	
Exon 3F	GTGAGCCCCGCAGGAACG	427
Exon 3R	CAGTGTGGCCTCACGGAAAGG	
Exon 4F	GTGTGCCTGGACTTCTGTGA	324
Exon 4R	GTGCAGCCCTCAGGGAGT	
Exon 5F	ACCCTCAAAATCTCCGACCT	287
Exon 5R	GAGTGTGCGTGTGGTGAGTG	
Exon 6F	TCAACCACCTTGACTGACCA	251
Exon 6R	ACACCCCCAACCCTACATTT	
Exon 7F	GGAGTGGAGTGGCCTCTGT	291
Exon 7R	CTCAACCAGCTGCCCACAT	
Exon 8F	TCCTGAGTGTGTGGCAGGTA	387
Exon 8R	GAAGCTGTCCTTGTTGCAGA	
Exon 9F	GGCATCCAGGCGTTGTCC	360
Exon 9R	AGCTGTAAGTGCGTCCCCGTGGT	

[a]F = forward primers, R = reverse primers of a pair for amplification. Primers for exons 3 and 9 from Bignell et al. *(26)*.

2.4. PCR Product Purification

1. QIAquick PCR purification kit (Qiagen, Valencia, CA).
2. Ethanol (99.5%).
3. Eppendorf tubes (1.5 mL).
4. Microfuge.

2.5. Automated Sequencing

1. ABI prism dye terminator cycle sequencing ready reaction kit (Perkin-Elmer Corp.).
2. ABI big dye terminator kit (Perkin-Elmer Corp.).
3. Long Ranger gel solution (FMC Bioproducts, Rockland, ME).
4. Urea.
5. Ammonium persulfate.
6. N,N,N',N'-Tetramethylethylene diamine (TEMED).
7. Primers (2 μM).
8. Sterile water.
9. 0.5 mL PCR tubes (Robbins).
10. Template (PCR product).

11. Tris-borate (TBE) buffer: 0.09 *M* Tris-borate, 0.002 *M* EDTA, pH 8.3.
12. Gel electrophoresis equipment (Perkin-Elmer Corp.) and power supply.
13. Applied Biosystems model 373A or 377 automated sequencer (Perkin-Elmer Corp.).

3. Methods

3.1. Blood Processing and DNA Extraction (see Note 1)

1. Take 5 mL of whole blood to the 15 mL polypropylene tube and add 5 mL of TKM-1+Nonidet buffer. Mix blood and buffer carefully and let them stay approximately 5 min in room temperature.
2. Centrifuge tubes at 1000*g* for 10 min at room temperature.
3. Pour the supernatant carefully away and wash the nuclei pellet with 10 mL of TKM-1 buffer. Centrifuge at 1000*g* for 10 min. Repeat this step if needed.
4. Pour the supernatant away and add 800 µL TKM-2 buffer. Transfer the nuclei pellet and buffer to 2-mL Eppendorf tube by Pasteur pipet. Break the nuclei pellet by pipeting.
5. Add 50 µL 20% SDS and vortex carefully.
6. Incubate tubes at + 55°C over night.
7. After incubation add 360 µL 5 *M* NaCl and mix well.
8. Centrifuge at 14,800*g* for 10 min at +4°C (in microfuge).
9. Pipet supernatant into 10 mL polypropylene tubes and add 5 mL of ice cold absolute ethanol. Turn tubes up and down until DNA precipitates.
10. Transfer DNA into 15 mL tube containing 10 mL of 70% ethanol. Wash DNA in a slow rotating wheel mixer over night.
11. Wind the DNA around a thin glass stick and let it dry until ethanol has evaporated. Dissolve the DNA in Tris-EDTA (pH 8.0) in cryo tubes (100–1500 µL).
12. Dissolve DNA by mixing it in rotating wheel mixer at +4°C (1–3 d).

3.2. Amplification of LKB1 Exons 1–9 (PCR)

1. The reactions are carried out in 50 µL reaction volume containing 100 ng of genomic DNA (*see* **Note 2**), 1X PCR reaction buffer, 200 µ*M* of each dNTP, each primer at 0.6 µ*M*, 1 unit of AmpliTaqGOLD polymerase. Use dimethylsulfoxide (DMSO) and additional amount of MgCl$_2$, in the following reactions: exons 1 and 6 2 m*M* MgCl$_2$; 5% DMSO, exons 5 and 8, 2 m*M* MgCl$_2$; exons 7 and 9, 10% DMSO.
2. Use the following cycling conditions: exons 1, 4, 5, 6: 10 min at 95°C, 35 cycles of 45 s at 95°C, 30 s at 59°C, 45 s at 72°C; exon 2: 10 min at 95°C, 35 cycles of 45 s at 95°C, 45 s at 58°C, 45 s at 72°C; exon 3: 10 min at 95°C, 3 cycles of 45 s at 95°C, 45 s at 68°C, 45 s at 72°C, 3 cycles of 45 s at 95°C, 45 s at 63°C, 45 s at 72°C, 5 cycles of 45 s at 95°C, 45 s at 60°C, 45 s at 72°C, 29 cycles of 30 s at 95°C, 45 s at 58°C, 1 min at 72°C; exons 7 and 8: 10 min at 95°C, 35 cycles of 45 s at 95°C, 45 s at 56°C, 30 s at 72°C; exon 9: 10 min at 95°C, 5 cycles of 45 s at 95°C, 45 s at 68°C, 45 s at 72°C, 5 cycles of 45 s at 95°C, 45 s at 62°C, 45 s at 72°C, 5 cycles of 45 s at 95°C, 45 s at 57°C, 45 s at 72°C, 25 cycles of 30 s at 95°C, 45 s at 55°C, 45 s at 72°C. Use final extension of 10 min at 72°C for all exons.

3.3. Agarose Gel Electrophoresis

1. Seal the edges of the plastic tray with tapes and put the comb 2.0–3.0 mm above the tray.
2. Prepare 3% agarose solution in 1X TBE buffer.
3. Cool the solution to 60°C, add EtBr solution to a final concentration of 0.5 μg/mL and mix thoroughly, pour the solution into the plastic tray.
4. Leave the gel for 45 min to solidify. After this has occurred remove the comb and the tapes.
5. Insert the tray with the gel in the electrophoresis tank filled with 1X TBE buffer.
6. Mix 5 μL of the PCR product with 1 μL of gel-loading buffer. Load the mixture into the well. Use 0.5 μg of φX DNA/*Hae*III marker.
7. Perform electrophoresis for 1.5 h at 100 V.
8. Check the specificity of the PCR product (*see* **Note 3**).

3.4. PCR Product Purification

If the PCR product is specific, purify the rest of the reaction product using QIAquick PCR purification kit according to the protocol provided by the manufacturer.

3.5. Sequencing

1. Mix 40 ng of the PCR product with 3.2 pmol of the sequencing primer in a volume of 12 μL. The PCR products are sequenced with the primers used in the PCRs. For exons 1 and 5 use only reverse primer (*see* **Note 5**).
2. Sequencing reactions are performed using ABI prism dye terminator cycle, sequencing ready reaction kit (373A automated sequencer) or ABI big dye terminator kit (377 automated sequencer) according to the manufacturer's instructions. Cycling conditions are indicated in the protocol provided by the manufacturer. Precipitate the sequencing reaction product with ethanol/sodium acetate according to the procedure in the manual.
3. Sequencing reactions are electrophoresed either on 6% Long Ranger gels, containing 8 *M* urea, or 5% Long Ranger gels, containing 6 *M* urea, and analyzed on an Applied Biosystems model 373A or 377 automated DNA sequencers, respectively (*see* **Notes 5** and **6**).

4. Notes

1. The above is especially true when searching for somatic mutations in tumor tissue, where contaminating normal cell DNA further reduces the proportion of the mutant allele in the template. Before tumor DNA extraction, the tumor percentage of the sample should be evaluated and recorded.
2. When performing the LKB1 exon PCRs always include a control mix lacking template, to detect contaminations by genomic or previously amplified DNA.
3. If after **Subheading 3.3.**, **step 8** you see the expected band, but also some unspecific amplification, you may consider optimizing the reaction. If this is not of

help, the correct band can be cut from the gel and DNA purified with QIAquick Gel Extraction Kit (QIAGEN, Valencia, CA). Note the possibility that a small genomic deletion may show as an extra band on the agarose gel.

4. Sequencing the samples to both forward and reverse directions increases mutation detection rate and is helpful in clarifying sequencing artifacts. For exons 1 and 5 only reverse primers gives high quality sequence in our hands.

5. *LKB1* germline mutations are typically heterozygous; software designed for mutation detection does not always pick these up. Evaluation by eye is also obligatory.

6. Further measures to clarify ambiguous results (typically a poorly reproducible double peak indicating a possible heterozygous one base change) include restriction enzyme digestion and allelic specific oligonucleotide analyses. These are rarely needed.

References

1. Peutz, J. L. (1921) [A very remarkable case of familial polyposis of mucous membrane of intestinal tract and accompanied by peculiar pigmentations of skin and mucous membrane] (Dutch). *Nederlands Tijdschrift voor Geneeskunde* **10,** 134–146.
2. Jeghers, H., McKusick, V. A., and Katz, K. H. (1949) Generalized intestinal polyposis and melanin spots of the oral mucosa, lips and digits. *N. Engl. J. Med.* **241,** 1031–1036.
3. Phillips, R. K. S., Spigelman, A. D., and Thomson, J. P. S. (eds.) (1994) *Familial adenomatous polyposis and other polyposis syndromes.* Edward Arnold, London.
4. Giardiello, F. M., Welsh, S. B., Hamilton, S. R., Offerhaus, G. J., Gittelsohn, A. M., Booker, S. V., et al. (1987) Increased risk of cancer in the Peutz-Jeghers syndrome. *N. Engl. J. Med.* **316,** 1511–1514.
5. Boardman L. A., Thibodeau, S. N., Schaid, D. J., Lindor, N. M., McDonnell, S. K., Burgart, L. J., et al. (1998) Increased risk for cancer in patients with the Peutz-Jeghers syndrome. *Ann. Intern. Med.* **128,** 896–899.
6. Wilson, D. M., Pitts, W. C., Hintz, R. L., and Rosenfeld, R. G. (1986) Testicular tumors with Peutz-Jeghers syndrome. *Cancer* **57,** 2238–2240.
7. Perzin, K. H. and Bridge, M. F. (1982) Adenomatous and carcinomatous changes in hamartomatous polyps of the small intestine (Peutz-Jeghers syndrome): report of a case and review of the literature. *Cancer* **49,** 971–983.
8. Patterson, M. J. and Kernen, J. A. (1985) Epithelioid leiomyosarcoma originating in a hamartomatous polyp from a patient with Peutz-Jeghers syndrome. *Gastroenterology* **88,** 1060–1064.
9. Hizawa, K., Iida, M., Matsumoto, T., Kohrogi, N., Yao, T., and Fujishima, M. (1993) Neoplastic transformation arising in Peutz-Jeghers polyposis. *Dis. Colon Rectum* **36,** 953–957.
10. Defago, M. R., Higa, A. L., Campra, J. L., Paradelo, M., Uehara, A., Torres Mazzucchi, M. H., and Videla, R. (1996) Carcinoma in situ arising in a gastric hamartomatous polyp in a patient with Peutz-Jeghers syndrome. *Endoscopy* **28,** 267.

11. Westerman A. M., Entius, M. M., de Baar, E., Boor, P. P., Koole, R., van Velthuysen, M. L., et al. (1999) Peutz-Jeghers syndrome: 78-year follow-up of the original family. *Lancet* **353,** 1211–1215.
12. Järvinen, H. J., Mecklin, J-P., and Sistonen, P. (1995) Screening reduces colorectal cancer rate in families with hereditary nonpolyposis colorectal cancer. *Gastroenterology* **108,** 1405–1411.
13. Hemminki, A., Markie, D., Tomlinson, I., Avizienyte, E., Roth, S., Loukola, A., et al. (1998) A serine/threonine kinase gene defective in Peutz-Jeghers syndrome. *Nature* **391,** 184–187.
14. Hemminki, A., Tomlinson, I., Markie, D., Järvinen, H., Sistonen, P., Björkqvist, A. M., et al. (1997) Localization of a susceptibility locus for Peutz-Jeghers syndrome to 19p using comparative genomic hybridization and targeted linkage analysis. *Nature Genet.* **15,** 87–90.
15. Knudson, A. G. (1971) Mutation and cancer: statistical study of retinoblastoma. *Proc. Natl. Acad. Sci.* **68,** 820–823.
16. Amos, C. I., Bali, D., Thiel, T. J., Anderson, J. P., Gourley, I., Frazier, M. L., et al. (1997) Fine mapping of a genetic locus for Peutz-Jeghers syndrome on chromosome 19p. *Cancer Res.* **57,** 3653–3656
17. Mehenni, H., Blouin, J. L., Radhakrishna, U., Bhardwaj, S. S., Bhardwaj, K., Dixit, V. B., et al. (1997) Peutz-Jeghers syndrome: confirmation of linkage to chromosome 19p13.3 and identification of a potential second locus, on 19q13.4. *Am. J. Hum. Genet.* **61,** 1327–1334.
18. Olschwang, S., Markie, D., Seal, S., Neale, K., Phillips, R., Cottrel, L. S., et al. (1998) Peutz-Jeghers disease: most families compatible with linkage to 19p13.3, but evidence for a second locus at a different site. *J. Med. Genet.* **35,** 42–44.
19. Nakagawa, H., Koyama, K., Tanaka, T., Miyoshi, Y., Ando, H., Baba, S., et al. (1998) Localization of the gene responsible for Peutz-Jeghers syndrome within a 6-cM region of chromosome 19p13.3. *Hum. Genet.* **102,** 203–206.
20. Nezu, J. (1996) Molecular cloning of a novel serine/threonine protein kinase expressed in human fetal liver (direct submission to GenBank, unpublished). In http://www.ncbi.nlm.nih.gov/irx/cgi-βin/birx_doc?genbank+65606.
21. Jenne, D. E., Reimann, H., Nezu, J., Friedel, W., Loff, S., Jeschke, R., et al. (1998) Peutz-Jeghers syndrome is caused by mutations in a novel serine threonine kinase. *Nature Genet.* **18,** 38–43.
22. Nakagawa, H., Koyama, K., Miyoshi, Y., Ando, H., Baba, S., Watatani, M., et al. (1998) Nine novel germline mutations of STK11 in ten families with Peutz-Jeghers syndrome. *Hum. Genet.* **103,** 168–172.
23. Mehenni, H., Gehrig, C., Nezu, J., Oku, A., Shimane, M., Rossier, C., et al. (1998) Loss of LKB1 kinase activity in Peutz-Jeghers syndrome, and evidence for allelic and locus heterogeneity. *Am. J. Hum. Genet.* **63,** 1641–1650.
24. Ylikorkala, A., Avizienyte, E., Tomlinson, I. P., Tiainen, M., Roth, S., Loukola, A., et al. (1999) Mutations and impaired function of LKB1 in familial and nonfamilial Peutz-Jeghers syndrome and a sporadic testicular cancer. *Hum. Mol. Genet.* **8,** 45–51.

25. Su, J.-Y., Erikson, E., and Maller, J. L. (1996) Cloning and characterization of a novel serine/threonine protein kinase expressed in early *Xenopus* embryos. *J. Biol. Chem.* **271,** 14,430–14,437.
26. Bignell, G. R., Barfoot, R., Seal, S., Collins, N., Warren, W., and Stratton, M. R. (1998) Low frequency of somatic mutations in the LKB1/Peutz-Jeghers syndrome gene in sporadic breast cancer. *Cancer Res.* **58,** 1384–1386.
27. Avizienyte, E., Roth, S., Loukola, A., Hemminki, A., Lothe, R., Salovaara, R., and Aaltonen, L. A. (1998) Somatic mutations in LKB1 are rare in sporadic colorectal and testicular tumors. *Cancer Res.* **58,** 2087–2090.
28. Wang, Z. J., Taylor, F., Churchman, M., Norbury, G., and Tomlinson, I. (1998) Genetic pathways of colorectal carcinogenesis rarely involve the PTEN and LKB1 genes outside the inherited hamartoma syndromes. *Am. J. Pathol.* **153,** 363–366.
29. Park, W. S., Moon, Y. W., Yang, Y. M., Kim, Y. S., Kim, Y. D., Fuller, B. G., et al. (1998) Mutations of the STK11 gene in sporadic gastric carcinoma. *Int. J. Oncol.* **13,** 601–604.
30. Avizienyte, E., Loukola, A., Roth, S., Hemminki, A., Tarkkanen, M., Salovaara, R., et al. (1999) LKB1 somatic mutations in sporadic tumors. *Am. J. Pathol.* **154,** 677–681.
31. Rowan, A., Bataille, V., MacKie, R., Healy, E., Bicknell, D., Bodmer, W., and Tomlinson, I. (1999) Somatic mutations in the Peutz-Jegners (LKB1/STKII) gene in sporadic malignant melanomas. *J. Invest. Dermatol.* **112,** 509–511.
32. Su, G. H., Hruban, R. H., Bansal, R. K., Bova, G. S., Tang, D. J., Shekher, M. C., et al. Germline and somatic mutations of the STK11/LKB1 Peutz-Jeghers gene in pancreatic and biliary cancers. *Am. J. Pathol.* **154,** 1835–1840.

18

Direct Sequencing for Cowden Syndrome Gene *PTEN* (*MMAC1*) Mutations

Lauri A. Aaltonen, Stina Roth, and Charis Eng

1. Introduction

Cowden syndrome is a rare dominantly inherited condition with predisposition to benign hamartomatous polyposis of the intestine, as well as malignant tumors of the breast and thyroid, and possibly some other cancer types. Other features include macrocephaly and dysplastic cerebellar gangliocytomatosis with ataxia, as well as predisposition to formation of trichilemmomas of the skin *(1)*. The latter are tumors of the hair root sheath.

It should be noted that, according to the present knowledge and unlike the other hamartomatous polyposis syndromes juvenile polyposis and Peutz–Jeghers syndrome, Cowden disease does not confer a clearly increased risk of colon cancer. Indeed, in the only population-based study, the risk of colon cancer was 3% *(2)*. The disease is so poorly recognized that it is difficult to estimate whether some risk is present; adenomatous polyps in Cowden disease have been described *(3)*. Clinical data of at least two Cowden syndrome families is compatible with colon cancer predisposition (Eng, unpublished).

Recently germline mutations of tumor suppressor gene *PTEN* (also known as *MMAC*1 or *TEP*1), a tumor suppressor gene on 10q23.3, have been shown to underlie the disease *(4)*. The gene was identified through deletion mapping in sporadic tumors *(5–7)*. *PTEN* acts as a tumor suppressor by negatively regulating the PI3K/PKB/Akt signaling pathway *(8)*.

Bannayan–Zonana (Bannayan–Riley–Ruvalcaba) syndrome, characterized by macrocephaly, pigmented macules of the glans penis and lipomas, in addition to hamartomatous intestinal polyposis *(1)*, appears to be allelic to Cowden syndrome *(9,10)*. Lhermitte-Duclos disease, which is an hamartomatous overgrowth of cerebellar tissue, is also associated with Cowden disease and

From: *Methods in Molecular Medicine, vol. 50: Colorectal Cancer: Methods and Protocols*
Edited by: S. M. Powell © Humana Press Inc., Totowa, NJ

germline *PTEN* mutations *(11)*. One report has associated *PTEN* mutations and juvenile polyposis *(12)* but this result has not been confirmed *(13)* and individuals with *PTEN* mutations should be considered as having Cowden disease, with increased risk of thyroid and breast cancer *(14,15)*.

PTEN is a relatively small gene comprising nine exons and encoding 403 amino acids. Thus we recommend genomic sequencing as the method of choice in the setting of clinical molecular diagnostics. Appropriate genetic counseling must be given before testing. In research environment consequences of missense changes to the phosphatase function can be evaluated *(16,17)*.

Somatic *PTEN* mutations or homozygous deletions have been detected in multiple sporadic tumor types. These include glioma *(18)* and melanoma *(19)*, tumors of the endometrium *(20–23)*, especially ones showing microsatellite instability *(24)*, prostate *(25–27)*, hepatocellular *(28,29)*, thyroid *(30)*, bladder *(31)*, breast *(32–34)*, colon *(35)*, head and neck *(36)*, and lung cancers *(37)*, as well as leukemia *(37)*, and B-cell non-Hodgkin's lymphomas *(38,39)*.

2. Materials
2.1. Blood Processing and DNA Extraction

1. EDTA anticoagulated blood tubes filled with whole blood (Vacuette, Greiner Labortechnik, Frickenhausen, Germany).
2. 15-mL polypropylene tubes (Greiner Labortechnik).
3. TKM 1 buffer: 10 mM Tris-HCl, pH 7.6, 10 mM KCl, 10 mM MgCl$_2$, 2 mM EDTA pH 7.6.
4. TKM 2 buffer: 10 mM Tris-HCl, pH 7.6, 10 mM KCl, 10 mM MgCl$_2$, 2 mM EDTA, pH 7.6, 0.4 M NaCl.
5. TKM1 + Nonidet buffer: 2.5 mL Nonidet in 100 mL TKM1.
6. Nonidet P-40 (Sigma Chemical, St. Louis, MO).
7. 20% SDS.
8. 5 M NaCl.
9. 10 mM Tris-HCl and 1 mM EDTA, pH 8.0.
10. Centrifuge.
11. 2-mL Eppendorf tubes.
12. Ethanol (99.5%).
13. Pasteur pipets.
14. Microfuge.
15. 1.8 mL cryo tubes (Greiner Labortechnik).

2.2. PCR Amplifications

1. Ampli*Taq* Gold DNA polymerase (Perkin Elmer Applied Biosystems Division PE/ABI, Foster City, CA).
2. 10X PCR reaction buffer (PE/ABI).
3. Oligonucleotides (*see* **Table 1**).

Table 1
Oligonucleotide Primers for Genomic Sequencing of the 9 *PTEN* Exons

Primer[a]	Sequence (5' → 3')	Product size, bp
Exon 1F	AGTCGCCTGTCACCATTTC	616
Exon 1R	ACTACGGACATTTTCGCATC	
Exon 2F	GTTTGATTGCTGCATATTTCAG	202
Exon 2R	TCTAAATGAAAACACAACATG	
Exon 3F	ATTTCAAATGTTAGCTCATTTTG	150
Exon 3R	TTTAGAAGATATTTCAAGCATAC	
Exon 4F	CATTATAAAGATTCAGGCAATG	205
Exon 4R	GACAGTAAGATACAGTCTATC	
Exon 5F	ACCTGTTAAGTTTGTATGCAA	379
Exon 5R	TCCAGGAAGAGGAAAGGAAA	
Exon 6F	CATAGCAATTTAGTGAAATAACT	274
Exon 6R	GATATGGTTAAGAAAACTGTTC	
Exon 7F	CAGTTAAAGGCATTTCCTGTG	252
Exon 7R	GGATATTTCTCCCAATGAAAG	
Exon 8F	CTCAGATTGCCTTATAATAGTC	558
Exon 8R	TCATGTTACTGCTACGTAAAC	
Exon 9F	AAGGCCTCTTAAAAGATCATG	375
Exon 9R	ATTTTCATGGTGTTTTATCCCTC	

[a]F = forward primer, R = reverse primer.

4. Sterile water.
5. dNTP-mix (Finnzymes, Espoo, Finland).
6. 15 mM $MgCl_2$ (PE/ABI, Foster City).
7. Thermocycler.
8. PCR tubes (Robbins Scientific, Sunnyvalley, CA).
9. Template (genomic DNA).
10. QIAquick PCR purification Kit (QIAGEN).
11. DMSO (Dimethyl sulfoxide, Sigma).

2.3. Gel Electrophoresis

1. Agarose (NuSieve, Bioproducts, Rockland, ME).
2. Tris-borate (TBE) buffer: 0.09 M Tris-borate, 0.002 M EDTA, pH 8.0.
3. Ethidium bromide (EtBr) solution in water (10 mg/mL).
4. Gel-loading buffer: 0.05% bromphenol blue, 0.05% xylene cyanole FF, 30% glycerol in water.
5. φX174 DNA/*Hae*III marker (Promega, Madison, WI).
6. Gel electrophoresis tank, accessories, and power supply.

2.4. PCR Product Purification

1. QIAquick PCR purification kit (Qiagen, Valencia, CA).
2. Ethanol (99.5%).
3. Eppendorf tubes (1.5 mL).
4. Microfuge.

2.5. Automated Sequencing

1. ABI prism dye terminator cycle sequencing ready reaction kit (Perkin-Elmer Corp.).
2. ABI big dye terminator kit (Perkin-Elmer Corp.).
3. Long Ranger gel solution (FMC Bioproducts, Rockland, ME).
4. Urea.
5. Ammonium persulfate.
6. N,N,N',N'-Tetramethylethylene diamine (TEMED).
7. Primers (2 μM).
8. Sterile water.
9. 0.5-mL PCR tubes (Robbins).
10. Template (PCR product).
11. Tris-borate (TBE) buffer: 0.09 M Tris-borate, 0.002 M EDTA, pH 8.3.
12. Gel electrophoresis equipment (Perkin-Elmer Corp.) and power supply.
13. Applied Biosystems model 373A or 377 automated sequencer (Perkin-Elmer Corp.).

3. Methods
3.1. Blood Processing and DNA Extraction (see Note 3)

1. Take 5 mL of whole blood to the 15 mL polypropylene tube and add 5 mL of TKM-1+Nonidet buffer. Mix blood and buffer carefully and let them stay approximately 5 min in room temperature.
2. Centrifuge tubes at 1000g for 10 min at room temperature.
3. Pour the supernatant carefully away and wash the nuclei pellet with 10 mL of TKM-1 buffer. Centrifuge at 1000g for 10 min. Repeat this step if needed.
4. Pour the supernatant away and add 800 µL TKM-2 buffer. Transfer the nuclei pellet and buffer to 2-mL Eppendorf tube by Pasteur-pipet. Break the nuclei pellet by pipeting.
5. Add 50 µL 20% SDS and vortex carefully.
6. Incubate tubes at +55°C over night.
7. After incubation add 360 mL 5 M NaCl and mix well.
8. Centrifuge at 14,800g for 10 min at +4°C (in microfuge).
9. Pipet supernatant into 10 mL polypropylene tubes and add 5 mL of ice-cold absolute ethanol. Turn tubes up and down until DNA is precipitating.
10. Transfer DNA into 15 mL tube containing 10 mL of 70% ethanol. Wash DNA in a slow rotating wheel mixer overnight.
11. Wind the DNA around the thin glass stick and let it dry until ethanol has evaporated. Dissolve the DNA in Tris-EDTA (pH 8.0) in cryo tubes (100–1500 µL).
12. Dissolve DNA by mixing it in rotating wheel mixer at +4°C (1–3 d).

3.2. Amplification of PTEN Exons 1–9 (PCR)

1. The reactions are carried out in 50 mL reaction volume containing 100 ng of genomic DNA (*see* **Note 1**), 1X PCR reaction buffer, 200 μ*M* of each dNTP, each primer at 0.8 μ*M*, 1 U of Ampli*Taq* Gold polymerase. Use dimethylsulfoxide (DMSO, 5%) in the following reactions: exons 3, 5, and 9. The MgCl$_2$ concentration was 2 m*M* in all reactions.
2. Use the following cycling conditions for: exons 1, 2, 3, 4, 5, 7, and 9: 10 min at 95°C, 40 cycles of 1 min at 95°C, 1 min at 55°C, 1 min at 70°C. For exons 6 and 8, use 10 min at 95°C, 40 cycles of 1 min at 95°C, 1 min at 56°C, 1 min at 72°C. Use final extension of 10 min at 72°C for all exons.

3.3. Agarose Gel Electrophoresis

1. Seal the edges of the plastic tray with tapes and put the comb 2.0–3.0 mm above the tray.
2. Prepare 3% agarose solution in 1X TBE buffer.
3. Cool the solution to 60°C, add EtBr solution to a final concentration of 0.5 μg/mL and mix thoroughly, pour the solution into the plastic tray.
4. Leave the gel for 45 min to solidify. After this has occurred remove the comb and the tapes.
5. Insert the tray with the gel in the electrophoresis tank filled with 1X TBE buffer.
6. Mix 5 μL of the PCR product with 1 μL of gel-loading buffer. Load the mixture into the well. Use 0.5 μg of ϕX DNA/*Hae*III marker.
7. Perform electrophoresis for 1.5 h at 100 V.
8. Evaluate the specificity of the PCR product (*see* **Note 4**).

3.4. PCR Product Purification

If the PCR product is specific, purify the rest of the reaction product using QIAquick PCR purification kit according to the protocol provided by the manufacturer.

3.5. Sequencing

1. Mix 40 ng of the PCR product with 3.2 pmol of the sequencing primer in a volume of 12 μL. The PCR products are sequenced with the primers used in the PCRs (*see* **Note 5**).
2. Sequencing reactions are performed using ABI prism dye terminator cycle sequencing ready reaction kit (373A automated sequencer) or ABI big dye terminator kit (377 automated sequencer) according to the manufacturer's instructions. Cycling conditions are indicated in the protocol provided by the manufacturer. Precipitate the sequencing reaction product with ethanol/sodium acetate according to the procedure in the manual.
3. Sequencing reactions are electrophoresed either on 6% Long Ranger gels, containing 8 *M* urea, or 5% Long Ranger gels, containing 6 *M* urea, and analyzed on an Applied Biosystems model 373A or 377 automated DNA sequencers, respectively (*see* **Notes 2** and **6**).

4. Notes

1. When performing the *PTEN* exon PCRs always include a control PCR mix lacking template, to detect contaminations by genomic or previously amplified DNA.
2. *PTEN* germline mutations are typically heterozygous; software designed for mutation detection does not always pick these up. Evaluation by eye is also obligatory.
3. The above is especially true when searching for somatic mutations in tumor tissue, where contaminating normal cell DNA further reduces the proportion of the mutant allele in the template. Before tumor DNA extraction, the tumor percentage of the sample should be evaluated and recorded.
4. If after **Subheading 3.3.**, **step 8** you see the expected band, but also some unspecific amplification, you may consider optimizing the reaction. If this is not of help, the correct band can be cut from the gel and DNA purified with QIAquick Gel Extraction Kit (QIAGEN, Valencia, CA). Note the possibility that a small genomic deletion may show as an extra band on the agarose gel.
5. Sequencing the samples to both forward and reverse directions increases mutation detection rate and is helpful in clarifying sequencing artifacts.
6. Further measures to clarify ambiguous results (typically a poorly reproducible double peak indicating a possible heterozygous one base change) include restriction enzyme digestion and allelic specific oligonucleotide analyses. These are rarely needed.

References

1. Phillips, R. K. S., Spigelman, A. D., and Thomson, J. P. S. (eds.) (1994) *Familial Adenomatous Polyposis and Other Polyposis Syndromes.* Edward Arnold, London, pp. 222,223.
2. Starink, T. M., van der Veen, J. P. W., Arwert, F., de Waal, L. P., de Lange, G. G., Gille, J. J. P., and Eriksson, A. W. (1986) The Cowden syndrome: a clinical and genetic study in 21 patients. *Clin. Genet.* **29,** 222–233.
3. Hover, A. R., Cowtherm, T., and McDanial, W. (1986) Cowden disease. *J. Clin. Gastroenterol.* **8,** 576–579.
4. Liaw, D., Marsh, D. J., Li, J., Dahia, P. L. M., Wang, S. I., Zheng, Z., Bose, S., et al. (1997) Germline mutations of the PTEN gene in Cowden disease, an inherited breast and thyroid cancer syndrome. *Nature Genet.* **16,** 64–67.
5. Li, J., Yen, C., Liaw, D., Podsypanina, K., Bose, S., Wang, S. I., et al. (1997) PTEN, a putative protein tyrosine phosphatase gene mutated in human brain, breast and prostate cancer. *Science* **275,** 1943–1947.
6. Steck, P. A., Pershouse, M. A., Jasser, S. A., Alfred Yung, W. K., Lin, H., Ligon, A. H., et al. (1997) Identification of a candidate tumour suppressor gene, MMAC1, at chromosome 10q23.3 that is mutated in multiple advanced cancers. *Nature Genet.* **15,** 356–362.
7. Li, D.-M. and Sun, H. (1997) TEP1, encoded by a candidate tumor suppressor locus, is a novel protein tyrosine phosphatase regulated by transforming growth factor β. *Cancer Res.* **57,** 2124–2129.

8. Stambolic, V., Suzuki, A., de la Pompa, J. L., Brothers, G. M., Mirtsos, C., Sasaki, T., et al. (1998) Negative regulation of PKB/Akt-dependent cell survival by the tumor suppressor PTEN. *Cell* **95,** 29–39

9. Marsh, D. J., Dahia, P. L. M., Zheng, Z., Liaw, D., Parsons, R., Gorlin, R. J., and Eng, C. (1997) Germline mutations in PTEN are present in Bannayan-Zonana syndrome. *Nature Genet.* **16,** 333–334.

10. Marsh, D. J., Coulon, V., Lunetta, K. L., Rocca-Serra, P., Dahia, P. L. M., Zheng, Z., et al. (1998) Mutation spectrum and genotype-phenotype analyses in Cowden disease and Bannayan-Zonana syndrome, two hamartoma syndromes with germline PTEN mutation. *Hum. Mol. Genet.* **7,** 507–515.

11. Koch, R., Scholz, M., Nelen, M. R., Schwechheimer, K., Epplen, J. T., and Harders, A. G. (1999) Lhermitte-Duclos disease as a component of Cowden's syndrome. Case report and review of the literature. *J. Neurosurg.* **90,** 776–779.

12. Olschwang, S., Serova-Sinilnikova, O. M., Lenoir, G., and Thomas, G. (1998) PTEN germline mutations in juvenile polyposis coli. *Nature Genet.* **18,** 12–14.

13. Marsh, D. J., Roth, S., Lunetta, K. L., Hemminki, A., Dahia, P. L., Sistonen, P., et al. (1997) Exclusion of PTEN and 10q22–24 as the susceptibility locus for juvenile polyposis syndrome. *Cancer Res.* **57,** 5017–5021.

14. Eng, C. and Peacocke, M. (1998) PTEN and inherited hamartoma-cancer syndromes. *Nature Genet.* **19,** 223.

15. Kurose, K., Araki, T., Matsunaka, T., Takada, Y., and Emi, M. Variant manifestation of Cowden disease in Japan: hamatomatous polyposis of the digestive tract with mutation of the PTEN gene. *Am. J. Hum. Genet.* **64,** 308–310.

16. Myers, M. P., Stolarov, J., Eng, C., Li, J., Wang, S. I., Wigler, M. H., et al. (1997) PTEN, the tumor suppressor from human chromosome 10q23, is a dual specificity phosphatase. *Proc. Natl. Acad. Sci.* **94,** 9052–9057.

17. Myers, M. P., Pass, I., Batty, I. H., van der Kaay, J., Storalov, J. P., Hemmings, B. A., et al. (1998) The lipid phosphatase activity of PTEN is critical for its tumor suppressor function. *Proc. Natl. Acad. Sci.* **95,** 13,513–13,518.

18. Dürr, E.-M., Rollbrocker, B., Hayashi, Y., Peters, N., Meyer-Puttlitz, B., Louis, D. N., et al. (1998) PTEN mutations in gliomas and glioneuronal tumours. *Oncogene* **16,** 2259–2264.

19. Guldberg, P., Straten, P., Birck, A., Ahrenkiel, V., Kirkin, A. F., and Zeuthen, J. (1997) Disruption of the MMAC1/PTEN gene by deletion or mutation is a frequent event in malignant melanoma. *Cancer Res.* **57,** 3660–3663.

20. Kong, D., Suzuki, A., Zou, T-T., Sakurada, A., Kemp, L. W., Wakatsuki, S., et al. (1997) PTEN1 is frequently mutated in primary endometrial carcinomas. *Nature Genet.* **17,** 143–144.

21. Tashiro, H., Blazes, M. S., Wu, R., Cho, K. R., Bose, S., Wang, S. I., et al. (1997) Mutations in PTEN are frequent in endometrial carcinoma but rare in other common gynecological malignancies. *Cancer Res.* **57,** 3935–3940.

22. Risinger, J. I., Hayes, A. K., Berchuck, A., and Barrett, J. C. (1997) PTEN/MMAC1 mutations in endometrial cancers. *Cancer Res.* **57,** 4736–4738.

23. Simpkins, S. B., Peiffer-Schneider, S., Mutch, D. G., Gersell, D., and Goodfellow, P. J. (1998) PTEN mutations in endometrial cancers with 10q LOH: additional evidence for the involvement of multiple tumor suppressors. *Gynecol. Oncol.* **71**, 391–395.

24. Gurin, C. C., Federici, M. G., Kang, L., and Boyd, J. (1999) Causes and consequences of microsatellite instability in endometrial carcinoma. *Cancer Res.* **59**, 462–466.

25. Cairns, P., Okami, K., Halachmi, S., Halachmi, N., Esteller, M., Herman, J. G., et al. (1997) Frequent inactivation of PTEN/MMAC1 in primary prostate cancer. *Cancer Res.* **57**, 4997–5000.

26. Gray, I. C., Stewart, L. M., Phillips, S. M., Hamilton, J. A., Gray, N. E., Watson, G. J., et al. (1998) Mutation and expression analysis of the putative prostate tumour-suppressor gene PTEN. *Br. J. Cancer* **78**, 1296–1300

27. Feilotter, H. E., Nagai, M. A., Boag, A. H., Eng, C., and Mulligan, L. M. (1998) Analysis of PTEN and the 10q23 region in primary prostate carcinomas. *Oncogene* **1**, 1743–1748.

28. Yao, Y. J., Ping, X. L., Zhang, H., Chen, F. F., Lee, P. K., Ahsan, H., et al. (1999) PTEN/MMAC1 mutations in hepatocellular carcinomas. *Oncogene* **18**, 3181–3185

29. Kawamura, N., Nagai, H., Bando, K., Koyama, M., Matsumoto, S., Tajiri, T., et al. (1999) PTEN/MMAC1 mutations in hepatocellular carcinomas: somatic inactivation of both alleles in tumors. *Jpn. J. Cancer Res.* **90**, 413–418.

30. Dahia, P. L., Marsh, D. J., Zheng, Z., Zedenius, J., Komminoth, P., Frisk, T., et al. (1997) Somatic deletions and mutations in the Cowden disease gene, PTEN, in sporadic thyroid tumors. *Cancer Res.* **57**, 4710–4713.

31. Aveyard, J. S., Skilleter, A., Habuchi, T., and Knowles, M. A. (1999) Somatic mutation of PTEN in bladder carcinoma. *Br. J. Cancer* **80**, 904–908.

32. Rhei, E., Kang, L., Bogomolniy, F., Federici, M. G., Borgen, P. I., and Boyd, J. (1997) Mutation analysis of the putative tumor suppressor gene PTEN/MMAC1 in primary breast carcinomas. *Cancer Res.* **57**, 3657–3659.

33. Freihoff, D., Kempe, A., Beste, B., Wappenschmidt, B., Kreyer, E., Hayashi, Y., et al. (1999) Exclusion of a major role for the PTEN tumour-suppressor gene in breast carcinomas. *Br. J. Cancer* **79**, 754–758.

34. Feilotter, H. E., Coulon, V., McVeigh, J. L., Boag, A. H., Dorion-Bonnet, F., Dubouz, B., et al. (1999) Analysis of the 10q23 chromosomal region and the PTEN gene in human sporadic breast carcinoma. *Br. J. Cancer.* **79**, 718–723.

35. Wang, Z. J., Taylor, F., Churchman, M., Norbury, G., and Tomlinson, I. (1998) Genetic pathways of colorectal carcinogenesis rarely involve the PTEN and LKB1 genes outside the inherited hamartoma syndromes. *Am. J. Pathol.* **153**, 363–366.

36. Okami, K., Wu, L., Riggins, G., Cairns, P., Goggins, M., Evron, E., et al. (1998) Analysis of PTEN/MMAC1 alterations in aerodigestive tract tumors. *Cancer Res.* **58**, 509–511.

37. Teng, D. H., Hu, R., Lin, H., Davis, T., Iliev, D., Frye, C., et al. (1997) MMAC1/PTEN mutations in primary tumor specimens and tumor cell lines. *Cancer Res.* **57**, 5221–5225.

38. Butler, M. P., Wang, S. I., Chaganti, R. S., Parsons, R., and Dalla-Favera, R. (1999) Analysis of PTEN mutations and deletions in B-cell non-Hodgkin's lymphomas. *Gen. Chromosom. Cancer* **24,** 322–327.

39. Dahia, P. L. M., Aguiar, R. C. T., Alberta, J., Kum, J., Caron, S., Sills, H., et al. (1999) PTEN is inversely correlated with the cell survival factor PKB/Akt and is inactivated by diverse mechanisms in haematologic malignancies. *Hum. Mol. Genet.* **8,** 185–193.

19

Genetic Analysis Using Microarrays

Wa'el El-Rifai and Sakari Knuutila

1. Introduction

A vast amount of genome sequencing data has become available over the past few years and methods to facilitate high-throughput analysis of large sets of genes and samples have been developed to localize novel genes related to human cancer. As advanced robotic applications have made it possible to manufacture high-precision microarrays on glass or membranes, pioneering scientists have introduced several variants of the "array" technology: oligonucleotide arrays *(1)*, DNA microarrays (CGH arrays) *(2)*, tissue microarrays *(3)*, and cDNA microarrays *(4,5)*. The array technology is based on fluorescently (glass-based arrays, chips) or radioactively (filter-based array) labeled nucleic acids that are hybridized to the microarray and imaged with a laser scanner or a phosphor imager, respectively. The images are then processed using microarray analysis software. These techniques have recently been reviewed in detail in *Nature Genetics* (vol. 21, Suppl. 1, 1999).

An oligonuclotide array is built up on a glass using a series of parallel oligonucleoside deposition steps. The oligonucleotide array is a powerful tool that allows rapid screening for mutations and sequence variations in genomic DNA. A single chip (1.6 cm^2 glass) made of 400,000 oligonucleotides can be used for resequencing ~50 kb of sequence. Thus it has been possible to design chips suitable for mutation screening in cancer-associated genes *TP53, BRCA1*, and *ATM* with detection sensitivity greater than 90% *(6,7)*. The GeneChip system developed by Affymetrix (www.affymetrix.com) is currently a fundamental element of this technology.

In DNA microarrays, hundreds of mapped DNA sequences can be printed on a glass slide. Based on the same principle as comparative genomic hybridization (CGH), the technique is dubbed CGH-arrays. Unlike CGH, DNA

From: *Methods in Molecular Medicine, vol. 50: Colorectal Cancer: Methods and Protocols*
Edited by: S. M. Powell © Humana Press Inc., Totowa, NJ

microarrays are not restricted by the resolution limits of metaphase chromosomes used in CGH. Vysis (www.vysis.com) have announced the release of GeneSensor Arrays and the first type (AmpliOnc I Array) will contain more than 50 different target genes which have been reported to be amplified in various human cancers. The upcoming versions of GeneSensor arrays will be updated with newly discovered amplicons. In addition, an array that incorporates all commonly reported tumor suppressor gene loci is already in the pipeline.

Tissue microarrays is a new technology that allows the study of hundreds of tumor specimens in a single experiment. Cylindrical biopsies from paraffin-embedded tissue sections are arrayed on a paraffin block and then transferred to a glass slide using an adhesive-coated tape sectioning system. At present 1000 tumors can be arrayed on one 45×20 mm glass slide. Fluorescent *in situ* hybridization is applied to the array using different probes. Candidate cancer genes are used as probes to study specimens from a large number of tumors at different stages of the disease to establish the diagnostic, prognostic, and therapeutic importance of these genes.

cDNA microarray technology allows the study of the expression of thousands of genes during a single experiment disclosing tumor-specific gene expression profiles. cDNAs of genes and sequence tags (ESTs) are robotically arrayed onto a glass slide or membrane (filter-based) and probed with fluorescence- or radioactively labelled cDNAs. By comparing the signal obtained with a probe from a tumor RNA to that obtained with a probe from another source (reference RNA), the relative expression of cDNA spots can be assessed and differentially expressed genes/ESTs can be identified (*see* **Fig. 1**). For the time being, the relatively high cost of glass-based arrays limits the use to few laboratories, whereas filter-based arrays are more affordable. In filter-based arrays minor RNA samples (0.1–2 µg of total RNA) can be used for a single experiment compared to 50–100 µg of total RNA needed for a fluorescent probe. However, a major disadvantage of filter arrays is that the comparison of expression profiles between two samples requires hybridization of each sample to a separate filter or sequentially to the same filter after stripping of the first hybridization. In fluorescent arrays the two samples can be labeled with two different fluorochromes and hybridized simultaneously to the same slide.

A wide range of cDNA arrays with relatively simple protocols is commercially available. Research Genetics (www.resgen.com) have introduced several releases of Human Gene filters, each release containing ~5000 genes/ESTs. The company provides a new release every few months in its ambitious goal to cover the whole genome. Clontech (www.clontech.com) have released a series of Atlas cDNA expression arrays (filter-based), where each array set contains ~600 known genes. Clontech have new filter-based Atlas releases (each con-

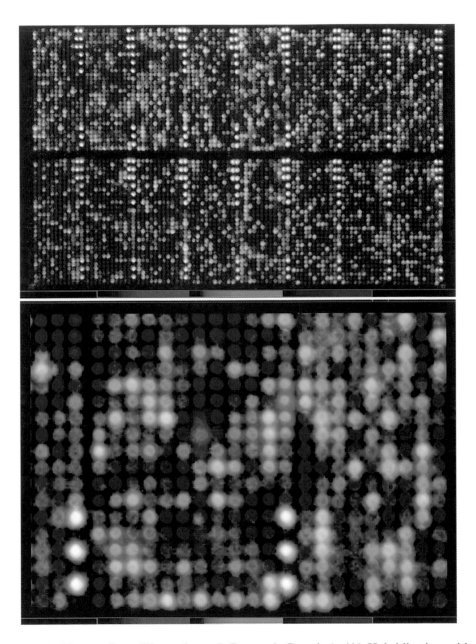

Fig. 1. Human Gene Filter release I (Research Genetics). (A) Hybridization with osteosarcoma cell line (green color) and normal osteoblast (reference, red color). The blue color is used to show the location of the 5000 cDNA spots on the filter. Yellow spots indicate genes that show balanced expression between tumor and reference. Spots with increased green intensities indicate over-expressed genes while increased red intensities indicate under-expressed genes in osteosarcoma. (B) Zooming one area in (A) showing clear green and red color variations. The intensities of the green and red were calculated using Pathway image analysis software (Research Genetics).

taining ~1000 genes) as well as glass-based microarrays. Genome Systems (www.genomesystems.com) have the filter-based Gene Discovery Array, which contains 18,000 redundant human cDNA clones, and the glass-based Human UniGEM V microarray, a recent release, which contains 4000 known human genes and up to 3000 ESTs. NEN Life Science (nenlifesci.com) have released the MICROMAX Human cDNA microarray system I. It contains two microarray slides, each pre-spotted with 2400 known genes.

Since the most current array-based studies focus on monitoring of RNA expression levels, we have chosen to describe here the filter-based cDNA microarray technique, currently adaptable in several laboratories.

2. Materials

2.1. RNA Isolation

1. Tumor tissue sample and reference sample.
2. RNeasy (Maxi) kit (Qiagen Inc., Santa Clarita, CA).
3. Oligotex mRNA kits (Qiagen).
4. Ethanol solution.

2.2. DNase Treatment of RNA

1. RNase-free DNase I (10 U/µL; Boehringer-Mannheim, Germany).
2. DNase I buffer: 400 mM Tris-HCl, pH 7.5, 100 mM NaCl, 60 mM MgCl$_2$.
3. 10X Termination mix: 0.1 M EDTA, pH 8.0, 1.0 mg/mL glycogen.
4. Phenol:chloroform:isoamyl alcohol (25:24:1).
5. 7.5 M NH$_4$OAc.
6. Ethanol solution.

2.3. cDNA Probe Synthesis

1. DNase-treated RNA
2. Alpha 33P dCTP at 10 mCi/mL concentration with specific activity of 3000 Ci/mmol (Amersham Pharmacia Biotech, Piscataway, NJ).
3. Superscript II Reverse Transcriptase (200 U/µL, Gibco-BRL, Gaithersburg, MD) or MMLV Reverse Transcriptase (50 U/µL, Gibco-BRL).
4. DTT (100 mM, Gibco-BRL).
5. dNTPs (100 mM, Amersham Pharmacia Biotech) and prepare 10X dNTP mix (5 mM each of dATP, dGTP, and dTTP).
6. Other reagents are supplied with the filter-array kit.

2.4. Hybridization and Washes

1. cDNA microarray filter, Human Gene filters (Research Genetics), Atlas Arrays (Clontech), or Gene Discovery Array (Genome Systems).
2. 20X SSC, pH 7 and 20% SDS to prepare washing solutions.
3. Hybridization oven (HYBAID [www.hybaid.co.uk]) and glass bottles (HYBAID).

4. Other hybridization reagents are included in the kit.
5. Whatman paper and nylon membranes.

2.5. Image Collection and Analysis

1. Autoradiography cassette.
2. Phosphor imaging, BAS 2500 (Fuji [www.home.fujifilm.com]). Other phosphor imager systems are produced by Molecular Dynamics (www.moleculardynamics. com) and Packard Instrument (www.packardinst.com).
3. Imaging plate, BAS-MP 2040S (Fuji).
4. A computer equipped with a software package capable of measuring and comparing intensities of two overlapping images (test and reference).

2.6. Stripping cDNA Spots from Array

1. Stripping solution I: 0.4 M NaOH, 0.1% SDS (20 mL 10 N NaOH, 2.5 mL 20% SDS, 477.5 mL H_2O).
2. Stripping solution II: 0.2 M Tris-HCl, pH 8.0, 1X SSC/0.1% SDS (100 mL Tris-HCl 1 M, 2.5 mL 20% SDS, 25 mL 20X SSC, and 375 mL H_2O).
3. Glass bottles (HYBAID) and hybridization oven (HYBAID).

3. Methods
3.1. RNA Extraction (see Note 1)

Several commercially available kits can be used for isolation of RNA. DNase treatment is necessary to ensure the purity of RNA.

1. Process your sample with Qiagen's RNeasy (Maxi) reagents according to the manufacturer's instructions.
2. Wash precipitated RNA pellet in 70% ethanol solution. Centrifuge for 30 min at 10,000g and carefully discard ethanol.
3. Air-dry the RNA pellet for approximately 15 min.
4. Resuspend RNA pellet in 100 µL of RNase-free DEPC-treated sterile water.
5. Proceed with DNase treatment (*see* **Subheading 3.2.**).
6. If arrays are to be done with mRNA, proceed with mRNA extraction according to Oligotex mRNA (Qiagen) extraction procedure.

3.2. DNase Treatment of Total RNA (see Note 2)

1. In a 2-mL Eppendorf mix 250 µL total RNA (1 mg/mL), 50 µL 10X DNase I buffer, 2.5 µL DNase I and 198 µL RNase-free sterile water.
2. Incubate at 37°C for 1 h.
3. Add 50 µL of 10X Termination and mix well.
4. Add 550 µL of phenol:chloroform:isoamyl alcohol (25:24:1), and vortex.
5. Spin in a microcentrifuge at 10,000g for 15 minutes.
6. Gently remove the tube and transfer the aqueous top layer to another Eppendorf.
7. Repeat **steps 4–6**.

8. Add 550 µL of chloroform:isoamyl alcohol (24:1) to the aqueous layer and vortex. Repeat **steps 5–6**.
9. Add 100 µL of 7.5 M NH$_4$OAc and 1.5 mL of absolute ethanol and vortex. Incubate at –20°C for minimum of 2 h to ensure precipitation of RNA.
10. Spin in a microcentrifuge at 10,000g for 30 min, and carefully discard supernatant (pellet may be loose).
11. Wash the RNA pellet with 70% ethanol solution and repeat **step 10**.
12. Air dry the pellet for approx 15 min.
13. Dissolve the RNA pellet in 100–250 µL of RNase-free DEPC water.

3.3. cDNA Array Procedure

3.3.1. cDNA Probe Synthesis and Purification (see **Note 3**)

1. Use 2 µg total RNA for cDNA synthesis. This is sufficient for most protocols.
2. Follow the protocol provided by your filter supplier.
3. Purify the probe to remove unincorporated 33P-labeled nucleotides and small (<0.1 kb) cDNA fragments using the protocol supplied with the filters.

3.3.2. Hybridization and Washing (see **Note 4**)

1. The first time you use a filter, it is recommended to wash it in 0.5% SDS at 55°C for 10 min with gentle agitation. This will clean the filter from any manufacturing residuals. From this step onwards, filters should not be allowed to dry.
2. In a HYBAID bottle, perform prehybridization blocking according to the filter supplier's instructions.
3. Place the filter in a clean HYBAID bottle containing 5 mL of hybridization mixture. Add your purified cDNA probe to the tube and mix well. Adjust the speed of the tube rotation inside the oven to 6–8 rpm and incubate for 12 h at the temperature recommended by the filter manufacturer. It is important that the tubes do not stop rolling during incubation.
4. Wash the filter following the manufacturer's instructions using 20X SCC and 20% SDS at different concentrations and temperatures. Washing is done in HYBAID bottles at 15–20 rpm using an ample amount of washing solution (100–200 mL) in each step to minimize background.
5. Cut a Whatman paper few cms larger than your filter and wet it with distilled water.
6. Carefully place your filter above the Whatman paper and wrap the filter in a nylon membrane. Avoid drying of the filter, air bubbles, and nonlinear wrapping.
7. Transfer the filter to an exposure cassette and place the image plate on it. Close the cassette firmly and apply adequate pressure on the cassette to ensure even transfer of the signals to the image plate. Exposure should last for an average of 48 h (24–96 h).

3.3.3. Image Collection and Analysis (see **Notes 5** and **6**)

1. Remove the filter from the cassette and scan the image plate using the BAS 2500 Fuji phosphor imager. Avoid exposing the plate to light.

2. Store the image as a 16-bit tif-format file.
3. Import the images to the analysis software. The software converts the two grey scale images into green (test) and red (reference) images. The two images are merged into a single image. Normalization of the images and background subtraction is done by the software. The relative hybridization intensities on each spot are determined in both tumor and reference to identify under- and over-expressed cDNA spots.
4. A report of the analysis of all spots can be produced.

3.3.4. Stripping of cDNA Probe (see **Note 7**)

The stripping protocol is performed as described earlier with some modifications.

1. Add 100 mL of prewarmed (65°C) solution I to a HYBAID bottle.
2. Unwrap the filter from the nylon and place it carefully inside the bottle.
3. Place the tube in the hybridization oven adjusted to 65°C and adjust speed to 15–20 rpm. Incubate for 30 min.
4. Discard the washing solution and add another 100 mL of solution I. Repeat **step 3**.
5. Discard the solution and add 100 mL of solution II. Repeat **step 3** at 50°C for 20 min.
6. Remove the filter from the bottle and wrap it in nylon as described under **Subheading 3.3.2.**
7. Check the efficiency of stripping by exposing the filter to the image plate for 24 h and scan it with phosphor imager. If stripping is not adequate, repeat the procedure.

4. Notes

1. The quality of RNA is the determining factor for a successful array experiment. We have observed that total RNA can give as smooth and clean array hybridization as mRNA, and it is more suitable when the tumor material is small. The comparison of test and reference RNAs requires that both samples are of the same type (total RNA vs total RNA or mRNA vs mRNA) and of similar quality.
2. The DNase treatment of RNA is crucial and, in addition to removing the DNA, it purifies the RNA and reduces background.
3. Use of ^{33}P dCTP in labeling gives a cleaner and sharper signal due to its lower energy compared to alpha ^{32}P dCTP. Because the array elements are physically close to one another, use of ^{32}P may result in diffuse signals that interfere with digital analysis and deteriorate detection of weak hybridization in surrounding spots.
4. The filters should be handled carefully and touched only by the edges. Because it is difficult to strip dry filters, the filters are to be kept moist during all processing stages. It is important to plan a project carefully in order to minimize variation within experiments. Due to variations in the microarray printing process, it is important to design a project utilizing multiple filters so that all filters are from

the same lot in order to minimize any differences introduced in the production process. If the number of filters can not be decided in advance, a hybridization with the reference sample has to be done for each lot, and test samples done on a particular lot can only be compared to a reference done on the same lot.

5. Phosphor imager systems replace standard autoradiography methods and provide spatial resolution suitable for array studies, producing very high image quality together with the highest sensitivity, quantitative accuracy, and speed. The imaging plate (Fuji) consists of a complex matrix that is excited by ionizing radiation. After scanning, the plate is erased using UV light for 1 h and it can be reused hundreds of times. The image plate should be kept dry through all stages of the process.

6. Hybridization images are to be stored as 16-bit tif-format images. Several software applications are available for the analysis. Of these, Pathway (Research Genetics) has been designed to analyze Human Gene filters. The program generates a custom-defined report of the analysis. Clontech have released AtlasVision, designed especially for analysis of the Atlas arrays. Normalization and background subtraction influence the results to a large extent. Images that show patches of background or irregular hybridization pattern in different areas of the filter can not be reliably analyzed. Normalization using all data points yields more accurate results. However, if spots show very high intensities, normalization using control data spots (housekeeping genes) is recommended.

7. Stripping should be done immediately after scanning. Long storage time makes it more difficult to strip the filters.

References

1. Pease, A. C., Solas, D., Sullivan, E. J., Cronin, M. T., Holmes, C. P., and Fodor, S. P. (1994) Light-generated oligonucleotide arrays for rapid DNA sequence analysis. *Proc. Natl. Acad. Sci. USA* **91,** 5022–5026.
2. Pinkel, D., Segraves, R., Sudar, D., Clark, S., Poole, I., Kowbel, D., et al. (1998) High resolution analysis of DNA copy number variation using comparative genomic hybridization to microarrays. *Nat. Genet.* **20,** 207–211.
3. Kononen, J., Bubendorf, L., Kallioniemi, A., Barlund, M., Schraml, P., Leighton, S., et al. (1998) Tissue microarrays for high-throughput molecular profiling of tumor specimens. *Nat. Med.* **4,** 844–847.
4. Schena, M., Shalon, D., Davis, R. W., and Brown, P. O. (1995) Quantitative monitoring of gene expression patterns with a complementary DNA microarray [see comments]. *Science* **270,** 467–470.
5. Shalon, D., Smith, S. J., and Brown, P. O. (1996) A DNA microarray system for analyzing complex DNA samples using two-color fluorescent probe hybridization. *Genome Res.* **6,** 639–645.
6. Hacia, J. G., Brody, L. C., Chee, M. S., Fodor, S. P., and Collins, F. S. (1996) Detection of heterozygous mutations in BRCA1 using high density oligonucleotide arrays and two-colour fluorescence analysis. *Nat. Genet.* **14,** 441–447.

7. Hacia, J. G., Sun, B., Hunt, N., Edgemon, K., Mosbrook, D., Robbins, C., et al. (1998) Strategies for mutational analysis of the large multiexon ATM gene using high-density oligonucleotide arrays. *Genome Res.* **8,** 1245–1258.
8. Pietu, G., Alibert, O., Guichard, V., Lamy, B., Bois, F., Leroy, E., et al. (1996) Novel gene transcripts preferentially expressed in human muscles revealed by quantitative hybridization of a high density cDNA array. *Genome Res.* **6,** 492–503.

20

Cyclooxygenase-2 (COX-2) Protein Expression by Western Blotting

Hossam M. Kandil and Raymond N. DuBois

1. Introduction

Most epidemiological studies *(1–7)* support a protective role of aspirin and nonsteroidal antiinflammatory drugs (NSAIDs) against colorectal cancer. People who (by their report) take aspirin regularly have about a 50% decrease in the incidence *(3,4)* and mortality *(1,2)* from colorectal cancer compared to those who reported no aspirin use. In addition, hospital-based case control studies suggest a protective effect of aspirin use on the development of large-bowel adenomas *(5–7)*. On the other hand, the Physician's Health Study failed to detect any protective effect for aspirin against the subsequent development of colorectal cancer over 12 years of follow up, although this may be due to the short period of follow up *(8,9)*.

Other evidence to support NSAID inhibition of colon tumorogenesis comes from studies on patients with familial adenomatous polyposis (FAP), where use of sulindac, is associated with a reduction in the number and size of adenomas *(11,12)*. Similar results are seen in mice with a mutated APC gene, which is the inherited defect in FAP patients. These mice spontaneously develop multiple intestinal neoplasms (*Min*) and treatment of *Min* mice with piroxicam resulted in a significant reduction of tumor burden *(13)*.

These studies suggest that inhibition of prostaglandins (PG) production and cyclooxygenase (COX) enzymes may be involved in the protective effect of NSAIDs on colon cancer *(14)*. Aspirin and other NSAIDs strongly inhibit PG synthesis via inhibition of COX, the key enzyme in the biosynthesis of PG via oxidative cyclization of arachidonic acid. At least two forms of COX are present in humans, COX-1 and COX-2. The former enzyme is constitutively expressed in most tissues and is thought to play an important role in maintain-

From: *Methods in Molecular Medicine, vol. 50: Colorectal Cancer: Methods and Protocols*
Edited by: S. M. Powell © Humana Press Inc., Totowa, NJ

ing the mucosal integrity, while the latter is inducible by a variety of agents including growth factors, cytokines and tumor promotors (15-19). Whether or not the inhibition of COX and prostaglandin synthesis is the main mechanism by which NSAIDs exert their effect on colon carcinomas is still under careful evaluation. For example, one of the 2 metabolites of sulindac which has no direct COX inhibitory activity (Sulindac Sulfone) has been shown to inhibit cell proliferation of colon adenocarcinoma cells in vitro *(20)*. However, in vivo studies indicate that the antitumor effect of sulindac in *Min* mice is mediated by the sulfide metabolite, but failed to demonstrate any antitumor effect for sulindac sulfone *(21)*. There is growing evidence to support a significant role of COX-2 expression in the development of colon cancer. Increased COX-2 levels were found in 85% of colorectal carcinomas compared with normal mucosa from the same individuals *(22–24)*. Similarly, increased COX-2 expression was seen in carcinogen-induced colon tumors in rats *(25)* and intestinal tumors in *Min* mice *(26,27)* compared to adjacent normal tissues. Oshima et al. *(28)* provided direct genetic evidence that COX-2 plays a key role in intestinal carcinogenesis. APC[D716] knockout mice that are nullizygous for COX-2 have a significant reduction in intestinal tumor burden compared to APC[D716] mice that are wild type for COX-2 *(28)*.

Another line of evidence to support a significant role for COX-2 in increasing the tumorigenic potential of epithelial cells comes from cell culture models. Rat intestinal epithelial cells engineered to overexpress COX-2 developed increased adhesion to extracellular matrix and became resistant to programmed cell death (apoptosis), which was reversed by NSAID treatment *(29)*. In addition, mouse xenograft studies show a significant inhibition of growth of carcinomas by treatment with selective COX-2 inhibitors *(30)*.

The mechanism by which NSAIDs reduce the risk of colorectal cancer has not been clearly established. The protective effect of NSAIDs cannot be explained only by regulation of epithelial cell proliferation. Studies by DeRobertis and Craven show increased proliferative activity of colonic epithelial cells by indomethacin and aspirin and that this effect is reversible by administration of exogenous PGE_2 analogue *(31,32)*. However, NSAIDs (indomethacin and NS-398, a specific COX-2 inhibitor) have been reported to exert anti-proliferative effects on gastric adenocarcinoma cells that overexpress COX-2 *(33)*. It has been recently suggested that NSAIDs modulate apoptosis and this could represent one of the mechanisms by which NSAIDs inhibit carcinogenesis *(20,29,34,35)*. The growth inhibitory effect of NSAIDs parallels their induction of apoptosis in colon adenoma cells *(20)*. Colonocyte suspension prepared from mucosal biopsies obtained from colon mucosa of FAP patients treated with sulindac displayed higher rates of apoptosis compared to colonocytes obtained prior to treatment *(34,35)*. Similarly, sulindac treatment of rat epithelial cells increases the rate of apoptosis *(29)*.

NSAIDs may also affect angiogenesis which is an important requirement for tumor growth and metastasis *(36)*. Previous studies have shown that NSAIDs inhibit angiogenesis *(37,38)*. Recent studies indicate that COX-1 and COX-2 can induce the production of angiogenic factors important for angio-genesis and colon-cancer growth and metastasis *(39)*. In an in vitro model sys-tem involving co-culture of endotheial cells with colon carcinoma cells, Tsujii et al. *(39)* demonstrated that COX-2 overexpression stimulates endothelial migration and tube formation. This effect was inhibited by treatment with a specific COX-2 inhibitor or aspirin. Of interest, COX-1 was shown to regulate angiogenesis in the endothelial cells under certain experimental conditions *(39)*. This suggests a new role that may explain how NSAID use reduces mor-tality from colon cancer *(1,2)*.

Patients with ulcerative colitis (UC) and Crohn's disease (CD), particularly those with long standing pancolitis, are at increased risk for developing colorectal cancer *(40–45)*. Increased tissue concentrations of prostaglandins have been reported in active UC and CD and their concentrations correlate with the level of inflammation *(46)*. Furthermore, it has been recently reported that, unlike normal colon where no COX-2 immunoreactivity was seen, COX-2 expression was increased in the epithelium in ulcerative colitis and Crohn's disease patients *(47)*. Whether or not COX-2 is involved in the development of colon cancer associated with chronic colitis remains to be determined.

2. Materials

1. Radioimmunoprecipitation assay buffer: 150 mM NaCl, 1% Nonidet P40 and 50 mM Tris-HCl, pH 8.0 containing 10 µg/mL aprotinin, 1 mmol/L sodium orthovanadate, and 100 µg/mL phenylmethylsulfonyl fluoride.
2. 7.5% polyacrylamide gels containing SDS.
3. Blocking solution: Tris-buffered saline containing 5% nonfat dried milk and 0.05% Tween-20.
4. Primary antiserum in Tris-buffered saline + 0.1% Tween-20 (TBST), pH 7.4.
5. Nitrocellulose membranes.
6. Secondary antibody: horseradish peroxidase-conjugated immunoglobulin.
7. Enhanced chemiluminescence system (Amersham Corp., Arlington Heights, IL).
8. X-Omat AR film (Kodak, New Haven, CT).

3. Method

1. Homogenize tissues at 4°C in radioimmunoprecipitation assay buffer.
2. Incubate on ice for 30 min and quick spin down at 4°C.
3. Determine protein concentrations using Bradford assay or Bio-Rad method.
4. Add equal amounts of protein (typically 50 µg) and loading buffer (*see* **Note 1**).

5. Prepare molecular weight markers with equal volumes of loading buffer.
6. Mix and boil for 5 min. Then centrifuge briefly at 10,000*g* to spin sample down.
7. Transfer molecular weight markers and samples to 7.5% polyacrylamide gels (*see* **Notes 2** and **3**) containing SDS and run at 200 volts until desired MW bands are separated (*see* **Note 4**).
8. Transfer proteins on gel to nitrocellulose membrane using Trans Blot SD at 20 V for about 60 min (*see* **Note 5**).
9. Place nitrocellulose membrane in Blotto on shaker for 1 h to overnight.
10. Incubate with primary antibody in TBST for 3 h or overnight at room temperature.
11. Wash membrane 3 times with TBST (10 min each).
12. Incubate membrane in secondary antibody in blotto on shaker for 45 to 60 min.
13. Wash membrane 3 times with TBST (10 min each).
14. Incubate membrane in enhanced chemiluminescence system for 1 min.
15. Expose membrane to X-Omat AR film for ~3 min, then develop the film.

4. Notes

1. Need at least 50 µg of protein per sample.
2. Use a maximum of 60 µL loading vol per lane (small gels).
3. Try to avoid outer lanes if possible.
4. Use 100 V when samples are in stacking buffer then 200 V.
5. Wet nitrocellulose membrane with methanol, wash with water, then soak in transfer buffer before use.

References

1. Thun, M. J,, Namboodiri, M. M., and Heath, C. W., Jr. (1991) Aspirin use and reduced risk of fatal colon cancer. *N. Engl. J. Med.* **325,** 1593–1596.
2. Thun, M. J., Namboodiri, M. M., Calle, E. E., Flanders, W. D., and Heath, C. W., Jr. (1993) Aspirin use and risk of fatal cancer. *Cancer Res.* **53,** 1322–1327.
3. Rosenberg, L., Palmer, J. R., Zauber, A. G., Warshauer, M. E., Stolley, P. D., and Shapiro, S. (1991) A hypothesis: nonsteroidal anti-inflammatory drugs reduce the incidence of large-bowel cancer. *J. Natl. Cancer Inst.* **83,** 355–358.
4. Giovannucci, E., Egan, K. M., Hunter, D. J., Stampfer, M. J., Meir, J., Colditz, G. A., et al. (1995) Aspirin and the risk of colorectal cancer in women. *N. Engl. J. Med.* **333,** 609–614.
5. Logan, R. F., Little, J., Hawkin, P. G., and Hardcastle, J. D. (1993) Effect of aspirin and non-steroidal anti-inflammatory drugs on colorectal adenomas: case-control study of subjects participating in the Nottingham faecal occult blood screening programme. *B. M. J.* **307,** 285–289.
6. Greenberg, E. R., Baron, J. A., Freeman, D. H., Jr., Mandel, J. S., and Haile, R. (1993) Reduced risk of large-bowel adenomas among aspirin users. *J. Natl. Cancer Inst.* **85,** 912–916.
7. Suh, O., Mettlin, C., and Petrelli, N. J. (1993) Aspirin use, cancer, and polyps of the large bowel. *Cancer* **72,** 1171–1177.

8. Giovannucci, E., Rimm, E. B., Stampfer, M. J., Colditz, G. A., Ascherio, A., and Willett, W. C. (1994) Aspirin use and the risk for colorectal cancer and adenoma in male health professionals. *Ann. Int. Med.* **121,** 241–246.

9. Sturmer, T., Glynn, R. J., Lee, I. M., Manson, J. A. E., Buring, J. E., and Hennekens, C. H. (1998) Aspirin use and colorectal cancer: Post-trial follow-up data from the Physicians' Health Study. *Ann. Int. Med.* **128,** 713–720.

10. Baganini-Hill, A., Hsu, G., Ross, R. K., and Henderson, B. E. (1991) Aspirin use and incidence of large-bowel cancer in California retirement community. *J. Natl. Cancer Inst.* **83,** 1182–1183.

11. Giardiello, F. M., Hamilton, S. R., Crush, A. J., Piantadosi, S., Hylind, L. M., Celano, P., et al. (1993) Treatment of colonic and rectal adenomas with sulindac in familial adenomatous polyposis. *N. Engl. J. Med.* **328,** 1313–1316.

12. Labayle, D., Fischer, D., Vielh, P., Drouhin, F., Pariente, A., Bories, C., et al. (1991) Sulindac causes regression of rectal polyps in familial adenomatous polyposis. *Gastroenterology* **101,** 635–639.

13. Jacoby, R. F., Marshall, D. J., Newton, M. A., Novakovic, K., Cole, C. E., Lubet, R. A., et al. (1996) Chemoprevention of spontaneous intestinal adenomas in the APC Min mouse model by the nonsteroidal anti-inflammatory drug piroxicam. *Cancer Res.* **56,** 710–714.

14. Gupta, R. A. and DuBois, R. N. (1998) Aspirin, NSAIDs, and colon cancer prevention: Mechanisms? *Gastroenterology* **114,** 1095–1100.

15. Vane, J. (1994) Towards a better aspirin. *Nature* **367,** 215,216.

16. Jones, D. A., Carlton, D. P., Mcintyre, T. M., Zimmerman, G. A., and Prescott, S. M. (1993) Molecular cloning of human prostaglandin endoperoxide synthase type II and demonstration of expression in response to cytokines. *J. Biol. Chem.* **268,** 9049–9054.

17. DuBois, R. N., Awad, J., Morrow, J., Roberts, M. J., and Bishop, P. R. (1994) Regulation of eicosanoid production and mitogenesis in rat intestinal epithelial cells by transforming growth factor-α and phorbol ester. *J. Clin. Invest.* **93,** 493–498.

18. Kargman, S., Charleson, S., Cartwrigh, M., Frank, J., Reindeau, D., Mancini, J., et al. (1996) Characterization of prostaglandin G/H synthase 1 and 2 in rat, dog, monkey and human gastrointestinal tracts. *Gastroenterology* **111,** 448–454.

19. Vane, J. R., Mitchell, J. A., Appleton, I., Tomlinson, A., Bishop-Balley, D., Croxtall, J., and Willoughby, D. A. (1994) Inducible isoforms of cyclooxygenase and nitric-oxide synthase in inflammation. *Proc. Natl. Acad. Sci. USA* **91,** 2046–2050.

20. Piazza, G. A., Rahm, A. K., Finn, T. S., Fryer, B. H., Li, H., Stoumen, A. L., et al. (1997) Apoptosis primarily accounts for the growth-inhibitory properties of sulindac metabolites and involves a mechanism that is independent of cyclooxygenase inhibition, cell cycle arrest and p53 induction. *Cancer Res.* **57,** 2452–2459.

21. Mahmoud, N. N., Boolbol, S. K., Dannenberg, A. J., Mestre, J. R., Bilinski, R. T., Martucci, C., et al. (1998) The sulfide metabolite of sulindac prevents tumors and restores enterocyte apoptosis in a murine model of familial adenomatous polyposis. *Carcinogenesis* **19,** 87–91.

22. Eberhart, C. E., Coffey, R. J., Radhika, A., Giardiello, F. M., Ferrenbach, S., and DuBois, R. N. (1994) Up-regulation of cyclo-oxygenase-2 gene expression in human colorectal adenomas and adenocarcinomas. *Gastroenterology* **107,** 1183–1188.

23. Kargman, S. L., O'Neill, G. P., Vickers, P. J., Evans, J. F., Mancini, J. A., and Jothy, S. (1995) Expression of prostaglandin G/H Synthase-1 and -2 protein in human colon cancer. *Cancer Res.* **55,** 2556–2559.

24. Kutchera, W., Jones, D. A., Matsunami, N., Groden, J., McIntyre, T. M., Zimmerman, G. A., et al. (1996) Prostaglandin H synthase 2 is expressed abnormally in human colon cancer: Evidence for a transcriptional effect. *Proc. Natl. Acad. Sci. USA* **93,** 4816–2820.

25. DuBois, R. N., Aramandala, R., Reddy, B. S., and Entingh, A. J. (1996) Increased cyclooxygenase-2 levels in carcinogen-induced rat colonic tumors. *Gastroenterology* **11,** 1259–1262.

26. Williams, C. S., Luongo, C., Aramandala, R., Zhang, T., Lamps, L. W., Nanney, L. B., et al. (1996) Elevated cyclooxygenase-2 levels in Min Mouse adenomas. *Gastroenterology* **111,** 1134–1140.

27. Shatuck-Brandt, R. L., Lamps, L. W., Heppner Goss, K. J., DuBois, R. N., and Matrisian, L. M. (1999) Differential expression of matrilysin and cyclooxygenase–2 in intestinal and colorectal neoplasms. *Mol. Carcinog.* **24,** 177–187.

28. Oshima, M., Dinchuk, J. E., Kargman, S. L., Oshima, H., Hancock, B., Kwong, E., et al. (1996) Suppression of intestinal polyposis in APC[D716] knockout mice by inhibition of cyclooxygenase 2 (cox-2). *Cell* **87,** 803–809.

29. Tsujii, M. and DuBois, R. N. (1995) Alterations in cellular adhesion and apoptosis in epithelial cells overexpressing prostaglandin endoperoxide synthase 2. *Cell* **83,** 493–501.

30. Sheng, H., Shao, J., Kirkland, S. C., Isakson, P., Coffey, R. J., Morrow, J., Beauchamp, R. D., DuBois, R. N. (1997) Inhibition of human colon cancer cell growth by selective inhibition of cyclooxygenase-2. *J. Clin. Invest.* **99,** 2254–2259.

31. DeRobertis, F. R., Craven, P. A., Saito, R. (1985) 16,16-Dimethyl prostaglandin E2 suppresses the increase of proliferative activity of rat colonic epithelium induced by indomethacin and aspirin. *Gastroenterology* **89,** 1054–1063.

32. Craven, P. A., Saito, R., and DeRobertis, F. R. (1983) Role of local prostaglandin synthesis in the modulation of proliferative activity of rat colonic epithelium. *J. Clin. Invest.* **330,** 156–160.

33. Sawaoka H., Kawano S., Tsuji S., Tsujii M., Murata H., and Hori M. (1996) Effects of NSAIDs on proliferation of gastric cancer cells in vitro: Possible implication of cyclooxygenase-2 in cancer development. *J. Clin. Gastroenterol.* **27(Suppl. 1),** S47–S52.

34. Pasricha, P. J., Bedi, A., O'Connor, K., Rashid, A., Akhtar, A. J., Zahurak M. L., et al. (1995) The effect of sulindac on colorectal proliferation and apoptosis in familial adenomatous polyposis. *Gastroenterology* **109,** 994–998.

35. Piazza, G. A., Kulchak-rahm, A. L., K rutzsch, M., Sperl, G., Shipp-Paranka, N., Gross, P. H., et al. (1995) Antineoplastic drugs sulindac sulfide and sulfone inhibit cell growth by inducing apoptosis. *Cancer Res.* **55**, 3110–3116.
36. Folkman, J. (1990). What is the evidence that tumors are angiogenesis dependent. *J. Natl. Cancer Inst.* **82**, 4–6.
37. Hudson, N., Balsitis, M., Wvweritt, S., and Hawkey, C. J. (1995) Angiogenesis in gastric ulcers: impaired in patients taking non-steroidal anti-inflammatory drugs. *Gut* **37**, 191–194.
38. Seed, M. P., Brown, J. R., Freemantle, C. N., Papworth, J. L., Colville-Nash, P. R., Willis, D., et al. (1997) The inhibition of colon-26 adenocarcinoma development and angiogenesis by topical diclofenac in 2.5% hyaluronan. *Cancer Res.* **57**, 1625–1629.
39. Tsujii, M., Kawano, S., Tsuji, S., Swaoka, H., Hori, M., and DuBois, R. N. (1998) Cyclooxygenase regulates angiogenesis induced by colon cancer cells. *Cell* **93**, 705–716.
40. Ekbom, A., Hermich, C., Zack, M., and Adams, H. O. (1990) Ulcerative colitis and colorectal cancer: a population based study. *N. Engl. J. Med.* **323**, 1228–1233.
41. Greenstein, A. J., Sachar, D. B., Smith, H., Pucillo, A., Papatestas, A. E., Kreel, I., et al. (1979) Cancer in universal and left-sided ulcerative colitis: Factors determining risk. *Gastroenterology* **77**, 290–294.
42. Ransohoff, D. F. (1988) Colon cancer in ulcerative colitis. *Gastroenterology* **94**, 1089–1091.
43. Sugita, A., Sachar, D. B., Bodian, C,, Ribeiro, M. B., Aufses, Jr. A. H., and Greenstein A. J. (1991) Colorectal cancer in ulcerative colitis: influence of anatomical extent and age at onset on colitis-cancer interval. *Gut* **32**, 167–169.
44. Sachar, D. B. (1994) Cancer in Crohn's disease. Dispelling the myths. *Gut* **35**, 1507, 1508
45. Greenstein, A. J., Sachar, D. B., Smith, H., Janowitz, H. D., and Aufses, Jr., A. H. (1980) Pattern of neoplasia in Crohn's disease and ulcerative colitis. *Cancer* **46**, 403–407.
46. Lauritsen, K., Laursen, L. S., Bukhave, K., Rask-Madsen, J. (1986) Effect of topical 5-aminosalicylic acid and prednisolone on prostaglandin E_2 and leukotrine B_4 levels determined by equilibium in vivo dialysis of rectum in relapsing ulcerative colitis. *Gastroenterology* **91**, 837–844.
47. Singer, I. I., Kawka, D. W., Schloemann, S., Tessner, T., Riehl, T., and Stenson, W. (1998) Cyclooxygenase 2 is induced in colonic epithelial cells in inflammatory bowel disease. *Gastroenterology* **115**, 297–306.

21

The Immunohistochemical Method

Lisa A. Cerilli and Henry F. Frierson, Jr.

1. Introduction

Immunohistochemistry involves the binding of an antibody to a cellular or tissue antigen of interest and then visualization of the bound product by a detection system. With the ever-increasing number of antibodies against cellular epitopes, immunohistochemistry is an extremely useful diagnostic tool as well as a means to guide specific therapies that target a particular antigen on neoplastic cells. As many antibodies are effective in fixed paraffin-embedded tissues, large retrospective studies of protein expression in a variety of human cancers can easily be performed.

There are several immunohistochemical staining methods that can be employed depending on the type of specimen under study, the degree of sensitivity required, and the cost. The most frequently used technique is the avidin-biotin immunoperoxidase complex (ABC) method. This chapter examines the technical aspects of immunohistochemistry, including a brief discussion of the principles of the various methods, and highlights the ABC procedure employed in our laboratory. Common technical issues related to specimen processing, fixation, reagents, and artifacts as well as potential pitfalls and means to avoid them are also addressed.

1.1. Immunohistochemical Technique

In the direct immunoassay, the enzyme-labeled primary antibody reacts with the specific epitope in the tissue (**Fig. 1**). Subsequent application of substrate and chromogen complete the reaction. As only one antibody is used, this method can be completed quickly with few nonspecific reactions. However, because of limited sensitivity, this method is rarely used today. Using the indirect immunoenzyme technique, the sensitivity is increased by devising a mul-

From: *Methods in Molecular Medicine, vol. 50: Colorectal Cancer: Methods and Protocols*
Edited by: S. M. Powell © Humana Press Inc., Totowa, NJ

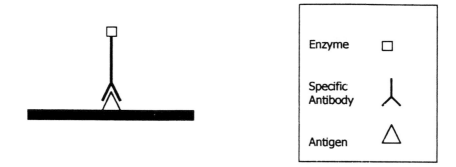

Fig. 1. Direct immunoenzyme technique.

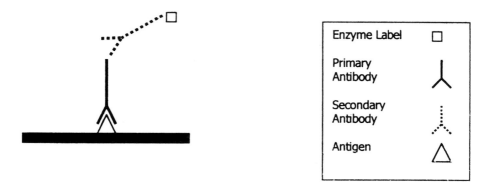

Fig. 2. Indirect immunoenzyme technique.

tilayered bridge which increases the amount of reaction product deposited at the site of the antigen (**Fig. 2**). The primary antibody is detected by a secondary enzyme-labeled antibody, which has specificity against immunoglobulin from the animal species which was the primary antibody source. Undesired reactions may occur if the secondary antibody cross-reacts with endogenous immunoglobulins in the tissue.

In the three-step method, a second enzyme-conjugated antibody is added to the previously described indirect technique. The primary and enzyme-conjugated secondary antibody are applied sequentially, followed by a third enzyme-conjugated antibody specific to the secondary antibody (i.e., if the secondary antibody was made in goat, the third antibody must be antigoat). The third layer of antibody serves to further amplify the signal, since more antibodies are bound to the secondary reagent. The peroxidase-antiperoxidase technique (PAP) utilizes a secondary antibody to form a bridge between the primary antibody and PAP complex (**Fig. 3**). The PAP complex consists of a combina-

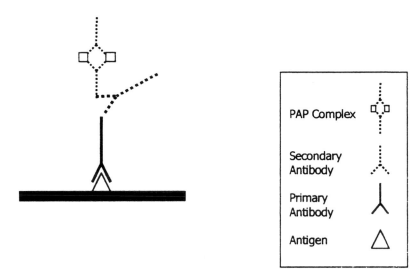

Fig. 3. Peroxidase-antiperoxidase (PAP) complex.

tion of antibody against horseradish peroxidase and several horseradish peroxidase molecules. The primary antibody may be highly diluted, thereby reducing background staining. Excellent commercial sources for rabbit, goat, and mouse PAP complex are currently available. Because the secondary antibody binds specifically to the Fc components of the primary and tertiary reagents, the PAP complex must be made from the same species used for preparation of the primary antibody.

A major technical advance in immunohistochemistry resulted from the knowledge that avidin has a very high affinity for biotin. The multistep staining procedure, the avidin-biotin immunoperoxidase complex technique (ABC method), yields high specificity and sensitivity, and has become the most widely accepted immunostaining procedure (**Fig. 4**). Important features contributing to the effectiveness of this method include: a) the irreversibility of the avidin-biotin binding reaction; b) the small size of the avidin-biotin peroxidase complex, thereby facilitating its tissue penetration; and c) the direct linkage of biotin to the secondary antibody, allowing it to be used in low concentrations. After the biotinylated secondary antibody step, avidin conjugated to peroxidase is added, localizing the enzyme to the site of the antigen-antibody complex.

1.2. Reagents

The primary antibody may be monoclonal (produced by murine hybridomas) or polyclonal (produced by immunization of animals, particularly rabbits). The advantages of using monoclonal antibodies in immunohistochemistry

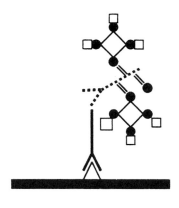

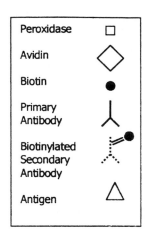

Peroxidase	□
Avidin	◇
Biotin	●
Primary Antibody	
Biotinylated Secondary Antibody	
Antigen	△

Fig. 4. The avidin-biotin immunoperoxidase complex.

over polyclonal reagents include high homogeneity, absence of nonspecific antibodies, ease of characterization, and no batch to batch variability. As monoclonal reagents recognize a limited number of epitopes, a higher level of protein sensitivity may be needed when particular epitopes are sparsely distributed. By combining several monoclonal antibodies into a "cocktail", this limitation can be minimized. Monoclonal reagents may also undergo apparent loss of epitope detection during fixation, may show weaker staining due to intrinsically lower affinity, and are more susceptible to degradation from repeated freezing and thawing (*1*). Therefore, although monoclonal reagents offer higher specificity, sensitivity may be reduced due to a variety of conditions.

It is recommended that all commercial and novel antibodies be subjected to testing for epitope specificity and sensitivity. The use of multitumor sausage blocks (MTSBs) provides an expedient way to aid in the assessment of epitopes in cells and tissues (*2*). With this technique, tissue from many types of tumors may be immunostained using a single MTSB slide, with the application of only a limited amount of antibody (*see* **Note 10**).

Of the enzymes used in the enzyme-substrate reactions, horseradish peroxidase (ABC method) and calf intestinal alkaline phosphatase (PAP method) are most commonly employed. Naturally occurring peroxidase in tissues can lead to binding of the avidin-biotin complex and cause misleading background staining. The endogenous peroxidase activity is largely limited to red and white blood cells. This problem may be obviated by either destroying the endogenous peroxidase using proteolytic enzymes or incubation with hydrogen peroxide and methanol, or by first using a chromogen the produces a different color reaction than the chromogen later applied to identify the epitope.

Chromogens are chemical electron donors that can form a particular colored product when reacted with an enzyme such as peroxidase. 3,3' diaminobenzidine tetrahydrochloride (DAB) is currently the most popular and produces a clearly visible brown reaction product. DAB is insoluble in alcohol, making it useful with a wide range of counterstains. In a comparative study of chromogens, it was suggested that DAB with imidazole is the most sensitive chromogen *(3)*. Although there is some conflicting data, DAB remains a suspected carcinogen, prompting some to use other reagents. The other commonly used chromogen is aminoethylcarbazole (AEC), which yields a red-brown reaction product. Unlike DAB, AEC is soluble in organic solvents and may not be used with dehydrated sections. Therefore, sections stained with AEC often fade over time *(4)*.

1.3. Tissue Processing

Immunohistochemistry can be performed on either fixed (formalin or other fixative) paraffin embedded tissue or cryostat-cut frozen sections. Cryostat (frozen) sections typically yield superior antigen preservation compared with that for paraffin-embedded sections; however, the morphological detail is considerably inferior, and the method of collecting specimens is often tedious (*see* **Note 5**). Fixatives stabilize the tissue and protect it from the harshness of subsequent processing and staining. By doing so, fixatives denature proteins and may cause conformational changes in the structure of proteins, altering the antigenic profile. Hence, fixation introduces problems of sensitivity because of "masking of epitopes." The extent of loss of immunoreactivity depends largely on the specific epitope to be detected and the antibody used. Discontinuous peptides (i.e., peptide sequences which depend on tertiary and quarternary folding of proteins to bring them into proximity) are more susceptible to masking of epitopes than those with sequences in the primary structure. Sensitivity may be reduced more for monoclonal than polyclonal antibodies, as there is less likelihood that all epitopes recognized by the polyclonal antibody are masked.

Among the practical factors that influence the choice of fixative are its availability, safety, cost, and appropriateness for the antigen of interest. Buffered 10% formalin is the most commonly used fixative in routine pathology laboratories. The deteriorating effects of formalin are most evident with certain proteins such as plasma proteins (e.g., immunoglobulins), alpha-feto protein, and factor VIII-related antigen *(5)*. The addition of zinc to formalin provides excellent antigen preservation as well as morphological detail and is used routinely in our laboratory. In automated tissue processing, 1% zinc sulfate is used in 3.7% unbuffered fomalin. Heavy metals act as potent protein precipitants forming insoluble complexes with polypeptides. Alcohol fixatives (e.g., ethanol, methanol) penetrate tissue rapidly; they provide optimal fixation for certain

Table 1
Optimization of Epitope Retrieval Pretreatment

Citrate buffer	pH 1–2	pH 6	pH 10–11
Microwave 100°C, 10"	Slide 1	Slide 2	Slide 3
Microwave or H$_2$O bath, 90°C, 10"	Slide 4	Slide 5	Slide 6

markers including intermediate filaments but cause significant tissue shrinkage and somewhat different tissue morphology *(6)*.

The obstacle of protein masking can often be circumvented by epitope retrieval, using the treatment of tissue sections with proteolytic enzymes or, more recently, the heating of sections at high temperature in water or in a variety of solutions prior to immunostaining *(7,8)*. Pretreatment with proteolytic enzymes is sometimes not ideal as enzymes also digest bonds in native proteins and may cause a reduction or absence in the intensity of staining. Heat induced epitope retrieval successfully increases sensitivity for many but certainly not all antibody reagents. The method of heating is not necessarily important, and a microwave oven, water bath or direct heat, wet autoclaving, pressure cooker, or a combination, can be used. For most antigens, the higher the temperature, the better the retrieval with short-term heating. At lower temperatures, heating must continue longer to give the same result.

Epitope retrieval using microwave heating is the most often employed method. For the majority of antibodies, citrate buffer at pH 6.0 provides the optimal heating solution. For the assessment of a new antibody reagent, use of a "test battery" of slides that have undergone pretreatment with a number of different combinations of temperature and pH may be helpful (*see* **Table 1**). In our laboratory, slides placed for 10–20 min in a 1200 W microwave oven in 10 m*M* citrate buffer yields optimal results. Sometimes decreasing the heating time is sufficient to optimize the reaction.

1.4. Interpretation of Results

Patterns of immunohistochemical labeling include cytoplasmic, surface membrane, and nuclear staining (**Fig. 5**). Since not all cells contain the same amount of antigen, staining in tissue may be absent, focal, or diffuse. The intensity of immunostaining can also be estimated. The percentage of stained cells times the degree of intensity can be used to indicate a staining score. Interpretation of immunohistochemically stained slides requires experience and skill, however. Reporting results of the degree of immunolabeling and percentage of positive cells may not always be reproducible or accurate, but can be improved by using image analysis systems.

1.5. Pitfalls of the Immunohistochemical Technique

Every step of the immunoperoxidase technique may harbor a problem (*see* **Table 2**). Suboptimal fixation, precipitate artifacts, and nonspecific binding are not uncommon problems. Underfixation may preserve an antigen, but the morphology may be distorted, while overfixation may mask or even destroy epitopes. For portions of tissue not exposed to fixative, nonspecific staining may occur. Loss of immunoreactivity for p53, bcl-2, and estrogen receptor, among others, has been reported in sections cut many months to years from paraffin blocks and stored routinely at room temperature. The degree and importance of this loss has not been thoroughly studied, however.

Various precipitates may be confused with positive DAB staining, but their tendency to be distributed randomly should provide a clue to their artifactual nature. The most common precipitate is formalin, which tends to produce a brown microcrystalline pigment when the pH of the formalin solution drops below 6.0. Treatment of the pre-stained sections with 1% sodium hydroxide in 70% ethanol results in removal of the formalin pigment without affecting the quality of immunostaining *(9)*. Other pigments that may be confusing include anthracotic pigment, malarial pigment, and melanin.

Misleading background and nonspecific staining can result from tissue sections that are cut too thick or are folded, as reagents may become trapped between the cell layers. Staining that occurs only along the free tissue edges or along knife marks is also usually nonspecific. Positive staining of crushed or necrotic cells is sometimes nonspecific, but some epitopes (such as keratin and leukocyte common antigen) can be detected even in completely infarcted tissue. If the specimen is very bloody or not washed properly before being processed, intense background staining may be observed if the antigen is present in high concentration in the serum.

Because of the wide tissue distribution of biotin, the avidin-biotin complex technique may result in nonspecific background staining due to endogenous biotin reactivity. Tissues containing a high endogenous biotin content include kidney, liver, pancreas, and adipose tissue. Binding is most pronounced using cryostat sections. Suppression of endogenous avidin binding activity, when necessary, is best accomplished by successive 20 min incubations of sections in 0.1% avidin and 0.01% biotin *(10)*. Because of the carbohydrate nature of the biotin moiety, it may also bind to lectin-like substances in tissues. An analogue to the carbohydrate on avidin such as 0.1 M alpha-methyl-D-mannodise is effective at blocking this binding *(11)*.

1.6. Immunohistochemistry as a Surrogate for Gene Mutation

Immunohistochemistry for p53 has frequently been used as a marker for p53 gene mutation, but harbors important interpretive pitfalls. Stabilization of the

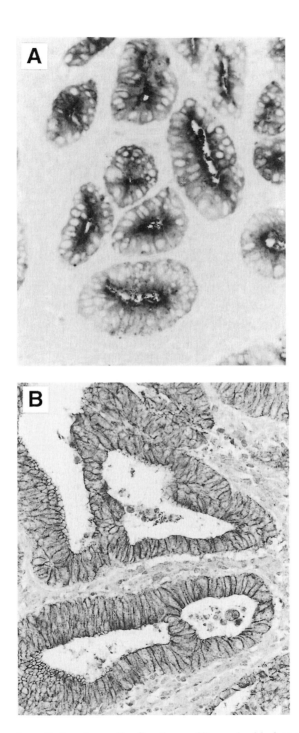

Fig. 5. Examples of zinc-formalin fixed paraffin-embedded sections of adenocarcinoma of the colon stained by the avidin-biotin immunohistochemical technique.
(**A**) diffuse strong cytoplasmic and surface staining for carcinoembryonic antigen

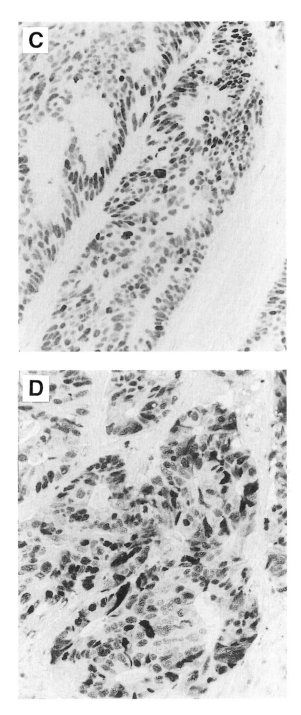

(CEA), **(B)** diffuse cytoplasmic membrane staining for E-cadherin, **(C)** variably intense diffuse nuclear staining for p53, and **(D)** variably intense nuclear staining for p27.

Table 2
Technical Difficulties Associated with Immunohistochemistry

Common problems	Possible causes
No staining	
In controls or specimen, except for counterstain	Omission of primary antibody or labeled reagent
	Use of alcohol-based counterstain or mounting medium with chromogens giving alcohol-soluble color products
	Incorrect preparation of substrate-chromogen mixture
	Incompatible buffer used for preparation of enzyme and substrate-chromogen reagents
	A mismatch of primary antibody and secondary antibody
No (or weak) specific staining	
In positive control and specimen, but both show at least some background staining	Primary antibody defective, excessively diluted, or, on occasion, excessively concentrated
	Proteolytic digestion or epitope retrieval omitted
	Incorrect buffer pH or ionic strength
	Excessive washing buffer or blocking serum remaining on tissue section prior to application or primary antibody, causing dilution of antibody
	Immunoreactivity diminished or destroyed during deparaffinization due to high oven temperature
	Use of inappropriate fixative
	Insufficient incubation time
	Incubation temperature suboptimal
In specimen only	Specimen fixed too long causing "masking" of antigenic determinants
	Sectioned portion of specimen not penetrated by fixative (unfixed tissue tends to bind all reagents nonspecifically)
	Specimen contains crushed or necrotic elements leading to false negative staining and intense background staining

	Antigen levels too low for detection; may be due to loss of antigenic determinants in some tumors
	Specimen incorrectly deparaffinized
High background	
In both specimen and both controls	Wrong blocking serum used (should come from same species for ABC method)
In specimen only	Specimen contains crushed or necrotic elements leading to false negative staining and intense background staining
	Excessive adhesive used on specimen slide
	Adhesive contaminated by bacterial growth
	Tissue section too thick
In positive control and specimen	Primary antibody insufficiently diluted
In negative control	Negative control serum inadequately diluted
	Negative control serum contaminated with bacterial growth
	Negative control serum contains antibody aggregates
In spots on controls, specimen, and glass slide	Undissolved granules of chromogen
In negative controls and specimen	Negative control serum contains antibodies biding nonspecifically to proteins from tissue donor
	Incomplete penetration of tissue specimen by fixative (penetrated area shows normal staining, but unfixed tissue tends to bind all reagents nonspecifically)
	Partial drying of tissue prior to fixation or during staining (unaffected areas show normal staining)
Miscellaneous problems	
Impaired morphology (loss of tissue integrity, frequently with excessive background)	Excessive proteolytic digestion
	Poor fixation
	Poor adherence of sections
	Necrosis of tissue
Endogenous avidin-biotin activity (liver, kidney, brain, lymph nodes, and adipose, usually; may encounter if used as controls)	Binding of avidin reagents (e.g., peroxidase-labeled avidin) to tissue biotin—need to quench biotin (see **Subheading 4.**)

wild-type protein results in positive immunohistochemistry but is false indication of the presence of p53 gene mutation, however. A negative immunohistochemical result also does not necessarily signify the absence of gene mutation. If the underlying mutation is a premature stop codon, the truncated protein may be unstable and not accumulate. Another possibility is that some missense point mutations do not stabilize the protein sufficiently for accumulation in the nucleus.

1.7. Evaluation of a New Antibody

In the event that a commercial antibody is not available to evaluate for expression of a particular protein, a novel antibody can be synthesized. For instance, a synthesized peptide sequence that corresponds to a portion of the protein of interest can be used to generate a rabbit polyclonal antibody. After purification, the specificity of the antibody should be accomplished using Western blot analysis of both positive and negative controls such as specific cell lines containing or lacking the epitope of interest. Cultured cells used as controls can readily be processed as frozen sections or placed in various fixative solutions, embedded in paraffin or agar, and treated as histological sections. A single immunoreactive protein band of the appropriate size should be seen. To also confirm the specificity, preincubation with the peptide used for immunization should result in a loss of the protein band. For immunohistochemistry, the antiserum preincubated with the competing peptide and, in a completely separate reaction, incubation with preimmune rabbit serum alone should result in no staining product. It may also be useful to compare the results of Western blots with mRNA expression. Finally, a cell line transfected with an appropriate cDNA expression vector is sometimes used for subsequent Western blot analysis for the transfected cell protein extract.

To optimize the immunohistochemical conditions, varying antibody concentration with and without epitope retrieval (for fixed cells) is paramount (*see* **Note 3**). After the technical details have been determined for cultured cells, important information regarding the cellular and tissue distribution of the epitope can then be gleaned by staining a series of all normal human tissues.

1.8. Tissue Microarrays

Large scale protein expression surveys may be performed quickly once tissue microarrays have been constructed. As many as 1000 cylindrical biopsies from paraffin-embedded tissues can be placed into a single tissue microarray *(12,13)*. In addition to analyzing protein expression in many tissues on a single slide, the microarray can also be used for *in situ* hybridization. Constructing the microarray, however, is tedious, requiring the identification and handling of many paraffin blocks and selection of appropriate microscopic foci for core "biopsy."

2. Materials

2.1. Deparaffinization and Rehydration of Tissue Sections, Blocking of Endogenous Peroxidase Activity

1. Reagent container tray. Twelve reservoirs with lids to be prepared as follows:
   a. Xylene in first 3 containers.
   b. Absolute ethanol in second 3 containers.
   c. 95% Ethanol in third 3 containers.
   d. Distilled water in last 3 containers.
2. Slide staining racks, each holding 20 or 25 slides.
3. Phosphate buffered saline.
4. Absolute methanol and 3% hydrogen peroxide.

2.2. Antigen Retrieval

1. 10 mM citrate buffer at pH 6.0.
2. Slide staining rack with metal handle removed.
3. Plastic container larger than staining rack.
4. Microwave.

2.3. Antibody Binding

1. Humid chamber lined with wet paper towel.
2. Plastic transfer pipets.
3. PAP pen.
4. Normal serum solution (corresponds to primary antibody type, i.e., mouse serum for mouse primary antibody).
5. Biotinylated secondary antibody solution.
6. Working ABC solution.
7. DAB chromogen solution (10 mg)—store at 4°C (suspected carcinogen, causes severe eye and skin irritation). To prepare stock solution:
   a. Allow bottle of DAB tablets to come to room temperature before opening.
   b. Place 10 mL of PBS into a test tube.
   c. Transfer 1 tablet to the tube and allow it to dissolve. Store at 4°C until ready.

2.4. Counterstaining

1. Gill's hematoxylin #3.
2. 0.5% Cupric sulfate.
   a. Stock solution: 5 g cupric sulfate added to 1000 mL volumetric flask and qs with distilled water. Stir until dissolved. Solution is stable for 1 yr at room temperature.
3. Volumetric flask.
4. 1% Lithium carbonate. Stock solution: 10 g lithium carbonate added to 1000 mL volumetric flask and fill to the top with distilled water (qs).

2.5. Rehydrating and Coverslipping

1. Permount.
2. Coverslips.
3. 4 × 4 gauze pads.
4. Plastic transfer pipets.

3. Methods

1. Prepare 5 μm sections from formalin-fixed tissue.
2. Allow tissue to affix overnight at 37°C or 1 h at 57°C.
3. Transfer fixed tissue slides to fresh xylene bath for 3 min. Repeat twice.
4. Transfer slides to fresh absolute ethanol for 3 min. Repeat.
5. Transfer slides to 95% ethanol for 3 min. Repeat.
6. Rinse gently under running water.
7. Slides may be stored in phosphate buffered saline, pH 7.6, for up to 24 h at 4°C.
8. Prepare a fresh solution of methanol:peroxide (130 mL of methanol and 15 mL of 3% hydrogen peroxide) in plastic staining container, and incubate slides for 30 min.
9. If antigen retrieval is required on any of the slides, load them in a separate rack. If not, proceed to immunostaining.

3.1. Antigen Retrieval

1. Transfer slides to a plastic slide rack that has had the metal handle removed.
2. Place the slide rack in a plastic container and fill to the rim with 10 mM citrate buffer.
3. Cover with plastic lid and place in the center of the microwave.
4. Incubate for 20 min on high and replace evaporated liquid with distilled water every 5 min.
5. Allow to cool at room temperature (no cold water bath) for 10–15 min in the citrate buffer. They should stay immersed in the buffer until ready to stain.

3.2. Antibody Binding

1. Wipe off excess buffer from slide, and using a PAP pen, draw a circle around the tissue.
2. Apply working normal serum solution that corresponds to the antibody being used on that slide (i.e., mouse for mouse primary antibodies).
3. Incubate at room temperature for 10 min.
4. Gently tap off excess serum. Do not rinse.
5. Apply enough primary antibody to cover the tissue.
6. Incubate at room temperature for the length of time appropriate for the particular antibody.
7. Rinse in PBS for 3 min.
8. Apply working biotinylated secondary antibody.
9. Incubate 10 min.

10. Rinse in PBS for 3 min.
11. Apply working ABC solution for 10 min.
12. Make a fresh batch of DAB solution from the stock solution. To prepare working solution:
    a. Transfer 2 mL DAB stock solution to another test tube.
    b. Add 15 µL of 3% hydrogen peroxide. Once prepared, working solution is only stable for 2 h.
13. Apply enough DAB working solution to cover tissue.
14. Incubate 7 min.
15. Rinse in running tap water for 5 min.

3.3. Counterstaining

1. Place slides in Gill's hematoxylin for 1 min.
2. Rinse briefly in tap water to remove excess stain.
3. Place slides in 0.5% cupric sulfate. Incubate for 3 min.
4. Rinse briefly with tap water.
5. Immerse slides in 1% lithium carbonate for 10 dips.

3.4. Rehydrating and Coverslipping

1. Dip slides in each reservoir of the reagent container tray beginning with distilled water and working backwards through 95% ethanol, absolute ethanol, and then xylene. Keep slides in xylene until ready to coverslip.
2. Place a small amount of Permount onto the tissue section using a plastic transfer pipet.
3. Drop the appropriate size coverslip onto the section and press down to allow air bubbles to float to outer edges of coverslip.
4. Turn slide over onto a 4 × 4 gauze pad and press to absorb excess Permount.
5. Dip briefly in xylene to remove any excess Permount or fingerprints. Air dry.

3.5. Interpretation

Cells which bear the antigen recognized by the antibody will display brown nuclear, membranous or cytoplasmic staining in addition to the blue counterstaining. Cells which do not bear the antigen will only display the counterstain.

4. Notes

1. Any reagent stored a 4°C must come to room temperature before use.
2. Use of the PAP pen to encircle the tissue on slides creates a hydrophobic barrier which acts to keep solutions on the specimen.
3. Usually the manufacturer offers prediluted reagents ready for use, or recommends dilution ranges. If this information is not available, optimal working dilutions must be determined by titration. A fixed incubation time must be selected, and then small volumes of series of experimental dilutions prepared. To determine the correct dilution for the primary antibody, hold the secondary antibody

concentration constant while varying the dilution. The objective is to dilute the primary antibody out as far as possible, and still achieve intense positive staining. A wide range of dilutions should be studied to avoid prozone-like problems. A good place to start is with dilutions of 1:100, 1:500, and 1:1000. The optimal dilution may vary depending upon the incubation time. Higher dilutions provide less nonspecific background staining but may require a longer incubation time.

4. Differences in the quality of the primary antibody strongly influence the quality of immunostaining. For example, substantial differences in the quality of the immunohistochemical staining have been observed for p53 depending on the particular primary anti-p53 antibody *(14)*. The various antibodies have different binding sites that influence the sensitivity. In order to optimize the conditions, selection of the primary antibody and use of antigen retrieval become important.

5. To prepare frozen (cryostat) tissue using liquid nitrogen, snap freeze 5 × 5 × 3 mm tissue in liquid nitrogen, cut 5 μm sections on cryostat, and dry at 6°C overnight. We have found that immersion in cold acetone (4°C) for 4 min after the tissue is cut is helpful. Fix in absolute ethanol for 15 min, then air dry. Proceed with immunostaining.

6. Occasionally, tissue sections may lift off of the slide as a result of long-term incubation and repeated washings. This problem is more likely to occur with paraffin-embedded tissues requiring overnight incubation and virtually never occurs with frozen tissue. The use of glycerin-albumin solution may alleviate this problem.

7. For quality assurance, use in-run positive and negative controls with the tissue under study. An ideal positive control contains not just the antigen of interest, but in small amounts that would be expected to correspond to the level of antigen in the studied tissue. Negative controls are tissue known to completely lack the antigen. An alternative negative control includes replacing the primary antibody with either non-immune serum or any other antibody of irrelevant specificity.

8. It is wise to retitrate the primary antibody when changing between lots of antibody aliquots.

9. It is advisable to put any tissue sections for immunohistochemistry on poly-L-lysine (Sigma Chemicals) coated or sialinated slides. The antigen retrieval method subjects tissue to harsh conditions. Tissues with a high collagen, lipid, or calcified content likely will lift off the slides. Titrating down the incubation time may help.

10. Multitumor sausage blocks (MTSB) are prepared from thin strips of tissue combined by dripping liquid paraffin onto them while they are rolled between the thumbs and forefingers, forming a tissue "log." As the paraffin cools, it binds the tissue strips. The tissue log is cut transversely at 0.3 cm intervals and is embedded into cassettes. It is easiest to cut sections while the log is still warm *(2)*.

Acknowledgment

We would like to thank Mark Clem and Lisa Gross for their technical assistance.

References

1. Bhan, A. K. (1995) Immunoperoxidase, in *Diagnostic Immunopathology* (Colvin, R. B., ed.), Raven New York, pp. 711–723.
2. Miller, R. T. and Groothuis, C. L. (1991) Multitumor "sausage" blocks in immunohistochemistry. *Am. J. Clin. Pathol.* **96,** 228–232.
3. Trojanowski, J. Q., Obrocka, M. A., and Lee, V. M. (1983) A comparison of eight different chromogen protocols for the demonstration of immunoreactive neurofilaments or glial filaments in rat cerebellum using the peroxidase-antiperoxidase method and monoclonal antibodies. *J. Histochem. Cytochem.* **31,** 1217–1223.
4. Tubbs, R. R. and Sheibani, K. (1981) Chromogens for immunohistochemistry. *J. Histochem. Cytochem.* **29,** 684.
5. Puchtler, H. and Meloan, S. N. (1985) On the chemistry of formaldehyde fixation and its effects on immunohistochemical reactions. *Histochemistry* **82,** 201–204.
6. Gown, A. M. and Vogel, A. M. (1984) Monoclonal antibodies to human intermediate filament proteins II. *Am. J. Pathol.* **114,** 3093–3312.
7. McNicol, A. M. and Richmond, J. A. (1998) Optimizing immunohistochemistry: antigen retrieval and signal amplification. *Histopathology* **32,** 97–103.
8. Werner, M., von Wasielewski, R., and Komminoth, P. (1996) Antigen retrieval, signal amplification and intensification in immunohistochemistry. *Histochem. Cell. Biol.* **105,** 253–260.
9. Leong, A. S.-Y., Wick, M. R., and Swanson, P. E. (1997) Principles of diagnostic immunohistochemistry, in *Immunohistology and Electron Microscopy of Anaplastic and Pleomorphic Tumors,* Cambridge University Press, UK and NY, pp. 7–31.
10. Wood, G. S. and Warnke, R (1981) Suppression of endogenous avidin-binding activity in tissues and its relevance to biotin-avidin detection systems. *J. Histochem. Cytochem.* **29,** 1196–1204.
11. Naritoku, W. Y. and Taylor, C. R. (1982) A comparative study of the use of monoclonal antibodies using three different immunohistochemical methods: an evaluatio of monoclonal and polyclonal antibodies against human prostatic acid phosphatase. *J. Histochem. Cytochem* **30,** 253–260.
12. Kononen, J., Bubendorf, L., Kallioniem, A., et al. (1998) Tissue microarrays for high-throughput molecular profiling of tumor specimens. *Nat. Med.* **4,** 844–847.
13. Moch, H., Schrami, P., Bubendorf, L., et al. (1999) High-throughput tissue microarray analysis to evaluate genes uncovered by cDNA microarray screening in renal cell carcinoma. *Am. J. Pathol.* **154,** 981–986.
14. Baas, I. O., Mulder, J.-M. R., Offerhaus, J. A., Vogelstein, B., and Hamilton, S. R. (1994) An evaluation of six antibodies for immunohistochemisty of mutant p53 gene product in archival colorectal neoplasms. *J. Pathol.* **172,** 5–12.

22

Immunohistochemical Detection and Quantitation of Cell Surface Receptors for Prostanoids

Rosana Cosme and James K. Roche

1. Introduction

The mucosa of the colon occupies 25% of the intestinal wall, from the *muscularis mucosa* to the lumen-lining epithelium, and contains a variety of cell types, predominantly B and T lymphocytes, but also monocytes, mast cells, and macrophages *(1,2)*. These cells secrete a variety of cytokines, including interleukins, leakotrienes, and prostaglandins. Most of these are locally active, diffuse throughout the mucosa, and do not substantially contribute to the concentration of cytokines in the blood.

For prostaglandins, generally regarded as ubiquitous and performing important cellular housekeeping functions to support normal physiological processes *(3)*, it has long been assumed that most cells bear cell surface receptors for most prostaglandins. In the case of the most plentiful prostaglandin in the colon (PGE_2), four receptors have now been discovered and cloned, designated EP_1, EP_2, EP_3, and EP_4 *(4)*.

Recently, long-term clinical trials of drugs that inhibit prostanoid synthesis suggest that prostanoids play an important role in the genesis of colonic epithelial cell tumors: persons who took 80 mg or more of aspirin per day, 16 d per month, for 10 yr experienced up to a 48% reduction in colonic tumors (including polyps) and a similar decrease in death due to cancer *(5)*. These findings increase the importance of determining which cells in the colon have receptors for PGE_2, and whether there was a difference in receptor density among cells, and between normal mucosa and that which is predisposed to colonic adenocarcinoma. Methodology to accomplish this involves: a) preparation of oriented tissue sections; b) optimal exposure to immunoglobulin reagents and substrate; and c) densitometric analysis of stained and control tissue using specifically designed software for imaging.

From: *Methods in Molecular Medicine, vol. 50: Colorectal Cancer: Methods and Protocols*
Edited by: S. M. Powell © Humana Press Inc., Totowa, NJ

2. Materials

2.1. Slides

1. Microscope slides (Fisherbrand microscope slides precleaned $25 \times 75 \times 1$ mm).
2. All slides coated with Vectabond reagent (Vector Laboratories).

2.2. Buffers

1. Dulbecco's phosphate-buffered saline 1X without $Ca^{2+}Cl_2$ or $MgCl_2$ (Gibco-BRL Life Technologies).
2. Substrate buffer for BCIP-NBT: 100 mM Tris-HCl, pH 9.5.
3. Substrate buffer for substrate red: 100 mM Tris-HCl, pH 8.6.
4. 0.1% BSA/PBS.

2.3. Immunohistochemical Reagents (All Acquired from Vector)

1. Normal goat serum (S-1000).
2. Bovine serum albumin immunohistochemical grade (SP-5050).
3. Secondary antibody—biotinylated antirabbit IgG (H+L) made in goat (BA-1000).
4. Alkaline phosphatase standard ABC-AP kit (AK-5000).
5. Alkaline phosphatase substrate kit—BCIP/NBT (SK-5400).
6. Alkaline phosphatase substrate kit—substrate red (SK-5100).

2.4. Primary Antibodies (All from Cayman Chemical)

1. EP_4 Receptor (human) polyclonal antiserum (cat. no. 101770, Lot 11976a).
2. EP_3 Receptor (human) polyclonal antiserum
3. EP_2 Receptor (human) polyclonal antiserum.
4. EP_1 Receptor (human) polyclonal antiserum.
   (**EP_3–EP_1 are available on a request basis, but not commercially sold.)
5. Normal rabbit serum (Sigma).

2.5. Chemicals

Trizma hydrochloride reagent grade (Tris[hydroxymethyl]aminomethane hydrochloride) (Sigma).

2.6. Mounting Medium

Cytoseal 60 mounting medium low viscosity (Stephens Scientific).

2.7. Software Equipment

1. Neurolucida software program (MicroBrightfield-Colchester, Vermont).
2. Leitz microscope equipped with a 12 V, 60 W tungsten halogen lamp, and a 40X/1.3 NA objective.

3. Methods

Please read **Notes 1–6** before starting.

1. In a staining dish, immerse the slides in (*see* **Note 6**):
   Xylene: twice for 7 min.
   100% Ethanol: twice for 3–5 min.
   95% Ethanol: once for 3–5 min.
   70% Ethanol: once for 3–5 min.
   50% Ethanol: once for 3–5 min.
   Distilled water: twice for 3–5 min.
   20% Acetic acid: twice for 2 min.
2. Pour out the acetic acid and immerse the slides 3 times in PBS (Dulbeco's phosphate buffered saline) for 5 min total. This process is referred to as a "wash" (*see* **Notes 7** and **8**).
3. Remove the slides from the staining dish and using a hand-held aspirator remove any excess PBS from around the sections. Pipet 100 µL of 10% normal goat serum/PBS around each section. Do not allow the bubbles to run together! Incubate at room temperature for 15–20 min (*see* **Notes 9** and **10**).
4. Using a hand held aspirator, remove the normal goat serum from the sections.
5. Pipet 100 µL of the primary antibody (made in 0.1% BSA/PBS) as a bubble around the tissues. If there are 4 sections on the slide, and 4 different immunoglobulins, then there should be 4 separate bubbles on the slide. Do not allow them to run together. Place the slides in a humidity chamber and incubate with the primary antibody for 45–60 min at 4°C (*see* **Note 11** and **Fig. 1**, *see* pp. 237).
6. Remove the primary antibody using the hand-held aspirator and pipet 100 µL of PBS onto each individual tissue. This is the most important wash of the experiment. Do not allow the PBS bubbles to run together. By dispensing and removing 100 µL of buffer with a pipet, wash the tissue 3 times for a total of 5 min (**Fig. 2**, *see* pp. 237).
7. Aspirate the PBS from each section and pipet 100 µL of the secondary biotinylated goat antirabbit IgG (made in 0.1% BSA/PBS) onto the sections and incubate for 30 min at room temperature.
8. At this time, make up the enzyme solution. The solution must stand for 30 min before use, so it is convenient to mix it during the incubation of the secondary antibody. Into the delivery bottle provided in the Alkaline phosphatase standard kit, add 2 drops of reagent A and B to 10 mL of PBS. Mix the solution thoroughly and allow to stand at room temperature (*see* **Note 12**).
9. After the incubation of the secondary antibody is complete, aspirate the liquid away, and wash the sections three times with PBS.
10. Using the delivery bottle, squeeze the premade enzyme solution over the tissue, making sure that the bubble covers the entire section.
11. Incubate the sections with the enzyme solution for 30–60 min at 4°C inside the humidity chamber.
12. Aspirate the enzyme bubbles away, and wash the sections 3 times with PBS. After the third wash, pipet the buffer solution on to the sections and leave the sections in the PBS.

13. At this time, mix the Alkaline phosphatase substrate solution in the plastic bottle provided in the vector kit. Pipet 5 mL of 100 m*M* Tris-HCl buffer into the bottle. Add 2 drops of reagent #1, reagent #2, and reagent #3 to the buffer solution and mix well. Make sure to add exactly 2 drops and follow the order of addition (*see* **Note 13**).

14. Aspirate the PBS and cover the sections with individual bubbles of the substrate solution for 10–20 min. Monitor the sections under a microscope to determine when to quench the reaction (*see* **Note 14**).

15. When the desired stain appears, stop the reaction by immersing the slides in a slide rack under running water for 5 min (**Fig. 3**, *see* pp. 237).

16. Remove the slide from the water and allow the water to evaporate. When all the sections are dry, add two or three drops of a nonaqueous mounting medium, and cover slip.

3.1. Densitometric Evaluation

The intensity of the immunohistochemical stain can be quantitated using a computer program. We have evaluated stained slides under a Leitz microscope with a 12 V, 60 W tungsten halogen lamp. The Neurolucida software and a Ludl motor-driven stage (MicroBrightField, Inc., Colchester, VT) are used for image analysis as previously described (*6*). A Leitz oil-immersion 40× objective is used. Five to ten visual fields representative of the staining pattern are chosen from each section. The relative brightness of immunoreactivity (revealed with black or red reaction product) of labeled cells is compared with the background in other cells within each section using the Neurolucida program. The measurements of brightness (units of pixel luminance in gray scale with black = 0 and white = 250) are performed with the same light intensity adjustment on the microscope on all sections to facilitate comparison between sections. With this scale, the background has the highest brightness values and the more intensely stained cells has the lowest brightness values. The areas of interest (individual lymphocytes or epithelia) are traced, and the brightness within the enclosed region is determined. Thus, the mean brightness of the immunoreactivity of the labeled cells, the background, and surrounding cells is determined for each section. Results are thus expressed as the reciprocal of the net brightness number (experimental minus control), where "experimental" represents the values obtained with specific antibodies; and "control," that obtained with an irrelevant immunoglobulin matched for concentration.

4. Notes

1. This protocol is written for paraffin embedded sections. The procedure requires proper access to embedding centers, flotation baths, and microtomes to cut the blocks. Avoid embedding the specimen in paraffin temperatures higher than 60°C. High temperatures will denature some antigens.

2. Using a microtome, cut the block into sections of desired width. Depending on the size of the tissue, at least four individual sections will fit on a slide. The thickness of the sections depends on the assay, but 5 μm is standard.

3. All slides should be precoated with a section adhesive to prevent the tissues from detaching. Vectabond reagent works well and coats up to 500 slides/bottle.

4. Dry the sections by placing them on a slide warmer with a temperature range of 50–55°C for 30 min. An overnight baking of the slides is preferred. Before starting the deparafination steps, the slides with tissue should be warmed on a slide warmer.

5. As soon as the deparaffination steps begin, do NOT allow the sections to dry out in any step of the experiment! Dry sections will increase the background stain and distort results at the end of the procedure.

6. During the deparaffination steps, most of the fixative and the paraffin itself should wash away from the sections. The duration of exposure to alcohol can vary to achieve this result. Any paraffin or fixative that remains on the tissue can distort the results of the assay. If the assay contains many slides, a large staining dish along with a glass slide rack proves convenient in the deparaffination procedure.

7. A "wash" refers to pouring or aspirating away any previous liquid and immersing the tissue in the PBS buffer solution for a set amount of time.

8. The remaining procedure uses the immunological reagents of Vector Laboratories. Their products exploit the high affinity ($10^{15}M^{-1}$) of a glycoprotein called avidin to a smaller molecule called biotin. The affinity of these two molecules far surpasses that of most antibodies to their antigens making avidin and biotin inseparable. Avidin also possesses four binding sites to biotin. Therefore, one can conjugate antibodies and enzymes with biotin molecules and create a molecular bridge between the antigen and the enzyme product.

    The technique involves an unlabeled primary antibody, followed by a biotinylated secondary antibody, followed by an alkaline phosphatase enzyme containing the avidin. The avidin molecules bind to all the sites where biotin resides. An enzymatic reaction by the alkaline phosphatase produces a colored precipitate indicating the presence of the antigen.

9. The exact volume needed to cover the tissue will vary depending on the size of the section. Usually, 100 μL is sufficient, although for large sections, 150 μL could be used.

    Various tissues possess endogenous alkaline phosphate activity that could result in erroneous staining at the end of the procedure. The researcher should use proper blocking techniques such as incubating the tissue with 10% normal goat serum and making all primaries and secondaries in 0.1% BSA/PBS.

10. For the remaining part of the experiment, the slides can be kept in a humidity chamber. These chambers are simple to construct: a small plastic box with a lid and a wet paper towel lying on the bottom to reduce evaporation of the bubbles during long incubation periods.

11. Antibody dilutions will vary depending on the type of tissue used. On colon tissue, a working dilution of EP_4 is 1:1000. For the goat antirabbit IgG, a favorable dilution is 1:600.

Proper control antibodies are used in the assay to ensure that the visible stain at the end of the procedure is not the product of an artifact. To determine the proper control antibody, one must know the host species of the experimental antibody. In the case of the EP_4 Antiserum, the host species is a rabbit. Normal rabbit serum serves as the primary control antibody in the assay. It undergoes the exact conditions as the experimental antibody and at the end of the procedure, there should be no stain in this section. If a stain appears in the control, then the assay is not valid. The final concentration of the control must match the final concentration of the experimental antibody by weight/volume (**Fig. 3**).

12. If the experiment includes only a small number of slides, then add only 1 drop of reagent A and B to 5 mL of PBS.

13. A variety of substrates are available for the alkaline phosphatase ABC kits: vector red, vector black, vector blue, and BCIP/NBT. In order to work properly, each substrate requires a 100 mM Tris-HCl solution of a specific pH. The BCIP/NBT substrate requires a pH of 9.5 while the Substrate Red requires a pH of 8.2–8.5. The buffers can be made ahead of time and stored at room temperature; however, they do require regular pH checks.

14. Knowing when to stop the alkaline phosphatase reaction can prove to be a little difficult. The desired stain must appear before the color of the background becomes too dark. Monitoring the sections in the first 10 min is crucial because if the reaction proceeds too quickly, everything will stain darkly and one cannot differentiate the stain from the background. A good rule to follow is to monitor the control sections. If any stain appears in these sections (cells or simply high background) then quench the reaction immediately! These sections should have no stain whatsoever. The EP_1, EP_2, EP_3, and EP_4 sera are specific to different areas of tissues. Experience with the antibodies and the tissue will increase your knowledge of a correct stain and increase your awareness of when to stop the reaction.

Fig. 1. Shown is the humidity chamber used for slides, so that the tissues remain humidified and do not dry. Tube caps are used to elevate the sections, and cotton swaps are saturated with water.

Fig. 2. Because the tissue is washed 2–3 times after each incubation, it is helpful to have an "aspirator," attached to a trap (prevents water from going into the vacuum system). The easiest aspirator to use is a small yellow pipet attached to a plastic disposable tube connected to a 1 L flask by two feet of tubing as shown.

Fig. 3. EP_4 prostanoid receptor expression on cells of normal human colon. Five micron-thick sections of histologically normal colon were incubated with a 1:1000 dilution of anit-EP_4 serum (**A**) or with normal rabbit serum (**B**), followed by secondary antibody and substrate. Arrowheads indicate EP_4-positive lamina propria mononuclear cells. Magnification, ×250.

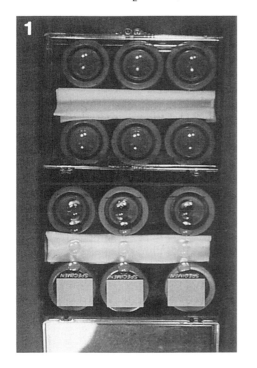

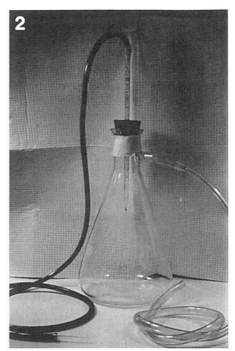

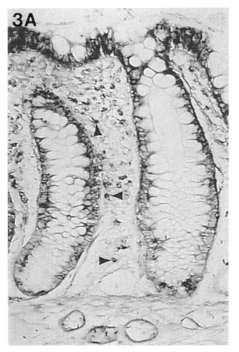

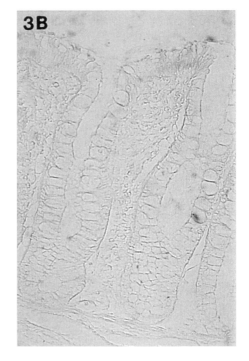

References

1. Fiocchi, C. (1990) Mucosal cellular immunity, in *Immunology and Immunopathology of the Liver and the Gastrointestinal Tract* (Target, S. R. and Shanahan, E., eds.), Igaqu-Shoin, New York, pp. 107–138.
2. Harvey, J., Jones, D. B., and Wright, D. H. (1989) Leucocyte common antigen expression on T cells in normal and inflamed gut. *Immunology* **68**, 13–17.
3. Eberhart, C. E. and Dubois, R. N. (1995) Prostanoids and the gastrointestinal tract. *Gastroenterology* **109**, 285–301.
4. Coleman, C. A., Smith, W. L., and Norumiya, S. (1994) Classification of prostanoid receptors: properties, distribution and structure of the receptors and their subtypes. *Phamacol. Rev.* **46**, 205–224.
5. Giovannucci, E., Egan, K. M., Hunter, D. J., Stampfer, M. J., Colditz, G. A., Willet, W. C., and Speizer, F. E. (1997) Aspirin and the risk of colorectal cancer in women. *N. Engl. J. Med.* **333**, 609–613.
6. Schreihofer, A. M. and Guyenet, P. G. (1997) Identification of C1 presympathetic neurons in rat rostral ventrolateral medulla by juxtracellular labelling *in vivo*. *J. Comp. Neurol.* **387**, 524–536.

23

Adhesion Signaling Through Integrins

Reid B. Adams and Joshua D. Rovin

1. Introduction

Tumor cell interactions with the local microenvironment influence a range of cellular activities. A ubiquitous and important "signal" for tumor cells is the surrounding protein stroma, the extracellular matrix (ECM). This protein network varies in composition and structure throughout the body and within tissues, having a profound effect on the cells interacting with it. Input from these proteins regulates normal and tumor cell functions including adhesion, motility, proliferation, apoptosis, and differentiation.

Cells interact with ECM primarily through integrins (1). These hetero-dimeric transmembrane receptors bind their specific ECM ligands, initiating a series of intracellular structural and biochemical changes that result in cytoskeletal reorganization and activation of other signaling cascades, such as the mitogen activated protein kinase (MAPK) pathways (2). Since integrins lack enzymatic activity, propagation of integrin signals requires cooperation with other intracellular molecules. A major partner for the initiation and trans-duction of integrin initiated signals is the nonreceptor protein tyrosine kinase, focal adhesion kinase (FAK) (3,4).

Focal adhesion kinase activation follows integrin engagement to the ECM or by integrin clustering. Cell adhesion, ligand engagement and integrin clus-tering stimulate autophosphorylation of FAK, predominantly on tyrosine 397. Phosphorylation at this site results in FAK activation and stimulates assembly of a multi-protein complex, focal adhesion formation, and propagation of fur-ther intracellular signals (4). As a consequence of FAK activation, several associated proteins become tyrosine phosphorylated and can be detected, fur-ther demonstrating the propagation of FAK initiated signals. Paxillin, a

From: *Methods in Molecular Medicine, vol. 50: Colorectal Cancer: Methods and Protocols*
Edited by: S. M. Powell © Humana Press Inc., Totowa, NJ

cytoskeletal protein, and p130Cas, a docking protein that recruits and binds the adaptor proteins Crk and Nck, are both recruited to focal adhesions, phosphorylated on tyrosine and bind to FAK in the multi-protein complex *(5–8)*. Further downstream, FAK effectors activate the MAPK pathway, and finally immediate-early genes such as c-Fos. Both can be detected and quantified following integrin engagement. These effectors represent some of the best-characterized molecules in this signaling cascade, but likely are only a fraction of those known or putatively involved. These integrin signals coordinate with those from growth factor receptors and together regulate progression through the cell cycle, growth, and the suppression of apoptosis *(9)*.

In normal cells, loss of cell adhesion results in rapid dephosphorylation of FAK on Tyr^{397}, loss of tyrosine phosphorylation on paxillin and p130Cas, and inactivation of MAPK. If reattachment does not occur in a timely fashion, apoptosis can ensue *(10)*. Attachment restores phosphorylation in a time dependent manner on FAK, paxillin and p130Cas, allows growth, progression through the cell cycle and prevents apoptosis, accounting for at least one of the pathways for anchorage dependence seen in normal cells *(11)*.

Adhesion signaling in tumor cells frequently behaves differently than normal cells *(12,13)*. Both matrix type and concentration requirements can differ, as can the signals mediated through the integrins. Anchorage independence is a hallmark of neoplastic cells and is manifest by the loss of "normal" adhesion signaling. When placed in suspension, tumor cells maintain Tyr^{397} phosphorylation on FAK, and thus continue to have robust kinase activity, despite the loss of adhesion. Such activation could account for the anchorage independent survival characteristics seen in tumor cells.

This chapter outlines experimental protocols designed to investigate the biochemical signals initiated following integrin binding of an appropriate ligand. Specifically, adhesion mediated activation of FAK can be evaluated by determining phosphorylation on Tyr^{397} and other tyrosine residues. Furthermore, propagation of FAK mediated signals can be assessed by detecting adhesion dependent tyrosine phosphorylation on paxillin and p130Cas.

Normal adhesion dependent signaling through FAK can be determined by examining the loss of tyrosine phosphorylation on FAK, paxillin and p130Cas following the placement of cells in suspension (loss of adhesion signal). Cells are then replated, allowing attachment and cell spreading. At the appropriate assay points, cells are harvested by RIPA lysis, detergent extracting the cellular proteins. Following protein quantification, the lysates are then assayed by direct immunoblotting with phospho-specific FAK antibodies or subjected to FAK, paxillin or p130Cas immunoprecipitation, followed by immunoblotting with phosphotyrosine specific antibodies.

Using these methods, time and matrix-dependent tyrosine phosphorylation of these focal adhesion proteins can be assayed and quantified. In addition, the kinetics of phosphorylation with respect to time can be determined, as can the ability of different extracellular matrices to stimulate FAK activation and signaling. Finally, the dose response of individual matrices necessary for maximal FAK activation can be resolved.

2. Materials (*see* Note 1)

2.1. Plate and Cell Preparation

2.1.1. Plate Preparation

1. 10 cm plastic (nontissue culture treated) Petri dishes (Fisher Scientific, Pittsburgh, PA).
2. Poly (2-hydroxyethylmethacrylate) [Poly-HEME], 2 mg/mL in 95% ethanol (*see* **Note 2**).
3. Phosphate buffered saline (PBS).
4. ECM solutions, at optimal concentrations as previously determined (*see* **Note 3**).
5. Blocking solution: Bovine serum albumin (fatty acid free) (BSA) 1% in PBS, (ICN Biomedicals Inc. Aurora, OH) (*see* **Note 4**).
6. Serum free cell culture media at 37°C (*see* **Note 5**).
7. Humidified 37°C chamber or 4°C cold room.

2.1.2. Cell Preparation

1. Cells of interest grown to 70% confluence (*see* **Note 6**).
2. PBS.
3. Detaching solution: trypsin-EDTA, 0.5% trypsin, 5.3 m*M* EDTA (10X) (Gibco-BRL, Rockville, MD).
4. Soybean trypsin inhibitor (STI), 1 mg/mL in PBS or serum free media.
5. Sterile 15 or 50 mL polystyrene conical tubes.
6. Low speed centrifuge for cell pelleting.
7. Hemocytometer.

2.2. Cell Spreading and Adhesion Signaling

1. Plates prepared in **Subheading 3.1.1.**
2. Cells of interest in suspension and counted.
3. Humidified 37°C incubator.

2.3. Protein Preparation and Quantification

1. Container with a bed of ice. Plates of cells will be placed on this.
2. PBS at 4°C.
3. RIPA lysis buffer at 4°C, 0.5–1.0 mL per 10 cm plate to be lysed (*see* **Note 7**).
4. Cell scrapers.
5. Eppendorf tubes, 1.5 mL, at 4°C.

6. Refrigerated microfuge at 4°C.
7. Protein assay system (BCA, Pierce Chemical Co, Rockford, IL).

2.4. Immunodetection of FAK with Phospho-Specific Antibodies

1. Electrophoretic apparatus and solutions for protein separation using SDS-PAGE.
2. Molecular weight markers (Gibco-BRL).
3. Cellular lysates of known protein concentrations from **Subheading 3.3.**
4. Laemmli sample buffer (2X): Tris-HCl 125 mM, pH 6.8, 4% SDS, 20% glycerol (JT Baker), 2% 2-mercaptoethanol, 0.003% bromphenol blue.
5. Apparatus and solutions for transferring proteins to nitrocellulose.
6. Nitrocellulose (Schleicher & Schuell, Keene, NH).
7. Rocking platform.
8. Tris buffered saline (TBS): 20 mM Tris base, 137 mM NaCl, pH to 7.6.
9. Tris buffered saline with Tween (TBS-T): TBS with 0.1% Tween-20.
10. Blocking solution: TBS-T with 5% nonfat dry milk. If blotting for phospho-tyrosine, block with TBS-T with 1% bovine serum albumin (Fraction V Heat Shock) (Boehringer Mannheim, Indianapolis, IN).
11. FAK phospho-specific antibodies (QCB, Biosource International, Camarillo, CA).
12. Secondary antibody (Protein A-HRP [for polyclonal Ab] or rabbit antimouse-HRP [for monoclonal Ab]) (Amersham Pharmacia Biotech, Piscataway, NJ).
13. Primary and secondary antibody solution: blocking solution plus antibody at recommended dilution.
14. Chemiluminescence detection reagents (ECL, Amersham).
15. X-OMAT LS or AR film (Kodak, Rochester, NY).
16. Stripping solution: 62.5 mM Tris-HCl, pH 6.7, 2% SDS, 100 mM 2-Mercaptoethanol.
17. Oven at 50°C.

2.5. Immunoprecipitation of Adhesion Proteins and Immunodetection of Tyrosine Phosphorylated Species

1. Cellular lysates of known protein concentrations from **Subheading 3.3.**
2. Eppendorf tubes, 1.5 mL, at 4°C.
3. Ice bath and/or cold room at 4°C.
4. Rocker or rotating platform at 4°C.
5. Refrigerated microfuge at 4°C.
6. TBS and RIPA base.
7. Rehydrated Protein A Sepharose CL-4B (*see* **Note 8**).
8. FAK (Upstate Biotechnology, Lake Placid, NY), paxillin (Transduction Laboratories, San Diego, CA), and p130Cas *(14)* specific antibodies.
9. Rabbit antimouse IgG antibodies (Jackson Immunoresearch Laboratories, West Grove, PA) (*see* **Note 9**).
10. Antiphosphotyrosine antibodies (RC20), (Transduction Laboratories).
11. Materials from **Subheading 2.4.** for immunoblotting.

3. Methods

3.1. Plate and Cell Preparation

3.1.1. Plate Preparation

1. Coat nontissue culture treated Petri dishes with the ECM of interest diluted in PBS to the appropriate concentration. Incubate on a rocker at 37°C for 1–2 h or at 4°C overnight. Aspirate solution from the dish, rinse twice with 5 mL of PBS, and then add 2 mL of BSA blocking solution. Incubate at 37°C for 1 h, aspirate BSA, wash twice with 5 mL of PBS and add 5 mL of culture media at 37°C.
2. To maintain cells in suspension, coat culture dishes with enough Poly-HEME to cover the entire dish (3–5 mL) and allow solution to evaporate in the tissue culture hood. After completely dry (60–90 min) repeat the coating with additional Poly-HEME. Allow plate to thoroughly dry (2 h). Do not expose to UV light. May keep coated dishes for several weeks.

3.1.2. Cell Preparation

1. Wash plates of cells with PBS. Use twice as many plates as you anticipate needing, to insure a sufficient number of cells. Aspirate PBS. Do not manipulate one plate of cells. Save this plate and do not detach the cells from the dish.
2. Place 1 mL of detachment solution in each 10 cm plate and incubate at 37°C until cells detach from plate. Collect cells in a 15- or 50-mL conical tube and centrifuge at 100*g* for 5 min at room temperature. Aspirate liquid and resuspend the cell pellet in STI, centrifuge at 100*g* for 5 min at room temperature to pellet cells.
3. Resuspend cells in serum free media and determine cell number by counting in a hemocytometer. Adjust cell concentration to 8×10^6 cells/mL.

3.2. Cell Spreading and Adhesion Signaling

1. Save one aliquot (5–10×10^6 cells) of cells for T = 0 (time zero) and place on ice.
2. Plate 5×10^6 cells/10 cm plate coated with either Poly-HEME or the ECM of interest. If immunoblotting only, 2 plates (10 cm) at each time point are usually sufficient. If immunoprecipitating and then immunoblotting, frequently 3–6 plates will be needed at each of the lower time points. Alternatively, several 15 cm plates can be used.
3. Place plated cells in an incubator.
4. Progress of attachment and spreading can be monitored and recorded at each time point by light microscopy or time-lapse video microscopy.

3.3. Protein Preparation and Quantification

1. The T = 0 aliquot of cells is pelleted and placed in ice. Wash once with 10 mL of cold PBS and repellet. Add 0.5–1 mL of cold RIPA. Aspirate several times and follow the remaining protocol.
2. Cells are harvested at sequential time points after plating, typically 10, 20, 30, and 60 min. Place the dish of cells on ice and aspirate the media. Add 10 mL cold

PBS, rinse cells, and aspirate PBS. Do this very gently, as cells are easily lost during this step. Add 0.5–1.0 mL cold RIPA per 10 cm dish. Swirl to cover entire dish. Scrape cells and then gently aspirate several times.

3. Place lysate into cold Eppendorf tubes, spin in microfuge, 4°C, at 15,000*g* for 10 min. Aspirate supernatant and place into cold Eppendorf tubes. Save 20 µL of each sample for protein quantification assay. Samples can be analyzed at this time or snap frozen in liquid nitrogen for storage and later analysis.

4. Quantify protein concentrations (BCA or other method of choice) for each sample according to the manufacturer's instructions.

3.4. Immunodetection of FAK with Phospho-Specific Antibodies

1. Aliquot 100–200 µg of protein lysate into an Eppendorf tube, add sample buffer and boil for 5 min. Load samples and molecular weight markers into gel lanes and separate proteins by SDS-PAGE. Transfer proteins to nitrocellulose.

2. Place nitrocellulose into enough blocking solution with 5% milk to cover blot. Incubate on a rocker for 1 h at room temperature (RT) (or overnight at 4°C). Remove blocking solution.

3. Cover blot with primary antibody solution (FAK phospho-specific Ab) and incubate for 1–2 h at RT. Wash with TBS-T: 5 times, 5 min per wash.

4. Remove last rinse, cover blot with secondary antibody solution and incubate for 1 h at RT. Repeat TBS-T washes as in **step 3**.

5. Detect bound antibody using ECL according to manufacturer's instructions.

6. To determine loading equivalency for each lane, strip the blot with stripping buffer according to ECL instructions. Reprobe with a primary antibody to FAK (*see* **Note 10**).

3.5. Immunoprecipitation of Adhesion Proteins and Immunodetection of Tyrosine Phosphorylated Species

3.5.1. Coupling Antibody to Protein A Sepharose (PAS) (see **Note 9**)

1. Place 100 µL of PAS slurry in a 1.5 mL Eppendorf tube. Add 10 µg of rabbit antimouse antibody.

2. Rotate for 1 h at 4°C. Spin in microfuge 15 s, remove supernatant and resuspend in 100 µL cold TBS. Repeat wash in TBS. After second wash, resuspend in cold RIPA base so that total volume of PAS and RIPA slurry is 100 µL.

3.5.2. Immunoprecipitation

1. Do all of this procedure at 4°C unless noted. Place 0.5-1.0 mg of protein lysate into Eppendorf tubes and dilute lysates with complete RIPA to achieve equal volumes in each Eppendorf.

2. Add antibody to protein of interest (FAK, paxillin, p130Cas). Use a mass ratio of protein to antibody of approx 50:1 to 100:1 (purified Ab or ascites). Rotate (mix) 1–4 h.

3. Add 100 µL of PAS (polyclonal Ab) or PAS coupled to rabbit antimouse Ab (mouse monoclonal Ab). Rotate 1–2 h.

4. Microfuge sample 15 s at 15,000*g*, decant supernatant, resuspend in complete RIPA, and briefly vortex to resuspend beads. Repeat these washes a total of 3 times in RIPA, 1 time in TBS, 100-200 μL per wash.
5. After last wash, remove supernatant, add 50 μL per tube of sample buffer and boil for 4–5 min. Spin down beads and load supernatants into gel lanes.
6. Do immunoblotting as outlined in Section 3.4. Apply antiphosphotyrosine antibody (RC20) as the initial primary antibody. Follow the manufacturer's instructions.
7. After completing this blot, strip it as described above and reblot for the protein of interest (FAK, paxillin, p130Cas) to determine loading equivalency.

4. Notes

1. All chemicals are from Sigma (St. Louis, MO) unless noted.
2. Poly-HEME coated plates prevent cell attachment and matrix deposition and serve as suspension (detached) controls. Cells growing continuously in culture (never having been detached) are used as controls to evaluate baseline, or stable, focal adhesion protein phosphorylation. The time to FAK inactivation should be determined for the cells of interest. Cells are placed in suspension in serum free media and at sequential time points aliquots are assayed for FAK tyrosine phosphorylation. Cells are used in experiments at the time point when FAK tyrosine phosphorylation has disappeared, generally after approximately 30 min in suspension.
3. Typical ECM proteins for experiments are fibronectin, collagen, laminin, and vitronectin. The optimal ECM type and concentration should be determined prior to experiments. Most are in the range of 10 μg/mL. Each cell type may have a different integrin repertoire and, therefore, may be able to bind only to a limited number of ECMs.
4. BSA should be endotoxin (LPS) and lysophosphatidic acid (LPA) free.
5. Serum free media is used, as serum contains ECM proteins that may interfere with experimental interpretation.
6. Optimal confluence for each cell line needs to be determined, but ranges from 60–75%.
7. RIPA lysis buffer–base: HEPES 50 m*M*, NaCl 150 m*M*, EDTA 2 m*M*, NP-40 1% (United States Biochemical, Cleveland, OH), combine and adjust to pH 7.2, add deoxycholic acid to 0.5%, store at 4°C. At the time of use, add protease inhibitors: leupeptin 100 μ*M* (Boehringer Mannheim), pepstatin 10 μ*M* (Boehringer Mannheim), aprotinin 0.05 TIU/mL, phenylmethylsulfonylfluoride 1 m*M*, benzamidine 1 m*M*, soybean trypsin inhibitor 0.02 mg/mL, and phosphatase inhibitors: Na_3VO_4 1 m*M*, Na pyrophosphate 10 m*M*, 4-nitrophenyl phosphate 40 m*M*, NaF 40 m*M*. Protease and phosphatase inhibitors can be made up as stock solutions and stored.
8. Rehydrating Protein A Sepharose (PAS). Place 1.5 g of PAS in a 50 mL conical tube, add 20 mL TBS and let stand for 2 h. Centrifuge at 200*g* for 5 min, decant supernatant, resuspend in 20 mL TBS, vortex to mix, and recentrifuge. Repeat

washes a total of 3 times. After the last spin, decant TBS and resuspend PAS 1:1 (vol:vol) in TBS. Store at 4°C. Cut off the very tip of the pipet to allow unimpeded aspiration of the PAS beads.

9. PAS does not effectively bind mouse monoclonal antibodies. To allow PAS capture of monoclonal antibody immunocomplexes, a rabbit antimouse IgG must be coupled to PAS.

10. It is important to do a loading control for each blot when immunoblotting for phosphoproteins. This will allow quantification relative to other cells and conditions. Stripping the phosphotyrosine blot and reprobing it for the protein of interest will allow each blot to serve as its own control. Proteins can be quantified by densitometry if the signal is within the linear response range for the film.

References

1. Hynes, R. O. (1992) Integrins: versatility, modulation, and signaling in cell adhesion. *Cell* **69**, 11–25.
2. Chen, Q., Kinch, M. S., Lin, T. H., Burridge, K., and Juliano, R. L. (1994) Integrin-mediated cell adhesion activates mitogen-activated protein kinases. *J. Biol. Chem.* **269**, 26,602–26,605.
3. Schaller, M. D., Borgman, C. A., Cobb, B. S., Vines, R. R., Reynolds, A. B., and Parsons, J. T. (1992) pp125FAK a structurally distinctive protein-tyrosine kinase associated with focal adhesions. *Proc. Natl. Acad. Sci. USA* **89**, 5192–5196.
4. Parsons, J. T. (1996) Integrin-mediated signalling: regulation by protein tyrosine kinases and small GTP-binding proteins. *Curr. Opin. Cell Biol.* **8**, 146–152.
5. Hildebrand, J. D., Schaller, M. D., and Parsons, J. T. (1995) Paxillin, a tyrosine phosphorylated focal adhesion-associated protein binds to the carboxyl terminal domain of focal adhesion kinase. *Mol. Biol. Cell* **6**, 637–647.
6. Richardson, A., Malik, R. K., Hildebrand, J. D., and Parsons, J. T. (1997) Inhibition of cell spreading by expression of the C-terminal domain of focal adhesion kinase (FAK) is rescued by coexpression of Src or catalytically inactive FAK: a role for paxillin tyrosine phosphorylation. *Mol. Cell. Biol.* **17**, 6906–6914.
7. Petch, L. A., Bockholt, S. M., Bouton, A., Parsons, J. T., and Burridge, K. (1995) Adhesion-induced tyrosine phosphorylation of the p130 src substrate. *J. Cell Sci.* **108**, 1371–1379.
8. Harte, M. T., Hildebrand, J. D., Burnham, M. R., Bouton, A. H., and Parsons, J. T. (1996) p130Cas, a substrate associated with v-Src and v-Crk, localizes to focal adhesions and binds to focal adhesion kinase. *J. Biol. Chem.* **271**, 13,649–13,655.
9. Giancotti, F. G. and Ruoslahti, E. (1999) Integrin signaling. *Science* **285**, 1028–1032.
10. Frisch, S. M. and Francis, H. (1994) Disruption of epithelial cell-matrix interactions induces apoptosis. *J. Cell Biol.* **124**, 619–626.
11. Frisch, S. M., Vuori, K., Ruoslahti, E., and Chan-Hui, P. Y. (1996) Control of adhesion-dependent cell survival by focal adhesion kinase. *J. Cell Biol.* **134**, 793–799.

12. Weiner, T. M, Liu, E. T., Craven, R. J., and Cance, W. G. (1993) Expression of focal adhesion kinase gene and invasive cancer. *Lancet* **342,** 1024–1025.

13. Xu, L., Yang, X., Craven, R. J., and Cance, W. G. (1998) The COOH-terminal domain of the focal adhesion kinase induces loss of adhesion and cell death in human tumor cells. *Cell Growth Differ.* **9,** 999–1005.

14. Bouton, A. H. and Burnham, M. R. (1997) Detection of distinct pools of the adapter protein p130CAS using a panel of monoclonal antibodies. *Hybridoma* **16,** 403–411.

24

Electrophoretic Mobility Shift Assay (EMSA)

Michael F. Smith, Jr. and Sandrine Delbary-Gossart

1. Introduction

Transcriptional regulation of gene expression is controlled through the binding of sequence-specific DNA-binding proteins (transcription factors) to the regulatory regions of genes. The exact gene expression program of a cell is determined by the spectrum of transcription factors present with the nucleus of a cell. The presence of these factors is dependent upon the cell type being examined and the stimulus to which the cell has been subjected. A knowledge of the transcription factors present during any given time can be important in generating a more thorough understanding of how a cell or tissue responds to its environment. Additionally, identifying the transcription factors required for the expression of a specific gene can provide a better understanding of the molecular mechanisms involved and suggest new therapies which may specifically target an individual gene or set of genes.

The electrophoretic mobility shift assay (EMSA), also known as gel retardation or band shift assay, is a rapid and sensitive means for detecting sequence-specific DNA-binding proteins *(1,2)*. This assay can be used to determine, in both a qualitative and quantitative manner, if a particular transcription factor is present within the nuclei of the cells or tissue of interest or to identify an unknown DNA binding protein which may control the expression of your gene of interest. The assay is based upon the ability of a transcription factor to bind in a sequence-specific manner to a radiolabeled oligonucleotide probe and retard its migration through a nondenaturing polyacrylamide gel. Either crude nuclear extracts or purified factors can be used as a source of the DNA-binding protein.

1.1. Critical Parameters

In theory, EMSA is a very simple and rapid assay. However, clean, successful gel shifts can require the optimization of a number of parameters which will

From: *Methods in Molecular Medicine, vol. 50: Colorectal Cancer: Methods and Protocols*
Edited by: S. M. Powell © Humana Press Inc., Totowa, NJ

influence the ability of many transcription factors to bind to their cognate DNA sequences. Binding reaction conditions and gel electrophoresis conditions are important to evaluate for each probe and/or factor studied. Critical parameters in the binding reaction which often must be determined empirically include: concentration of mono- and divalent ions, pH, type and concentration of non-specific competitor DNA, amount of nuclear extract included, and concentration of glycerol. When assessing these parameters it is important to take into account the amount of nuclear extract included in the reaction since it can provide a significant amount of the buffer components. The most typical component of the binding buffer to titrate is the concentration of KCl. Typical concentrations range from 50–150 mM. The other single most important factor to consider is the nonspecific competitor DNA. Most transcription factors have binding affinities for their specific DNA sequences that are many fold higher than those for DNA in general. For a set amount of nuclear extract it is important to titrate the amount of nonspecific DNA included. Too low of a concentration and all the probe will be bound nonspecifically, too high of a concentration and no probe will be bound. The type of competitor DNA used is also an important factor. In general very simple synthetic copolymers such as poly (dI-dC) provide the best results. Use of more complex DNAs, such as sonicated salmon sperm DNA, runs the risk of providing binding sites for your factor of interest.

Likewise, parameters in the nondenaturing gel stage which may be altered include percentage of acrylamide used (we typically use 4–6% acrylamide), *bis* to acrylamide ratios, and buffer composition. Most commonly Tris-acetate (TAE) or Tris-borate (TBE) buffer at 0.25X to 0.5X are used. In some cases inclusion of glycerol and/or Mg^{2+} in the gel can also improve DNA/protein complex resolution.

The choice of specific DNA probe also must be considered. Fragments of DNA ranging in size from 20 to 200 bp can successfully be used in this assay. It is important to remember that the longer the fragment of DNA that you are working with, the more likely you will be to observe multiple DNA/protein interactions. In addition, longer probe lengths make distinction of shifted complexes from unreacted probe more difficult.

The procedure outlined in this chapter is that which is routinely used in our laboratory and works well for a variety of different transcription factors *(3)*. However, for best results, conditions as described above and in the notes may need to be optimized for other factors.

1.2. Determination of Specificity of the DNA/Protein Interaction

Two common approaches are used to determine the specificity of DNA/protein interaction as well as to identify the protein involved in complex for-

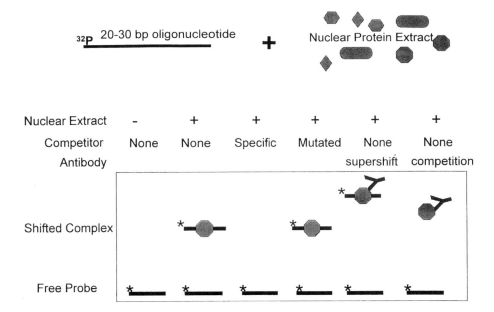

Fig. 1. Hypothetical autoradiograph of an EMSA experiment showing the effects of competition with oligonucleotides specific for the factor of interest and mutated in the critical DNA sequences required for factor binding. Also shown are two potential outcomes when antibodies specific for the factor are included in the reaction: "supershift" and competition with the DNA probe for a binding site on the transcription factor. *▬▬ represents the radiolabled DNA probe.

mation: competition with unlabeled competitor DNA and antibody supershifts. These are demonstrated in the hypothetical autoradiograph shown in **Fig. 1**.

1.2.1. Unlabeled Competitions

This is the most common test of specificity. Prior to the addition of radiolabeled probe DNA, a 50–100-fold molar excess of unlabeled competitor DNA is added to the reaction mix. Individual reactions are performed with oligonucleotides containing the target DNA sequence and oligonucleotides which have been specifically mutated within the target sequence. Specific binding is indicated by a loss of factor binding to the radiolabeled probe. The alteration of conserved bases within the binding site can abolish the ability of a transcription factor to bind to its cognate DNA. Thus for site-directed mutant competitions, binding of the radiolabeled probe is preserved. In addition, competitions should also be performed with well characterized consensus DNA sequences specific for the factor of interest.

1.2.2. Antibody Supershifts

In this modification of the EMSA, antibodies specific to the putative DNA binding protein are incubated with in the binding reaction prior to addition of radiolabeled probe. If the antibody recognizes the target protein two results are possible. If the antibody does not inhibit binding it will create a higher molecular weight complex which will be observed as a "supershift" on the autoradiograph. Alternatively, the antibody may prevent DNA/protein interactions by preventing the binding of the protein to the DNA probe thus resulting in a loss of the specific complex.

2. Materials

2.1. Preparation of Nuclear Extract

Based upon the procedure of Dignam et al. *(3)*.

1. Approximately $3 - 5 \times 10^7$ cells cultivated in 150 mm dish for 24 h, in the appropriate medium + 10% fetal bovine serum, at 37°C and 5% CO_2.
2. 1X Phosphate-buffered saline solution (PBS) (Gibco-BRL).
3. Buffer A:10 mM HEPES, pH 7.9, 1.5 mM MgCl$_2$, 10 mM KCl, 0.5 mM DTT (dithiothreitol), 1 µg/mL leupeptin, 2 µg/mL aprotonin, 1 µg/mL pepstatin A, 0.5 mM PMSF (phenyl methyl sulphonyl fluoride), 10 mM β-glycerophosphate, 1 mM sodium orthovanadate.
4. Buffer B: 20 mM HEPES, pH 7.9, 25% glycerol, 0.42 M NaCl, 1.5 mM MgCl$_2$ 0.2 mM EDTA, 1 µg/mL leupeptin, 2 µg/mL aprotonin, 1 µg/mL pepstatin A, 0.5 mM PMSF, 0.5 mM DTT, 1 mM sodium orthovanadate, 10 mM β-glycerophosphate.
5. 15 mL Polypropylene tubes, 1.5 mL microfuge tubes.
6. Rocker and centrifuge.

2.2. Assay for Protein Concentration

Bio-Rad protein assay kit (Bio-Rad).

2.3. Synthesis of the DNA Oligonucleotide Used as Probe for Gel Retardation Assay

Two complementary single-stranded oligonucleotides of 20 to 30 bases are chosen from a specific DNA sequence (located in the 5'-promoter region) according the nature of the investigation and are commercially synthesized (Integrated DNA Technologies, Coralville, IA). For labeling by fill-in reaction, oligonucleotides should be designed such that they contain a short 3' overhang which can be filled in using DNA polymerase and α^{32}P-dNTP.

2.4. Annealing of the DNA Oligonucleotide

1. DNA Oligonucleotides (250 mg/mL stock diluted in sterile water).
2. 10X Klenow DNA polymerase buffer.

3. Sterile water.
4. Microfuge tubes.

2.5. Labeling of DNA Probe

1. Double-stranded oligonucleotide.
2. α-^{32}P-dCTP (3000 Ci/mmol, Amersham Pharmacia Biotech.) for filling-in 3' overhanging dGTP.
3. 10X T7 DNA polymerase Buffer (Amersham Life Science).
4. Sterile water.
5. DTT (0.5 M stock).
6. dATP, dGTP, dTTP stock (2.5 mM each diluted in sterile water).
7. EDTA (0.5 M stock).
8. TE: 10 mM Tris-HCl, 1 mM EDTA, pH 8.0 T7 DNA polymerase (Amersham Life Science).
9. Sephadex G-50 columns.
10. Water bath.

2.6. Binding Reactions

1. Poly d[I-C] (Boehringer Mannheim Corp., 1 mg/mL stock).
2. Binding buffer: 20 mM HEPES, pH 7.9, 1 mM DTT, 0.1 mM EDTA, 50 mM KCl, 5% glycerol, 200 mg/mL bovine serum albumin (Fraction V). Make fresh or aliquot and store at –20°C.
3. α-^{32}P labeled DNA probe (~0.5 ng/mL).
4. Nuclear extracts diluted at 1 mg/mL in binding buffer.
5. Sterile water.
6. Microcentrifuge tubes.

2.7. Nondenaturing Polyacrylamide Gel, Electrophoresis and Autoradiography

1. 4–6% nondenaturing polyacrylamide gel 1.5 mm thick:
   a. Acrylamide and bis N,N'-methylene-bis-acrylamide (29:1 acrylamide:bis ratio).
   b. 5X TBE (0.445 M Tris-borate, 0.445 M boric acid, 0.01 M EDTA).
   c. Sterile water.
   d. 10% Ammonium persulfate.
   e. TEMED.
2. Electrophoresis buffer: 0.25X TBE.
3. Gel electrophoresis rig, accessories and power supply.
4. Gel dryer and blotting paper.
5. Autoradiography film, exposure cassettes, developer and processor.

3. Methods

3.1. Preparation of Nuclear Extracts

Adapted from Dignam et al. (*3*).

Samples should be kept on ice at all times.

1. Remove media, wash cells with 10 mL PBS, harvest cells and centrifuge in polypropylene tubes at 400*g* for 10 min, at 4°C.
2. Lyse cells by resuspending in 5 vol Buffer A.
3. Incubate on ice for 10 min. If lysis is incomplete, cells can be broken using a dounce homogenizer fitted with a loose pestle to release the nuclei.
4. Centrifuge at 800*g* for 10 min at 4°C to pellet the nuclei.
5. Remove the supernatant and resuspend the pellet in 2 packed nuclear volumes buffer B.
6. Extract 30 min at 4°C, gently on rocker.
7. Centrifuge at 13,000*g* for 30 min at 4°C.
8. Aliquot the supernatant and store the nuclear extracts at –70°C.

3.2. Assay for Protein Concentration

The determination of the concentration of protein in the extracts is similar to the method of Bradford, which allows comparing the same amounts of proteins from the different extracts. Follow protocol as suggested by the manufacturer.

3.3. Design of the DNA Oligonucleotide Used as Probe

The type and size of the probe used depends on the nature of the investigation. In the case of a previously identified DNA binding site to be studied, a synthetic oligonucleotide probe should be usually used. Synthetic binding sites are made by choosing two complementary single-stranded DNA oligonucleotides including the sequence of interest and then annealing together. These oligonucleotides are designed to possess overhanging ends at the 3'-extremity when annealed. (*See* **Note 2**).

3.4. Annealing of the DNA Oligonucleotide

1. Mix 10 µL of equimolar amounts of the 2 oligonucleotides A and B (diluted at 250 µg/mL), 5 µL of 10X Klenow buffer and 25 µL of sterile water.
2. Heat to 65°C for 5 min.
3. Slowly cool the oligonucleotides to room temperature. This is easily done by allowing a beaker containing approximately 250 mL of 65°C water to equilibrate to room temperature.
4. Store annealed products at –20°C until labeling.

3.5. Labeling of DNA Probe

1. Take 1 µL of annealed DNA oligonucleotide (from **Subheading 3.4.**).
2. Add:

    5 µL 10X T7 buffer
    2.5 µL α-^{32}P-dCTP
    40 µL sterile water

0.5 µL DTT (0.5 *M*)

1 µL dNTP (dCTP)

1 µL T7 Sequenase DNA polymerase (*see* **Note 3**)

3. Incubate 10 min at 37°C.
4. Add 2 µL 0.5 *M* EDTA and 148 µL TE.
5. Remove unincorporated dNTPs by centrifuge 2 times over Sephadex G-50 columns, at 1600*g* for 5 min, room temperature (*see* **ref. 4**).
6. Determine specific activity and store labeled DNA oligonucleotide at −20°C until use.

3.6. Binding Reactions

1. Mix all components except labeled probe in a final volume of 19 µL.

    5 µg of nuclear extracts (1 mg/mL stock) = 5 µL (from **Subheading 3.1.**)

    7.5 µL of binding buffer

    1.25 µL poly d[I-C] (*see* **Note 4**)

    5.25 µL sterile water

    Total: 19 µL (without the labeled DNA probe).

2. Incubate 20 min at 4°C.
3. Add 1 µL of labeled DNA probe (from **Subheading 3.5.**), and incubate at room temperature for an additional 20 min (*see* **Note 5**).

3.7. Nondenaturing Gel Electrophoresis and Autoradiography

1. Prepare a 4–6% nondenaturing polyacrylamide gel: for 45 mL of 4% polyacrylamide 1.5 mm thick gel, mix:

    6 mL 30% acrylamide/bis (29:1 acrylamide:bis ratio)

    4.5 mL 5X TBE

    300 µL 10% ammonium persulfate

    30 µL TEMED

    34.5 mL H_2O.

2. After adding ammonium persulfate and TEMED, pour the gel immediately.
3. Add comb and let the gel polymerize for approx 1 h at room temperature.
4. Remove comb and set up gel in electrophoresis apparatus in appropriate buffer (0.25X TBE for this example).
5. Prerun the gel for 20 min prior loading the samples.
6. Load the samples (20 µL, from **Subheading 3.6.**) onto the gel while it is running at about 25 V.
7. Also load a few µL of gel loading buffer containing dyes to an unused lane as a marker.
8. Run the gel at constant voltage (approx 100–150 V) until the bromophenol blue is about 2–3 cm from the bottom.
9. Take down apparatus and place the gel on Whatman paper, cover with plastic wrap and dry on gel dryer at 80°C for approx 60 min.
10. Place the dried gel in a film cassette, expose overnight at −70°C and develop film.

4. Notes

1. Protein extracts may be prepared from whole cells or nuclei. The amount of nuclear extract required may need to be varied depending on the protein concentration of the extracts and the amount and affinity of the transcription factor to be studied.

2. Often, the oligonucleotides are designed to possess the overhanging ends of a restriction enzyme site when annealed which permit them to be cloned into a variety of plasmid vectors.

3. The labeling of fragment probes depends on the nature of DNA ends. In the case of fragments with 3'-overhanging ends, T7 DNA polymerase, which possesses a 5' to 3' polymerase activity is used for labeling. An alternative method for the labelling of oligonulceotides is to add a ^{32}P to the 5' end using T4 polynucleotide kinase and γ^{32}P-ATP. In this case, the oligonucleotides are designed with blunt ends.

4. Poly d[I-C] is added to the binding reaction as a competitor for nonspecific DNA binding protein. You can also use sonicated salmon sperm DNA (ssDNA), however, in general, the very simple copolymers provide the best results. Concentration and combination of poly d[I-C] and ssDNA often needs to be determined empirically. A good starting point might be 1 µg d[I-C] and 0.5 µg ssDNA.

5. Competition analysis with unlabeled an DNA fragment (same sequence as for the labeled probe) can be used to test the specificity of the complex formation to the DNA sequence. Approximately 50–100-fold molar excess of an unlabeled DNA fragment is added to the binding reaction, 20 min prior to the labeled probe. Binding of the unlabeled competitor DNA to the transcription factor of interest will result in a decrease in the amount of protein available for binding to the probe. This will lead to an attenuation or elimination of the band corresponding to the complex formed by that protein. Alternatively, competition with unlabeled oligonucleotides which have mutations within the critical sequences required for transcription factor binding would not be expected to compete with the labeled probe.

   To positively identify the proteins which complex to the DNA-binding sites, antibodies against known transcription factors are included in the binding reaction, before adding probe at 4°C. These antibodies may bind to the complex, causing an alteration in the mobility of the complex, characterized by a supershift of the DNA-protein complex or it can completely inhibit the complex formation by binding to an essential site on the transcription factor required for DNA binding, resulting in the absence of the DNA-protein complex on the gel.

References

1. Fried, M. and Crothers, D. M. (1981) Equilibria and kinetics of *lac* repressor-operator interactions by polyacrylamide gel electrophoresis. *Nucleic Acids Res.* **9,** 6505–6525.
2. Garner, M. M. and Revzin, A. (1981) A gel electrophoresis method for quantifying the binding of proteins to specific DNA regions: application to components of

the *Escherichia coli* lactose operon regulatory system. *Nucleic Acids Res.* **9,** 3047–3060.

3. Smith, M. F., Jr., Carl, V. S., Lodie, T. A., and Fenton, M. J. (1998) Secretory interleukin-1 receptor antagonist gene expression requires both a PU.1 and a novel composite NF-kB/PU.1/GA-binding protein binding site. *J. Biol. Chem.* **273(37),** 24,272–24,279.

4. Dignam, J. D., Lebovitz, R., and Roeder, R. G. (1983) Accurate transcription initiation by RNA polymerase II in a soluble extract from isolated mammalian nuclei. *Nucleic Acids Res.* **11,** 1475–1489.

5. Maniatis, T., Fritsch, E. F., and Sambrook, J. (1982) Spun column procedure, in *Molecular Cloning: A Laboratory Manual* (Maniatis, T., Fritsch, E. F., and Sambrook, J., eds.), Cold Spring Harbor Laboratory, Cold Spring Harbor, NY, pp. 466–467.

25

Transfection Assays for Transformation of Model Colonic Cell Lines

Mark T. Worthington and Roger Qi Luo

1. Introduction

The recognition of cancer as a genetic disease has changed the approach investigators take to understanding the mechanisms of carcinogenesis. The discovery of oncogenes, and the recognition of the inactivation of tumor suppressor genes, DNA repair enzymes, and of apoptotic pathways have provided a clearer picture of the dysregulation which is required for a cell to become a cancer.

One method of understanding the function of genes identified in carcinogenesis is through the use of model cell lines. Unfortunately, many of the commonly employed colonic cell lines are derived from cancers that have already accrued mutations in genes of potential interest, lost typical cell surface markers, and have been selected by the organism growth in a hostile environment, such as evading normal immune surveillance. Early mutations responsible for the pathogenesis of the disease may be overshadowed by more global mutations when the disease is clinically apparent, such as those arising from large deletions or widespread mismatch repair errors.

A reasonable in vitro model would mimic the multistep process of carcinogenesis from normal mucosa, to adenoma, and then to carcinoma. This would allow introduction of mutant genes and inactivation of native ones, and could be assayed using conventional in vitro means for proliferation, apoptosis, etc., all features of tissue culture cell lines. In particular, a desirable model would have one normal cell line which mimics the features of normal colonic mucosa—TGF-alpha growth stimulation, TGF-beta growth inhibition, and "anoikis," the property of colonic cells to ordinarily undergo apoptosis when separated from their basement membrane matrix (*1–3*). An additional stage in progression would be a cell line from the same organism that loses the proper-

From: *Methods in Molecular Medicine, vol. 50: Colorectal Cancer: Methods and Protocols*
Edited by: S. M. Powell © Humana Press Inc., Totowa, NJ

ties of TGF-beta growth inhibition and apoptosis—like an adenomatous polyp—but retain anchorage-dependent growth in vitro. A final stage would be to progress to anchorage-independent growth and tumor formation in athymic nude mice. For optimal usefulness, these cell lines should be easily transfected with plasmid DNA or infected with retroviruses, which could be used to introduce exogenous or inactivate endogenous genes. A final criterion would be easy propagation and storage.

A reasonable model for this sort of system for colon cancer has been developed from the Immorto mouse by the Whitehead laboratory *(1,2)*, which carries a temperature-sensitive SV40 T-antigen in its genome and grow vigorously. Cells from tissues from this mouse can be readily propagated at 34°C, but undergo growth arrest at 39°C and assume the phenotype of the native tissue. This laboratory has derived two cell lines, one from a normal mouse colon (YAMC) and one derived from crossing the Immorto mouse with the Min mouse (IMCE) that is a presumptive model of adenomatous polyp formation. The Min mouse develops tens to hundreds of ademomatous polyps in its gastrointestinal tract due to a mutation in the adenomatous polyposis coli (APC) gene, and is a rodent model of the human disease familial adenomatous polyposis coli (FAP). FAP carriers have a myriad of colonic polyps and a near 100% colon cancer rate over a lifetime. The IMCE cell line displays anchorage independent growth and tumors in nude mice when transformed with a mutant ras oncogene, resulting in further phenotypic progression of the disease, suggesting progression to frank carcinogenesis. The YAMC cells are not susceptible to transformation by *ras*, confirming that the loss of APC is a critical step in colon cancer progression *(4)*. Not all IMCE cells transform with *ras* and whether the second APC mutation is required for this process has not to our knowledge been characterized. Small intestinal cells are available (MSIE cells) from the same mouse strain as the YAMC cells.

The properties of these cell lines are as follows:

Cell line	34°C properties	39°C properties	Growth pattern	Tumors in nude mice
YAMC	Proliferation	Apoptosis	Contact inhibited, growth inhibited by TGF-β	No
IMCE (+/– APC)	Proliferation	No apoptosis	Contact inhibited, no inhibition by TGF-β	No
IMCE + mutant Ras	Proliferation	No apoptosis	Anchorage independent growth, cells pile up on tissue culture plate and can grow in soft agar	Yes

These cells have the temperature-sensitive tsA58 mutant of the SV40 large T antigen under the control of an interferon-inducible Class I major histocompatibility promoter. This T antigen is active at the growth permissive temperature, but inactive at the nonpermissive temperature (*see* **Note 1**). Mouse γ-interferon is required in the medium for expression of the T antigen, but can be removed from the medium for other experiments. We have propagated the cells, removed the interferon, raised the temperature, and performed subsequent experiments with good results.

The defined and readily manipulatable growth and apoptotic properties of these cells provide a good foundation for the study of genes involved in colon cancer progression. Similar cell lines have been derived from gastric, liver, small intestinal, cardiac, pancreas, renal, and adipocyte tissues. The mouse with the temperature-sensitive T antigen in its genome (Immorto) can be purchased from Jackson laboratories if the investigator wishes to attempt cell lines from other tissues.

Other potential uses exist. Since IMCE cells can be transformed with an activated *ras* to change the growth potential of the cells, these cells can be potentially transfected with a human colon cancer expression library which is known not to have a *ras* mutation to identify new genes in colon carcinogenesis (*see* **Note 2**). Individual clones can be identified based upon changes in growth pattern and phenotype. The fact that the MSIE and YAMC cells are derived from the same mouse raises the possibility that genes that are preferentially expressed from one tissue of origin could be identified. Genes in these cells could be randomly inactivated by retroviral integration or other means to identify important genes in carcinogenesis.

2. Materials

2.1. Cells and Plasmids

The YAMC and IMCE cells can be obtained by contacting Dr. Robert Whitehead at the Ludwig Cancer Institute, Melbourne, Australia. We obtained the activated K-ras plasmid, pMLC12, from Dr. Manuel Perucho at the Burnham Institute, La Jolla, California. pMLC12 contains a genomic *K-ras* with an activating mutation and like activated H-ras, is capable transforming in the IMCE cells. The lacZ mammalian expression plasmid pYN3214 was a kind gift from Dr. Yusaku Nakabeppu, Medical Institute for Bioregulation at Kyushu Univeristy, Fukuoka, Japan.

2.2. Growth Media and Tissue Culture

1. Complete media (for propagation): RPMI1640 medium with 5% fetal bovine serum, 1:100 Pen/Strep (all Life Technologies), to which is added 5 U/mL of murine

γ-interferon just before use (*see* **step 2**, below). Make up the RPMI with all additives except interferon in advance and sterilize by passage through a sterilizing 0.22 μ filter apparatus. Interferon is added to an aliquot just before use. Store at 4°C for up to one month.

2. Murine γ-interferon. Required for these cells to proliferate. Reconstitute lyophilized murine γ-interferon (R & D Systems) to 500 U/mL and filter through a low-protein binding, low volume sterilizing syringe filter. Store in aliquots at –70°C to minimize inactivation by freeze/thawing, and add 1:100 volume to the otherwise complete, sterile RPMI media when needed.

3. Tissue culture flasks or dishes, pipets, laminar flow tissue culture hood.

4. Tissue culture incubators, one set to 34°C for propagation and set to 39°C for nongrowth conditions. These should be capable of maintaining 5% CO_2 and accurate temperature, for obvious reasons. The permissive temperature for propagation of YAMC and IMCE cells is 33–34°C; the nonpermissive is 39°C. We use 34°C for propagation and for transfections.

5. Phosphate buffered saline, sterile, without magnesium or calcium (Life Technologies).

6. Trypsin (Life Technologies).

7. Mr. Frosty Freezing Unit (Nalgene).

8. Superfect transfection reagent (Qiagen, Chatsworth, CA).

9. Transfection quality DNA.

10. X-gal in DMF, potassium ferricyanide, potassium ferrocyanide, 25% glutaraldehyde (for X-gal staining).

3. Methods

3.1. Splitting YAMC and IMCE Cells

1. Remove growth media with a sterile pipet, and wash three times with 3 mL phosphate buffered saline in a 60 mm dish.

2. Add 0.8 mL trypsin and allow cells to incubate for 10 min. Remove cells to a sterile 50 mL conical tube and centrifuge at 500 g for 10 min.

3. Resuspend cells in 5 mL PBS or media and spin again.

4. Split cells 1:4 and plate on tissue-culture coated flasks with complete RPMI media, including γ-interferon. Incubate at 34°C until cells are attached.

3.2. Long-Term Storage of YAMC and IMCE Cells

1. Trypsinize cells and wash as above. Do not suspend in complete media.

2. Resuspend cells at $2 - 5 \times 10^6$ cells/mL in Freezing Solution (sterile complete RPMI media with 10% fetal bovine serum and 10% tissue culture grade DMSO) and place 1–1.5 mL of this in a cryovial.

3. Freeze at 1°C/min in a Mr. Frosty freezing container, following the manufacturer's instructions. Remove to a liquid nitrogen freezer the next morning for storage.

3.3. Thawing YAMC and IMCE Cells After Liquid Nitrogen Storage

1. Remove from liquid nitrogen and thaw quickly in 37°C water bath. Spray the exterior of the tube with 70% ethanol to sterilize and perform further manipulations in a laminar flow tissue culture hood.
2. Aseptically transfer the contents of the vial into a 25 cm^2 tissue culture flask with double the usual amount of complete media to dilute out the DMSO (8 mL).
3. Change medium after cells have attached, usually 4–24 h. Wash three times with 3 mL PBS, then add the usual volume of complete medium with interferon (3 mL).
4. It is recommended that these cells not become confluent, to avoid a change in growth potential.

3.4. Transfection of IMCE Cells in a 60 mm Dish

These instructions are for a 60 mm dish and for IMCE cells:

1. Prepare transfection-quality plasmid DNA using traditional means. We use the Nucleobond Plasmid DNA purification kit (Clontech, Palo Alto, CA) following the manufacturer's instructions, but see no reason which other standard methods should not work. The plasmid DNA is resuspended at 1 µg/µL.
2. Split the cells and plate at 20–60% confluence under permissive conditions (33–34°C). The cells should be evenly dispersed and not in clumps. Allow cells to attach for several h to overnight.
3. Take 5 µg of plasmid DNA and add RPMI1640 to 150 µL (without the fetal bovine serum). Add 30 µL Superfect reagent and incubate at room temperature for 10 min. Add the complexes to cells and incubate 3–5 h in a 34°C, 5% CO_2 incubator. Replace with fresh complete medium at that time (*see* **Note 3**).
4. Assay for desired phenotype at the desired timepoint.

3.5. Focus Assay

After transfection with an activated Ras plasmid, 7–10 d of incubation at 34°C is necessary to see transformed foci, up to 50 per plate. The cells are identified by their change in growth properties. Cells will pile up and will no longer be in a monolayer when transformed, forming mounds of transformed cells. With prolonged incubation, these mounds of cells will rise out of the tissue culture plate and can be several cells thick (*see* **Note 4**).

3.6. Beta-Galactosidase Transfection and Staining (5)

We transfect an *E. coli* beta-galactosidase reporter plasmid under control of a strong mammalian promoter to establish transfection efficiency. Similar plasmids are commercially available. Typically >50–75% of the cells will turn blue when stained with X-gal, suggesting that they have taken up the reporter DNA. A mock transfected dish (a plasmid without the beta-galactosidase gene) is assayed in parallel (*see* **Note 5**).

The protocol for X-gal staining of cells in a 60 mm dish is:

1. Remove medium and add 0.05% glutaraldehyde in PBS for 5 min at room temperature. We perform this assay in a fume hood. Glutaraldehyde is toxic and protective gloves, lab coats, and eyewear should be worn. Ask your institution about glutaraldehyde disposal.
2. Discard fixative solution and wash cells three times with PBS.
3. Add X-gal solution just to cover cells. Incubate from 1–18 h at 37°C. X-gal solution is prepared in PBS: 35 mM potassium ferricyanide, 35 mM potassium ferrocyanide, 1 mM MgCl$_2$ (this stock is stable for months at room temperature). Just before use, add X-gal to 1 mg/mL from a 40X stock in N, N dimethylformamide (*see* **Note 6**). Store the X-gal stock protected from light at –20°C.
4. Remove X-gal solution when some cells are perceptibly blue, add PBS to cover, and count the numbers of blue vs nonblue cells with an inverted microscope.

4. Notes

1. At the permissive temperature, the presence of a functional T antigen would be expected to amplify plasmids which contain an SV40 origin of replication, but to our knowledge, this has not been investigated. This may be important for potentially toxic genes.
2. The original manuscript used an *H-ras* expressing retrovirus to transform IMCE cells. The benefit of potentially higher efficiencies has to be weighed vs the potential risks of having a potent oncogene in viral form.
3. Depending upon the experiment, experiment after transfection may require incubation at the nonpermissive temperature and/or in medium without interferon to avoid T-antigen or cytokine effects. We transfect at the lower temperature, then raise the temperature the next morning and substitute medium without interferon, then assay at 48 h.
4. Other assays, such as growth in soft agar, can be performed with these cells, if desired *(4)*.
5. The glutaraldehyde fixation in the X-gal staining step kills the cells in that assay. Investigators should keep this in mind when designing experiments if a co-transfection with a reporter gene is required.
6. X-gal can be resuspended in DMSO with essentially similar results.

Acknowledgments

This work was supported by an American Digestive Health Foundation Industry Research Scholar Award and NIH Grant to Mark T. Worthington. Special thanks to Theresa T. Pizarro, PhD for use of equipment and helpful discussions.

References

1. Whitehead, R. H., VanEeden, P. E., Noble, M. D., Ataliotis, P., and Jat, P. S. (1993) Establishment of conditionally immortalized epithelial cell lines from

both colon and small intestine of adult H-2Kb-tsA58 transgenic mice. *Proc. Natl. Acad. Sci. USA* **90(2),** 587–591.

2. Whitehead, R. H. and Joseph, J. L. (1994) Derivation of conditionally immortalized cell lines containing the min mutation from the normal colonic mucosa and other tissues of an "Immortomouse"/min hybrid. *Epithelial Cell Biol.* **3(3),** 119–125.
3. Grossmann, J., Maxson, J. M., Whitacre, C. M., Orosz, D. E., Berger, N. A., Fiocchi, C., and Levine, A. D. (1998) New isolation technique to study apoptosis in human intestinal epithelial cells. *Am. J. Pathol.* **153(1),** 53–62.
4. D'Abaco, G. M., Whitehead, R. H., and Burgess, A. W. (1996) Synergy between Apc min and an activated ras mutation is sufficient to induce colon carcinomas. *Mol. Cell. Biol.* **16(3),** 884–891.
5. Cepko, C. (1992) Preparation of a specific retrovirus producer cell line, in *Current Protocols in Molecular Biology,* John Wiley & Sons, New York, pp. 9.10.1–9.10.13.

26

Assessment of Intestinal Stem Cell Survival Using the Microcolony Formation Assay

Kimberly S. Tustison, Joanne Yu, and Steven M. Cohn

1. Introduction

The microcolony assay originally described by Withers and Elkind in 1970 *(1)* has been a useful method for investigating the effects of radiation and various other genotoxic and cytotoxic damaging agents on the intestinal epithelial stem cell population and to assess the ability of a variety of compounds to protect the epithelial stem cell population from the lethal effects of chemical and physical agents (e.g., *2–7*). Epithelial stem cells are located near the base of each intestinal crypt and play an important role in normal epithelial renewal and differentiation, epithelial injury-repair, and in neoplastic transformation *(8–11)*. In the adult mouse small intestine these functionally anchored clonogenic stem cells divide rarely to produce a daughter stem cell (self renewal) as well as a more rapidly replicating transit cell. Transit cells, in turn, undergo a number of rapid cell divisions in the proliferative zone located in the lower half of each crypt. Their progeny subsequently differentiate into the mature epithelial cell types found in the small intestine as they migrate away from the proliferative zone in each intestinal crypt *(8–11)*. Following intestinal injury and disruption of the epithelium, epithelial cells adjacent to the wound first migrate over the injured area to reestablish continuity of the epithelium. Stem cells subsequently proliferate to increase their numbers and to give rise to the more rapidly proliferating transit cell population. The transit cell population then expands rapidly to form a regenerative crypt. If the injury has completely destroyed some crypts, the surviving regenerative crypts can subsequently branch and divide to restore near normal numbers of viable crypts *(3)*.

From: *Methods in Molecular Medicine, vol. 50: Colorectal Cancer: Methods and Protocols*
Edited by: S. M. Powell © Humana Press Inc., Totowa, NJ

The microcolony assay is a functional assay for quantifying stem cell survival following acute cytotoxic injury based on the capacity of the surviving clonogenic stem cells to regenerate crypt-like foci of cells, termed microcolonies *(1,3)*. Although this assay can be used to study epithelial regeneration in response to any cytotoxic insult the response of the gastrointestinal epithelium to acute radiation injury in the mouse has been the most extensively characterized model. The actively proliferating transit cell population undergo apoptosis or cell cycle arrest following γ-irradiation or other genotoxic injury. Since cell migration from the crypt onto the villus epithelium continues, the crypts are rapidly depleted of the replicating transit cell population. If one or more of the anchored clonogenic stem cells within a crypt survives irradiation, it will go on to replicate and form a focus of regenerating epithelial cells which first appear about three days after irradiation. The number of these regenerative cryptlike foci can then be scored on histologic cross-sections of intestine. Thus, the number of surviving crypts in each cross-section can be used as a surrogate measure of the survival of crypt epithelial stem cells in the intestine. We have modified the original microcolony assay to include BrdUrd-labeling of regenerating, S-phase epithelial cells prior to sacrificing animals for analysis and subsequent immunohistochemical detection of incorporated BrdUrd in intestinal cross-sections *(7,12,13)*. This allows the investigator to easily distinguish viable regenerative crypts within the microscopic section based on the presence of S-phase cells within these foci.

2. Materials

1. 5-Bromo-2'-deoxyuridine (BrdUrd) 8 mg/mL in sterile water or saline (Sigma, St. Louis, MO); or labeling reagent from kit.
2. 5-Fluoro-2'-deoxyyuridine (FdUrd) 0.8 mg/mL in sterile water or saline (Sigma).
3. Accustain Bouin's solution (Sigma).
4. Bacto agar (Difco, Detroit, MI).
5. 10% Neutral buffered formalin (Fisher Scientific, Pittsburgh, PA).
6. SuperFrost plus charged and precleaned slides (Fisher Scientific).
7. Xylenes (Sigma).
8. Absolute ethanol, 95% ethanol, 90% ethanol, 70% ethanol.
9. Methanol.
10. Cell proliferation kit (anti-BrdUrd staining reagents for immunohistochemistry; RPN 20 available through Amersham Pharmacia Biotech).
11. Humidified slide incubation chamber.
12. Staining dishes with slide racks.
13. PAP pen (Research Products International Corp.).
14. Phosphate buffer: Na_2HPO_4, 5.75 g; $NaH_2PO_4 \cdot 2H_2O$, (1.48 g); distilled H_2O to 1 L.
15. PBS: Na_2HPO_4 (11.5 g), $NaH_2PO_4 \cdot 2H_2O$ (2.96 g), NaCL (5.84 g), distilled H_2O to 1 L.

16. PBS blocking buffer: bovine serum albumin (1.0 g), powdered skim milk (0.2 g), Triton X-100 (0.3 mL), PBS to 100 mL.
17. Sigma Fast 3,3' diaminobenzidene (DAB) tablet sets (D4293, Sigma).
18. Hematoxylin (Richard Allan Scientific, Kalamazoo, MI).
19. Acid alcohol: 500 μL HCl (12 *M*) diluted into 200 mL 70% ethanol.
20. Ammonia water: 600 μL ammonium hydroxide (14.8N) diluted in 200 mL distilled H_2O.
21. Brightfield microscope with 10×, 20×, and 40× objectives.

3. Methods

3.1. Tissue Preparation

1. Expose the mice to varying doses of the test damaging agent. We routinely use 5–6 mice per group.
2. Let mice recover 82 h.
3. Administer 0.12 mg BrdUrd per gram of mouse weight and 0.012 mg FdUrd per gram of mouse weight by intraperitoneal injection.
4. Sacrifice mice 2 h after injection.
5. Excise the intestine from the stomach to the ileal-cecal junction. Stretch out the entire intestine and measure and cut five cm below stomach.
6. Divide the remaining length of small intestine into thirds removing as much digested matter and extraneous tissue as possible. The first third, closest to the stomach, is the proximal jejunum, the second third is the distal jejunum, and the last third section is the ileum.
7. Cut through the proximal jejunum perpendicular to its longitudinal axis approximately every cm. Put these sections in 5–10 mL of 10% neutral buffered formalin or Bouin's fixative (*see* **Note 1**). Repeat the same processes with the distal jejunum and ileum.
8. After the tissue samples have fixed for 12 h pour off the fixative solution and pipet out any remaining drops.
9. Add 10 mL of 70% ethanol to the tissue and allow it to soak at least overnight at room temperature.
10. Replace with an equal volume of fresh 70% ethanol for several h then again replace with 10 mL of fresh 70% ethanol.

3.2. Slide Preparation

1. Melt 2 g of agar in 50 mL distilled H_2O in a boiling water bath and bring the solution to 60°C. Add 50 mL of prewarmed 10% neutral buffered formalin to yield a final concentration of 2% agar and 5% formalin. Keep the agar mix at 55–60°C in a water bath while preparing the tissues for orientation and embedding.
2. When ready to mount tissues, remove 1 cm intestine sections from ethanol and trim off the curled ends of each segment with a razor blade, cutting the segment perpendicular to the longitudinal axis of the intestine.
3. Stand each 1 cm segment of intestine up on end on a glass slide so that several segments of intestine are side by side on the slide. The last 1 cm segment of

intestine is placed on its side (so that it will be sectioned along the longitudinal axis) next to the segments to be cut in cross section. This is done so that one can correct for changes in the probability of sectioning through a regenerative crypt due to changes in crypt dimensions induced by the test agent (*see* **Note 2**).

4. Carefully infiltrate the warm agar around the tissue segments to hold them in a fixed orientation. This is done to maintain the orientation of tissues during subsequent paraffin embedding so that cross-sections of multiple tissue segments, each of which remains perpendicular to the longitudinal axis of the intestine, can be produced from a single paraffin block. When the agar has fully solidified trim off the excess agar surrounding the cluster of intestinal segments.
5. Slide the agar fixed tissue off the slide into a cassette and snap it closed. Label the cassette in pencil, and soak it in 70% ethanol.
6. Embed in paraffin blocks.
7. Cut 5 μm paraffin sections perpendicular to the long axis of the intestine and mount on Superfrost plus charged slides. This cut should result in a section containing several donut shaped intestinal cross-sections.
8. Dry paraffin sections in 60°C oven for 1–2 h.

3.3. Slide Staining

1. Deparaffinize slides in xylene 5 min.
2. Wash in xylene for 5 min.
3. Rehydrate slides by washing two times in 100% ethanol for 5 min each, once in 95% ethanol for 5 min, once in 70% ethanol for 5 min, and once in tap water for 5 min.
4. Quench endogenous tissue peroxidase activity by incubating the slides in 2–3% H_2O_2 in methanol for 15 to 30 min.
5. Rinse in tap water then wash in PBS three times (5 min with each wash).
6. Dab off excess fluid from around the tissue section and draw a circle around the tissue section with a PAP pen.
7. Cover the tissue for 30 min with PBS blocking buffer (about 100 μL).
8. Tap off blocking the buffer from the slide and add 75–100 μL of mouse anti-BrdUrd diluted 1:100 in reconstituted nuclease mixture from the kit (*see* **Note 1**). Incubate for 1 h at room temperature.
9. Wash three times in PBS at room temperature (5 min each wash).
10. Cover tissue section with freshly diluted peroxidase antimouse IgG2a (75–100 μL). Incubate for 30 min at room temperature.
11. Wash three times in PBS at room temperature.
12. Incubate for 5–10 min in excess freshly prepared DAB substrate solution (*see* **Note 3**).
13. Wash three times in distilled water at room temperature (3 min each wash).
14. Counterstain lightly in hematoxylin for 10–30 s. Wash in slowly running tap water until the effluent runs clear.
15. Dip 3–4 times in acid alcohol solution.
16. Rinse in slowly running tap water for 5 min.

17. Dip 3–4 times in ammonia water.
18. Rinse in slowly running tap water for 5 min.
19. Dehydrate sections through 70% ethanol, 90% ethanol, 95% ethanol, 2 changes of absolute ethanol, and 2 changes of xylenes. Coverslip with Permount or other suitable clear mounting media.

3.4. Data Analysis

Examine each cross-section under the microscope. Only well oriented, complete cross-sections are scored. A crypt is considered to be a viable surviving crypt if it has five or more S-phase, BrdUrd-labeled cells in the crypt. The number of surviving crypts is scored in each cross-section and the mean number of surviving crypts per cross-section is determined for each animal (*see* **Note 2**). Fractional crypt survival is the mean number of surviving crypts per cross-section in treated animals divided by the total number of crypts per cross-section in the same segment of intestine from uninjured control animals. Crypt survival data are usually expressed as a log-linear plot of fractional crypt survival versus dose of damaging agent (**Fig. 1**). The fractional crypt survival curve plotted in this manner consists of an initial plateau followed by an exponential decline in crypt survival with increasing dose. The magnitude of the initial plateau appears to be related to the intrinsic repair capacity of individual clonogenic cells within the injured crypt and to the number of clonogenic epithelial cells present in the crypt. A comprehensive description of the response of the crypt epithelium to radiation injury and the statistical analysis of fractional crypt stem cell survival curves is beyond the scope of this chapter and has been reviewed in detail by C.S. Potten (*see* **ref. 4**).

4. Notes

1. Bouin's fixative can be used as an alternative to 10% neutral buffered formalin. Nuclease digestion is frequently not required when using Bouin's fixative. In this case the mouse anti-BrdUrd antibody may be diluted 1:100 in PBS blocking buffer instead of the nuclease solution.
2. Since the size of the regenerating crypt may not be the same for each treatment group the probability of a section passing through a regenerative crypt may vary depending on the experimental conditions. If this is the case, the number of surviving crypts per cross-section must be corrected for crypt size to control for the effect of treatment on the probability of observing a regenerative crypt within a section (**14**). The width of fifteen representative crypts for each animal is measured in longitudinal sections of proximal jejunum at the widest point in each crypt, and the mean surviving crypts per circumference is corrected for the variation in crypt size. Under most circumstances the correction factor, $C.F. = D_c/D_t$ where D_c is the mean crypt diameter in the longitudinal axis from untreated animals and D_t is the mean crypt diameter in treated animals, can be employed. For a more extensive discussion of conditions effecting this correction *see* **ref. 14**.

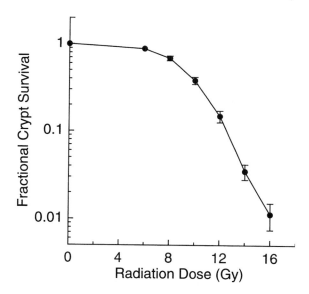

Fig. 1. Fractional crypt survival as a function of radiation dose. FVB/n mice (10–12 wk old) were γ-irradiated with the indicated dose and animals were euthanized for analysis at 84 h after irradiation. All animals received 120 mg/kg BrdUrd and 12 mg/kg FdUrd by intraperitoneal injection 2 h prior to sacrifice. The number of surviving crypts containing 5 or more BrdUrd-labeled nuclei per cross-section were scored at each radiation dose and divided by the mean number of crypts per cross-section in unirradiated animals to calculate fractional crypt survival. Data are shown as the mean fractional crypt survival ±SEM for groups of 6 mice.

3. DAB substrate, diluent, and intensifier are provided in the Amersham Pharmacia kit. 3,3' diaminobenzidene is a suspected carcinogen and caution should be exercised to avoid inhalation or contact with skin or mucous membranes when weighing or handling this reagent. Sigma Fast 3,3' diaminobenzidene tablet sets may be used as an alternative to avoid having to weigh the DAB powder. The timing of slide incubation in the DAB substrate solution should be determined empirically to provide sufficient deposition of the brown reaction product over the Brd-Urd-labeled nuclei without excess, nonspecific background staining.

References

1. Withers, H. R., and Elkind, M. M. (1970) Microcolony survival assay for cells of mouse intestinal mucosa exposed to radiation. *Int. J. Radiat. Biol.* **117,** 261–267.
2. Hanson, W. R. and Thomas, C. (1983) 16, 16-dimethyl prostaglandin E_2 increases survival of murine intestinal stem cells when given before photon radiation. *Radiat. Res.* **96,** 393–398.
3. Potten, C. S. (1990) A comprehensive study of the radiobiological response of the murine (BDF1) small intestine. *Int. J. Radiat. Biol.* **58,** 925–973.

4. Potten C. S. (1995) Interleukin-11 protects the clonogenic stem cells in murine small-intestinal crypts from impairment of their reproductive capacity by radiation. *Int. J. Cancer.* **62,** 356–361.
5. Potten, C. S., Booth, D., and Haley, J. D. (1997) Pretreatment with transforming growth factor beta-3 protects small intestinal stem cells against radiation damage in vivo. *Br. J. Cancer* **75,** 1454–1459.
6. Khan, W. B., Shui, C., Ning, S., and Knox, S. J. (1997) Enhancement of murine intestinal stem cell survival after irradiation by keratinocyte growth factor. *Radiat. Res.* **148,** 248–253.
7. Cohn, S. M., Schloemann, S., Tessner, T., Seibert, K., and Stenson, W. F. (1997) Crypt stem cell survival in the mouse intestinal epithelium is regulated by prostaglandins synthesized through cyclooxygenase-1. *J. Clin. Invest.* **99,** 1367–1379.
8. Cheng, H. and Leblond, C. P. (1974) Origin, differentiation and renewal of the four main epithelial cell types in the mouse small intestine. V. Unitarian theory of the origin of the four epithelial cell types. *Am. J. Anat.* **141,** 537–561.
9. Gordon, J. I. and Hermiston, M. L. (1994) Differentiation and self-renewal in the mouse gastrointestinal epithelium. *Curr. Opin. Cell Biol.* **6,** 795–803.
10. Potten, C. S., Booth, C., and Pritchard, D. M. (1997) The intestinal epithelial stem cell: the mucosal governor. *Int. J. Exp. Path.* **78,** 219–243.
11. Hauft, S. M., Kim, S. H., Schmidt, G. H., Pease, S., Rees, S., Harris, S., et al. (1992) Expression of SV-40 T antigen in the small intestinal epithelium of transgenic mice results in proliferative changes in the crypt and reentry of villus-associated enterocytes into the cell cycle but has no apparent effect on cellular differentiation programs and does not cause neoplastic transformation. *J. Cell Biol.* **117,** 825–839.
12. Cohn, S. M. and Lieberman, M. W. (1984) The use of antibodies to 5-bromo-2'-deoxyuridine for the isolation of DNA sequences containing excision-repair sites. *J. Biol. Chem.* **259,** 12,456–12,462.
13. Houchen, C. W., George, R. J., Sturmoski, M. A., and Cohn, S. M. (1999) FGF-2 enhances intestinal stem cell survival and its expression is induced after radiation injury. *Am. J. Physiol.* **276,** G249–G258.
14. Potten, C. S., Rezvzni, M., Hendry, J. H., Moore, J. V., and Major, D. (1981) The correction of intestinal microcolony counts for variations in size. *Int. J. Radiat. Biol* **40,** 321–326.

27

Gene Transfer into the Colonic Mucosa

Başak Çoruh and Theresa T. Pizarro

1. Introduction

Somatic gene therapy is based on the principle of transferring recombinant genes efficiently into somatic tissues and achieving expression of the gene product in order to replace genetically defective gene functions or alter pathological disease processes. The development of a gene therapy model system that can stably produce and deliver bioactive target proteins into the intestinal microenvironment may represent an important advance in the treatment of several gut-related diseases including inflammatory bowel disease (IBD) and colon cancer. Ideally, transfection of the gut epithelia and their progenitor stem cells (i.e., epithelial crypt cells), would enable the local and targeted production of the desired gene product into the intestinal milieu. Furthermore, such genetically altered cells would have the ability to replicate the transfected gene and continue to produce and secrete its specifically encoded protein without interfering with the function of the tissue in which they reside.

The intestinal epithelium is an attractive target for gene therapy because it is readily accessible by relatively noninvasive procedures, has a large tissue mass, and contains a progenitor cell in the crypts, which are immortal and are capable of sustained proliferation in vivo. Although few studies have targeted the intestinal epithelium for gene transfer, reports have suggested that both crypt and villus epithelial cells can be transduced in vivo by exposure to retroviral vectors instilled into the lumen of the gut (1,2). In fact, retroviral gene transfer, overall, is one of the most efficient ways to introduce stable and heritable genetic material into mammalian cells. The intrinsic retroviral transduction machinery allows stable integration of the cloned target gene into the host genome of almost all mitotically active cells, such as intestinal epithelial crypt progenitor cells (3,4).

From: *Methods in Molecular Medicine, vol. 50: Colorectal Cancer: Methods and Protocols*
Edited by: S. M. Powell © Humana Press Inc., Totowa, NJ

The development of cell lines with the ability to package retroviral RNAs into infectious viral particles, while at the same time produce replication incompetent virus, has established current safety measures for retroviral gene transfer technology (*5,6*). These so-called "packaging cell lines" are also responsible for expressing the viral *env* gene, which encodes the envelope protein that determines the cellular host range of the packaged virus. This retroviral envelope protein facilitates infection of various target cell types via specific surface-expressed receptors. Amphotropic packaging cell lines are most commonly used because the amphotropic retrovirus receptor exhibits a broader host range than most other cell lines (*7*). In the context of the gut, however, the cloning of the rat ecotropic retroviral receptor (EcoR) and studies of its expression in intestinal tissues revealed that EcoR was present along the entire length of the rat small intestine and colon. In addition, EcoR was more abundant in nondifferentiated epithelial cells and declined as the cells underwent differentiation (*8*). These patterns of EcoR expression indicate that ecotropic retroviruses should be suitable vectors with which to attempt gene transfer into the intestinal epithelium in either the rat or mouse host. The exact localization of the rat ecotropic retroviral receptor on the polarized gut epithelium, however, has not been established. Likewise, the amphotropic retroviral receptor, which allows retroviral infection in a wider range of host species, has not been extensively investigated in the intestinal mucosa. The differential expression of these receptors on polarized intestinal epithelial cells has important ramifications on the efficacy of retrovirally-mediated transfection delivered from the apical versus the basolateral surface. In addition, the issue of vectorial secretion of the transfected gene product from the polarized gut epithelium is also an important consideration.

Our group has developed a model system that can successfully and specifically transduce colonic epithelial cells with the ability to locally produce and deliver recombinant proteins into the colonic microenvironment (*9*). Utilizing this model, we previously demonstrated that successful transduction of the colonic mucosa could be attained by retention enema delivery of a retrovirally encoded reporter gene following experimentally-induced intestinal inflammation. This locally induced gut damage initiates crypt progenitor stem cells to actively divide in order to reconstitute normal epithelial barrier function. Since retroviruses transduce only actively replicating cells, the retrovirally encoded gene specifically targets to these progenitor cells which give rise to all other intestinal epithelial cell types (i.e., enterocytes, goblet cells, Paneth cells) so that they, in turn, have the ability to produce the desired gene protein product. In subsequent studies, we determined the therapeutic value of this model system using a retroviral vector encoding the antiinflammatory cytokine, IL-1 receptor antagonist (IL-1ra), to treat experimentally-induced colitis (*10*). We demonstrated that the retroviral IL-1ra treatments significantly decreased acute colonic inflammation compared to controls (retroviral backbone treatment) in colitis animals, and reached those levels measured in baseline (noncolitic) control animals *(10)*. Therefore, transduction of the intestinal epithelium using retrovirally-based gene therapy can be used to locally deliver factors (i.e., antiinflammatory mediators), to the colonic microenvironment and may serve as a novel therapy for the treatment of gut-based diseases. The following gene therapy methodologies have been used for the treatment of animal models of colitides, but also have the potential for use in colon cancer-based animal model systems.

2. Materials

2.1. Preparation of Retrovirus

1. Gene of interest cloned into retroviral vector (*see* **Note 1**).
2. Packaging cell line (*see* **Note 1**).
3. Dulbecco's Modified Eagle's Medium (DMEM) (Sigma, St. Louis, MO).
4. Fetal bovine serum (FBS) (Sigma).
5. L-glutamine (200 mM) (Sigma).
6. Penicillin/streptomycin solution (10,000 U/mL penicillin and 10,000 μg/mL streptomycin) (Sigma).
7. Dulbecco's phosphate buffered saline (D-PBS) (Sigma).
8. BES-buffered saline (2X) (*see* **Note 2**).
9. $CaCl_2$ (2.5 M) (*see* **Note 3**).
10. Trypsin-EDTA (Sigma).
11. G418 (Geneticin) (50 mg/mL) (Gibco-BRL, Gaithersburg, MD).
12. Polybrene (hexadimethrine bromide) (Sigma).
13. Target cells, such as NIH3T3 (ATCC, Rockville, MD).
14. 100 mm tissue culture plates.
15. 15 mL conical tubes.
16. Cloning cylinders (PGC Scientific, Frederick, MD).
17. 6-well plates.

2.2. In Vivo Retroviral Transduction of the Gut Epithelium

1. Experimental animals (*see* **Note 4**).
2. Rabbit antihuman IgG fraction (Sigma).
3. Rabbit antihuman whole serum fraction (Sigma).
4. Human serum albumin (HSA) (5%) (Sigma).
5. Ketamine HCl (Aveco Co., Fort Dodge, IA).
6. Rompum/xylazine (Bayer, Shawnee Mission, KS).
7. Acepromazine/atropine sulfate (Fujisawa, Deerfield, IL).
8. Lubricant (i.e., Surgilube) (E. Fougera & Co., Melville, NY).
9. Paraformaldehyde (16% solution) (Electron Microscopy Science, Ft. Washington, PA).

10. Protamine sulfate (Sigma).
11. 10 mL polypropylene tubes with cap.
12. Glass rods (approx 6 in.).
13. 10 mL syringe attached to 15 cm catheter (*see* **Note 5**).

3. Methods
3.1. Preparation of Retrovirus

1. Clone desired gene of interest into chosen retroviral vector (*see* **Note 6**).
2. Prepare complete medium by combining DMEM (500 mL), FBS (50 mL), L-Gluta-mine (10 mL of stock; 4 mM final concentration), and penicillin/streptomycin solution (5 ml; 100 U/mL and 100 mg/mL final concentrations of penicillin and streptomycin, respectively).
3. Plate packaging cells at a density of $5–7 \times 10^5$ cells/100 mm plate and incubate at 37°C in an atmosphere of 5% CO_2 for 12–24 h. Wash cells twice with D-PBS and replace with 10 mL fresh complete medium 1–2 h before transfection (*see* **Note 7**).
4. Mix 10–15 mg plasmid DNA from **Subheading 3.1, step 1** with 0.5 mL of 0.25 M $CaCl_2$, add 0.5 mL of 2X BES-buffered saline, and incubate for 20 min at room temperature.
5. Carefully add mixture in a dropwise fashion to plated packaging cells, gently swirling to insure complete and even distribution throughout the plate. Incubate the cultures for 18–24 h at 37°C in an atmosphere of 5% CO_2.
6. Aspirate medium and wash cells twice with D-PBS. Add 10 mL of fresh complete medium and incubate for 24–48 h at 37°C in an atmosphere of 5% CO_2.
7. Remove medium and wash cells with D-PBS. Add 1–2 mL of trypsin-EDTA solution for approximately 1 min to remove cells from plate, and add 5–10 mL of complete medium to stop trypsinization.
8. Collect cells, transfer to a 15 mL conical tube, and centrifuge for 10 min at 1500g. Remove supernatant and resuspend cells gently, but thoroughly, in 1–2 mL of selection medium (i.e., complete medium containing 0.5 mg/mL of G418) (*see* **Note 8**).
9. Add resuspended cells to a 100 mm plate and bring up volume to a total of 10 mL selection medium. Culture for one week at 37°C in an atmosphere of 5% CO_2 (*see* **Note 9**).
10. One day prior to viral particle collection, plate target cells (i.e., NIH3T3) at $0.5–1 \times 10^5$ cells/well in a 6-well plate.
11. Collect virus-containing medium from packaging cells. Add polybrene to medium at a final concentration of 4 µg/mL and filter through a 0.45 µm filter (*see* **Note 10**).
12. To titer virus, take an aliquot of the virus-containing medium and dilute into 6 10-fold serial dilutions using fresh complete medium containing 4 mg/mL polybrene. Remaining virus-containing medium can be frozen at –80°C until needed for in vivo retroviral transduction protocols.

13. Continue with viral titer assessment by adding serial dilutions of virus-containing medium to plated target cells from **Subheading 3.1.**, **step 10** (4 mL/well) and incubate for 48 h at 37°C in an atmosphere of 5% CO_2.
14. Aspirate medium, wash twice with D-PBS and subject cells to appropriate antibiotic selection (0.5 µg/mL) for one week and assay by an appropriate method (*see* **Note 11**).
15. Count colonies present at the highest dilution and multiply by the dilution factor to calculate the titer of retrovirus (*see* **Note 12**).

3.2. In Vivo Retroviral Transduction of the Gut Epithelium

1. Prepare Solution A for immune complexes (calculate 1 mL/rabbit) by combining 1 part rabbit antihuman IgG fraction, 1 part rabbit antihuman whole serum fraction, and 2 parts human serum albumin (0.5 mg/mL) in a polypropylene tube.
2. Cap, shake, and incubate mixture at 37°C for one h. Following incubation, place Solution A in 4°C overnight.
3. Make Solution B by preparing HSA at 6 mg/mL in sterile LPS-free water.
4. Fast rabbits 12–16 h prior to experimental procedure by removing food the night before retention enema/immune complex delivery.
5. Prepare anesthetic solution (approx 0.6 mL/rabbit) by combining ketamine/ketasil (60%), rompum (30%), and acepromazine (10%).
6. Anesthetize rabbits by intramuscular injection (0.6 mL) of anesthetic solution.
7. Move rabbits onto their right side and gently insert a lubricated glass rod into the rectum and up into the distal colon to facilitate introduction of rubber catheter with attached syringe (*see* **Note 5**).
8. To initiate the induction of inflammation in the distal colon, slowly deliver 4.0 mL of formalin solution (or saline for control animals)/rabbit by intrarectal enema using catheter/syringe apparatus. Delivery should be slow (i.e., over a 30 s time period) and care should be taken to not leak solution from the rectum.
9. Before immune complex injection, make a mark on tube containing Solution A (from **Subheading 3.2.**, **step 2**) delineating total volume. Subsequently remove supernatant from settled immune complex solution and replace this volume with Solution B, filling up to mark made on tube. Vortex immune complex mixture well.
10. Exactly 2 h after the delivery of the formalin retention enema solution, administer 0.9 mL of immune complex mixture/rabbit intravenously through ear vein injection. Animals can be returned to appropriate housing after waking up from anesthetic.
11. Deliver a total of five retroviral enemas over the next 72 h (*see* **Note 13**).
12. To prepare retrovirus for retention enema delivery, virus-containing medium (from **Subheading 2.2.**, **step 12**) should be quick-thawed and adjusted to a concentration of 6×10^5 cfu/mL. Add protamine sulfate to the virus-containing medium at a final concentration of 10 µg/mL (a total volume of 4.0 mL solution/rabbit will administered for experimental animals). This preparation should be freshly done immediately before each retroviral retention enema delivery. Retroviral solution must be kept on ice prior to intrarectal administration and remaining fluid should be discarded.

13. To administer retroviral as well as appropriate control retention enemas (4.0 mL total volume/rabbit), follow exact methods described under **Subheading 3.2, steps 5–8**, replacing formalin enema with retroviral or control enemas.
14. After completion of all five retroviral retention enemas, animals will be allowed to recover for a period of seven days until the resolution of inflammation in the distal 10 cm of the colon is fully attained (*see* **Note 14**).

4. Notes

1. Retroviral gene transfer is based on the complimentary design of the backbone retroviral vector and the packaging cell line. Currently, there are a number of commercially available retroviral backbone vectors as well as packaging cell lines. One reliable source is Clontech's Retro-X System, including various Retro-X Vectors and the RetroPack PT67 packaging cell line.
2. 2X BES-buffered saline (50 m*M* BES (*N, N*-bis[2-hydroxyethyl]–2-amino-ethanesulfonic acid), 280 m*M* NaCl, and 1.5 m*M* Na$_2$HPO$_4$·2H$_2$O) is made by dissolving 1.07 g BES, 1.6 g NaCl and 0.027 g Na$_2$HPO$_4$ in a total volume of 90 mL distilled H$_2$O, adjusting the pH to 6.96 and bringing up the volume to 100 mL. Solution is then filter sterilized using a 0.22-micron filter and can be aliquoted and stored at –20°C.
3. 2.5 *M* CaCl$_2$ is made by dissolving 13.5 g of CaCl$_2$·6H$_2$O in 20 mL of distilled H$_2$O. Solution is filter sterilized using a 0.22-micron filter and can be aliquoted and stored at –20°C.
4. The materials and methods detailed in **Subheadings 2.2.** and **3.2.**, respectively, are specifically designed for the in vivo gene transfer into the colonic mucosa of rabbits (approximate weight of 2.2–2.5 kg). These methodologies are a modification of an established model of experimental colitis, which has been previously described in detail *(11)*. Further modifications can be made to the protocol to accommodate the use of other animal species.
5. Makeshift catheters for enema delivery can be made using closed-ended rubber tubing. Tubing is cut to be 15 cm in total length and a 10 cm mark, from closed end, should be permanently delineated. Pin-sized holes are made along the entire length of catheter within the 10 cm mark. Tubing should also chosen to fit end of syringe securely.
6. Use standard molecular biology techniques to clone your desired target gene into the retroviral backbone vector *(12)*.
7. We routinely use the standard calcium-phosphate coprecipitation procedures for retroviral transfection into packaging cells. However, other techniques, such as electroporation, are also commonly used for both stable and transient transfections.
8. In order to obtain stable-virus producing cell lines, the packaging cells are plated in selection medium after transfection with the desired retroviral plasmid contruct. Most retroviral contructs carry the neomycin (Neo^R) gene as a selectable marker. Retroviral vectors carrying other selectable markers can also be used to obtain stable virus producing cell lines, in which case the appropriate antibiotic should be utilized for selection.

9. For in vivo protocols, we have found that using high titer clones optimizes the infection of target cells. Therefore, individual clones can be isolated using cloning cylinders or limited dilution techniques and propagated in complete medium. Selection medium is not required for their propagation at this time.

10. The filter can be cellulose acetate or polysulfonic, but not nitrocellulose. Nitrocellulose has the potential to destroy the retrovirus by binding membrane-bound viral proteins.

11. Colonies can be simply counted or stained for alkaline phosphatase expression if using a control vector such as pLAPSN (Clontech).

12. For example, if there are 6 colonies in the 1:100,000 dilution, then the calculated viral titer would be 6×10^5 cfu.

13. The standard time line we use is delivery of the first retroviral retention enema the same day of the initial experimental procedure, (i.e., approximately 6–8 h following the formalin enema/immune complex administration). Thereafter, retroviral retention enemas are delivered twice daily for the next two days. Prior to each enema, animals are anesthetized as described in **Subheading 3.2, steps 5 and 6**). In addition, a modification of the protocol described in Chapter 26, "Assessment of Intestinal Stem Cell Survival Using the Microcolony Formation Assay," can be performed to specifically identify and localize colonic cell populations that are targeted for retroviral transduction using the gene transfer procedure outlined in the present chapter. By following the methods detailed in Chapter 26, beginning at **Subheading 3.1., step 3**, it is possible to specifically identify actively replicating cell populations (in S-phase) in the colonic mucosa with the potential for retroviral transduction (**Fig. 1**).

14. At this point, the colonic epithelium should be stably transduced with retrovirus and has the ability to produce the desired target gene product. This can be assessed by routine immunohistochemical techniques and protein measurements to detect the presence of the retrovirally encoded gene product (protein). Routine β-galactosidase (β-gal) staining is also often utilized to verify and localize retrovirally-encoded gene expression when a control β-gal retrovirus is employed. However, caution should be taken when using a construct containing β-gal for transduction into the intestinal milieu since high background staining often results in the gut due to the endogenous presence of β-gal. Aside from evaluating the resulting gene expression in the intestinal mucosa, animals are now ready for experimental protocols to challenge or determine the therapeutic value of the retrovirally encoded gene product.

Acknowledgments

This work was supported in part by a Crohn's and Colitis Foundation of America Student Research Award (to Paul L. Alabanza) and by the National Institutes of Health/NIAID through grant R29-AI40303 (to Theresa T. Pizarro).

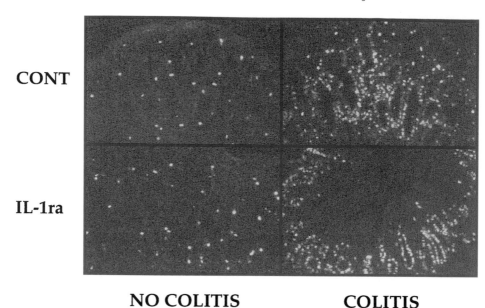

Fig. 1. Identification of colonic mucosal cells as potential targets for retroviral transduction. In order to induce colonic inflammation, New Zealand rabbits (2.2–2.5 kg)
were treated with either a dilute formalin (16%) (right panels) or a saline control (left
panels) enema (4.0 mL total volume), followed 2 h later by an iv immune complex
injection. Five intrarectal administrations of either retrovirally-encoded IL-1Ra (bottom panels) or control backbone vector (top panels) were delivered over a 3 d period.
All animals received 120 mg/kg BrdUrd and 12 mg/kg FdUrd by ip injection 2 h
prior to sacrifice. Anti-BrdUrd staining demonstrates actively replicating cells (in
S-phase) within the colonic mucosa. Induction of inflammation increases epithelial
progenitor crypt cell replication (right panels) with the potential to serve as targets for
retroviral transduction.

References

1. Noel, R. A., Shukla, P., and Henning, S. J. (1994) Optimization of gene transfer
   into intestinal epithelial cells using a retroviral vector. *J. Ped. Gastroenterol.
   Nutri.* **19**, 43–49.
2. Lau, C., Soriano, H. E., Ledley, F. D., Finegold, M. J., Wolfe, J. H., Birkenmeier,
   E. H., and Henning, S. J. (1995) Retroviral gene transfer into the intestinal epithelium. *Human Gene Ther.* **6**, 1145–1151.
3. Ausubel, F., Brent, R., Kingston, R. E., Moore, D. M., Seidman, J. G., Smith, J.
   A., and Struhl, K. (1994) *Current Protocols in Molecular Biology.* Green Publish-
   ing Associates, Inc., and John Wiley & Sons, Inc.
4. Coffin, J. M. and Varmus, H. E. (1996) *Retroviruses.* Cold Spring Harbor Laboratory, Cold Spring Harbor, NY.

5. Mann, R., Mulligan, R. C., and Baltimore, D. (1989) Construction of a retrovirus packaging mutant and its use to produce helper-free defective retrovirus. *Cell* **33,** 153–159.

6. Miller, A. D. and Buttimore, C. (1986) Redesign of retrovirus packaging cell lines to avoid recombination leading to helper virus production. *Mol. Cell. Biol.* **6,** 2895–2902.

7. Miller, A. D. and Chen, F. (1996) Retrovirus packaging cells based on 10A1 murine leukemia virus for production of vectors that use multiple receptors for cell entry. *J. Virol.* **70,** 5564–5571.

8. Puppi, M. and Henning, S. J. (1995) Cloning of the rat ecotropic retroviral receptor and studies of its expression in intestinal tissues. *Proc. Soc. Exp. Biol. Med.* **209,** 38–45.

9. Pizarro, T. T., Casini-Raggi, V., Gordon, M., and Cominelli, F. (1995) Transduction of the colonic mucosa by retention enema delivery of a retroviral reporter gene following experimentally-induced rabbit colitis. *Gastroenterology* **108(4),** A894.

10. Alabanza, P. L., Woraratanadharm, J., Kozaiwa, K., Huybrechts, M. M., Fox, L. M., Nast, C. C., and Pizarro, T. T. (1999) Anti-inflammatory effects of IL-1 receptor antagonist (IL-1ra) gene therapy in experimental rabbit colitis. *Gastroenterology* **116(4),** A660.

11. Cominelli, F., Nast, C. C., Llerena, R., Dinarello, C. A., and Zipser, R. D. (1990) Interleukin 1 suppresses inflammation in rabbit colitis. Mediation by endogenous prostaglandins. *J. Clin. Invest.* **85,** 582–586.

12. Sambrook, J., Fritsch, E. F., and Maniatis, T. (1989) *Molecular Cloning: A Laboratory Manual.* Cold Spring Harbor Laboratory, Cold Spring Harbor, New York.

Index

From: *Methods in Molecular Medicine*, vol. 50: *Colorectal Cancer: Methods and Protocols*
Edited by: S. M. Powell © Humana Press Inc., Totowa, NJ